NO TIME TO LOSE

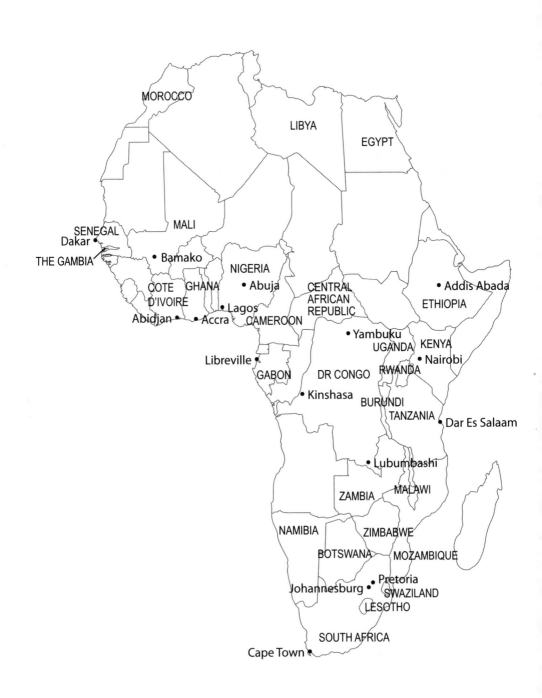

MOROCCO

LIBYA

EGYPT

MALI

SENEGAL
Dakar •
THE GAMBIA

• Bamako

NIGERIA

COTE
D'IVOIRE

GHANA

• Abuja

CENTRAL
AFRICAN
REPUBLIC

• Addis Abada

ETHIOPIA

Abidjan •

• Accra

• Lagos

CAMEROON

• Yambuku

UGANDA

KENYA

Libreville •

GABON

DR CONGO

RWANDA

• Nairobi

• Kinshasa

BURUNDI

TANZANIA

• Dar Es Salaam

• Lubumbashi

MALAWI

ZAMBIA

NAMIBIA

ZIMBABWE

BOTSWANA

MOZAMBIQUE

Pretoria
Johannesburg • •

SWAZILAND

LESOTHO

SOUTH AFRICA

Cape Town •

NO TIME TO LOSE

A Life in Pursuit of Deadly Viruses

PETER PIOT

WITH RUTH MARSHALL

W. W. NORTON & COMPANY

NEW YORK · LONDON

For information about permission to reproduce selections from this book,
write to Permissions, W. W. Norton & Company, Inc.,
500 Fifth Avenue, New York, NY 10110

For information about special discounts for bulk purchases, please contact
W. W. Norton Special Sales at specialsales@wwnorton.com or 800-233-4830

Manufacturing by Courier Westford
Book design by Brooke Koven
Production manager: Louise Mattarelliano

Library of Congress Cataloging-in-Publication Data

Piot, Peter, 1949–
No time to lose : a life in pursuit of deadly viruses / Peter Piot. — 1st ed.
p. ; cm.
Life in pursuit of deadly viruses
Includes index.
ISBN 978-0-393-06316-5 (hardcover)
I. Title. II. Title: Life in pursuit of deadly viruses.
[DNLM: 1. Piot, Peter, 1949– 2. Joint United Nations Programme on HIV/AIDS.
3. Virology—Belgium—Autobiography. 4. Virology—England—Autobiography.
5. Acquired Immunodeficiency Syndrome—history—Belgium. 6. Acquired
Immunodeficiency Syndrome—history—England. 7. Hemorrhagic Fever, Ebola—
history—Belgium. 8. Hemorrhagic Fever, Ebola—history—England. 9. History,
20th Century—Belgium. 10. History, 20th Century—England. 11. History,
21st Century—Belgium. 12. History, 21st Century—England. 13. International
Cooperation—Belgium—Autobiography. 14. International Cooperation—
England—Autobiography. WZ 100]

616.9'101—dc23

2012011911

W. W. Norton & Company, Inc.
500 Fifth Avenue, New York, N.Y. 10110
www.wwnorton.com

W. W. Norton & Company Ltd.
Castle House, 75/76 Wells Street, London W1T 3QT

1 2 3 4 5 6 7 8 9 0

Our responsibility is historic, for when the history of AIDS and the global response is written, our most precious contribution may well be that at the time of plague we did not flee; we did not hide; and we did not separate.

—JONATHAN MANN

Rust roest.

—FLEMISH PROVERB

In the course of human history, there has never been a greater threat than the HIV/AIDS epidemic. Our attention to this issue cannot be distracted or diverted by problems that are apparently more pressing. History will surely judge us harshly if we do not respond with all the energy and resources that we can bring to bear in the fight against HIV/AIDS.

—NELSON MANDELA, *closing ceremony of the XV International AIDS Conference, Bangkok, Thailand, July 16, 2004*

CONTENTS

PREFACE

S IXTY-TWO MAY BE a bit young for writing a memoir. However, I felt that the distance between events and writing was long enough, but yet not too hazy, to tell my story of two of the most extraordinary adventures of our time: the discovery of Ebola hemorrhagic fever and AIDS and the world's response to them. I was a privileged witness and actor in the history of two previously unknown viruses— enough material for two different books. Whereas the unraveling of the first known epidemic of Ebola hemorrhagic fever in Africa was my initiation into scientific discovery, even life-threatening adventure, and into the world of what is now called global health, the AIDS epidemic forced me to confront the extreme complexity of health and disease, and to learn the hard way the realities of big and small politics. Already as a child I wanted to discover the world beyond my village, and combined with a deep curiosity for all kinds of scientific inquiry, this led to paths that I could not have imagined at the beginning of my adult life, which at times was a whirlwind.

Both epidemics show the enormous potential and real limitations of science to solve today's health problems, such as through the discovery of life-saving antiretroviral drugs, but also the failure to produce a vaccine over twenty-five years after the discovery of the human immunodeficiency virus—not to forget the major role that societal determinants and lifestyle play in emerging diseases, be they infectious in origin such as Ebola and HIV or the current tsunami of obesity, diabetes, and cardiovascular disease. Who would have predicted that the end of the last millennium would see the emergence of new pathogens and epidemics, when the medical world thought it had it all under control—at least in the wealthier part of the world? Both Ebola and HIV infection continue to exist, probably for generations to come, and in contrast to some overoptimistic scenarios, I don't believe the end of AIDS is in sight. The story of new viruses is also not over, and it is safe to predict that more pathogens will emerge and affect us in always faster and more global ways.

In the Belgian surrealist tradition of painter Rene Magritte naming his painting of a pipe *Ceci n'est pas une pipe*, "ceci n'est pas une autobiographie," this is not an autobiography—as my journey is hopefully not finished yet—nor is this a doctoral thesis about the history or the politics of the two epidemics with hundreds of bibliographic references. This is a memoir of discovery, selected moments, people, and developments, seen through one lens—my own experiences—with no ambition to give a complete picture. Scholars not as involved as I are better placed to write those books.

At times I was an outbreak detective in the heart of Africa, a scientist studying antimicrobial resistance in bacteria or the genetic diversity of HIV, a desperate clinician caring for patients when there was no antiretroviral treatment, a researcher and public health practitioner designing prevention and treatment programs, a UN official leading a complex multilateral organization in eighty countries and spearheading UN reform, a patient diplomat negotiating political resolutions and price reductions of antiretroviral drugs, a stubborn campaigner reaching out to the powerful of this world and bringing AIDS awareness to unexpected places, a frustrated fighter of bureaucrats, an activist from the beginning . . . and so often all of the above simultaneously, always in connection with numerous other actors. My memoir reflects on all these incarnations.

This book is also a personal chronicle of the still unfolding AIDS pandemic—the most devastating epidemic in modern times. It narrates how the face of AIDS has changed dramatically thanks to science, politics, and the efforts of thousands of people, putting in perspective the suffering of more than 60 million who are living with HIV or lost their lives from AIDS. It gives an inside view of the daily life and struggles in the United Nations system, where as head of UNAIDS I served under three very different secretaries-general. I saw how the UN can be at its best and be effective when it convenes multiple countries and players around a very concrete project such as confronting AIDS, but also how the UN can be synonym of inefficiency when its more than 190 member states or its organization or civil servants do not want action or let process dominate.

Perhaps most important, I have seen over and over again how a catastrophe like AIDS brings out the best and the worst in the human species—regardless of whether a person is well educated or illiterate. I had to deal with physicians refusing to care for AIDS patients; clergy rejecting them from churches or campaigning against condoms; homophobic politicians and public health officials; drug control authorities declaring war on drug users, not on drugs; and midlevel UN system bureaucrats who were only interested in their own turf. However, above all, I met incredibly passionate and compassionate men and women trying to save lives, fighting for justice, and searching for scientific solutions. I had the privilege to work with so many unsung heroes of the AIDS struggle: groups of people living with HIV, visionary politicians, generous philanthropists, pharmaceutical innovators, caring clergy, and my tireless fellow scientists, activists, clinicians, and program managers across the world—my global community for the last thirty years. These experiences largely compensated for the numerous brain-killing meetings I had to endure during my tenure at UNAIDS, where I learned not to be guided by that modern plague—the quarterly result, the short-term view—but to focus on the ultimate goal of saving as many lives as possible. And along the way I got this big bonus, as I continued to discover myself a bit. That is why this memoir is in the first instance about people and their institutions and movements, not just about viruses.

• PART ONE •

CHAPTER I

A Blue Flask of Virus

O N THE LAST Tuesday in September 1976 my boss at the microbiology lab was alerted that a special package was on its way to us from Zaire. It was flying in from Kinshasa: samples of blood from an unusual epidemic that seemed to be stirring in the distant Équateur region, along the river Congo.

Nothing quite like this had happened in the two years I had so far been working in a junior position at the lab in Antwerp, Belgium. But I knew it was part of the job. We sometimes took in strange samples of bodily fluids and tried to work out what they were. Our lab was certified to diagnose all kinds of diseases, including arbovirus infections like yellow fever, and the working hypothesis for this epidemic was reported to be "yellow fever with hemorrhagic manifestations."

I never actually worked with any suspected yellow fever. It wasn't every day we received samples from as far away as equatorial Zaire. And it was clear this was an unusual sample, and that something pretty curious had occurred, because several Belgian nuns apparently died of the disease even though their vaccinations were completely up to date.

The next day—September 29—the package arrived: a cheap plastic thermos flask, shiny and blue. I settled down with Guido Van Der Groen—a shy, funny, fellow Belgian aged about thirty, a few years older than I—and René Delgadillo, a Bolivian postdoc student, to open it up on the lab bench. Nowadays it makes me wince just to think of it. Sure, we were wearing latex gloves—our boss insisted on gloves in the lab but we used no other precautions, no suits or masks of any kind.

We didn't even imagine the risk we were taking. Indeed, shipping those blood samples in a simple thermos, without any kind of precautions, was an incredibly perilous act. Maybe the world was a simpler, more innocent place in those days, or maybe it was just a lot more reckless.

Unscrewing the thermos, we found a soup of half-melted ice: it was clear that subzero temperatures had not been constantly maintained. And the thermos itself had taken a few knocks, too. One of the test tubes was intact, but there were pieces of a broken tube—its lethal content now mixed up with the ice water—as well as a handwritten note, whose ink had partially bled away into the icy wet.

It was from Dr. Jacques Courteille, a Belgian physician who worked at the Clinique Ngaliema in Kinshasa. He described the thermos's contents as two vials, each containing 5 milliliters of clotted blood from a Flemish nun who was too ill to be evacuated out of Zaire.* She was suffering from a mysterious epidemic that had so far evaded identification, possibly yellow fever.

I was still trying to find my way in the labyrinth of infectious diseases research, and this kind of thing made my heart beat faster. As a kid, growing up in the flat countryside of Flanders—the coastal plain between Holland and France—I was always drawn to tales of exotic adventures far away. I read the comic-strip explorations of Tintin, a Belgian boy with a quiff and a little dog made world famous by Steven Spielberg. There were also the Karl May books—great florid escapades set in the American Far West—and the swashbuckling sci-

*Once a Belgian colony known as the Belgian Congo, the country was named Zaire in 1971, before being renamed the Democratic Republic of Congo in 1997.

entific fantasies of Jules Verne. I devoured biographies of the great nineteenth-century explorers: Henry Morton Stanley, who explored Africa, and Robert Burke, who led an expedition of camels across Australia in 1860, and Richard Burton and John Speke, who went to the Great Lakes of Africa to search for the source of the Nile.

I was a bit of a loner as a kid. Although we lived in a then small farming village first mentioned in 1036, Keerbergen, where everyone spoke the local Flemish dialect, my parents insisted that we speak standard Dutch at home—what is known, in Flanders, as "general civilized Dutch." My father was a staunch supporter of Flemish nationalism, and he felt that indulging in separate dialects would divide the Flemish people and prevent us from rising from the mud. We needed to unite and become as smart as the *French*-speaking Belgians, who had dominated the country since its independence in 1830. But very few Flemish kids ever grew up speaking standard Dutch; that was a literary, formal language, used only for school. So sure, it gave me an advantage with matters academic, but it also meant that my siblings and I grew up rather separate from our peers.

I often cycled, alone, the three miles from Keerbergen to the village of Tremelo, where a white, L-shaped farmhouse with green shutters had been transformed into a small museum. This was the birthplace of Father Damien, a Catholic missionary who was the local claim to fame, because of his heroic work with lepers in the islands of Hawaii in the nineteenth century. In those days leprosy was thought to be highly contagious, and it was incurable. Thousands of Hawaiians who contracted the disease were removed to an isolated peninsula on Molokai where they eked out a brief existence in squalor and pain. Father Damien volunteered to serve them, though this potentially was a death sentence; and he sent back hundreds of artifacts and images before dying from leprosy himself. On those cold afternoons, with the rain lashing down on the fields outside, I stared mesmerized at pictures of leprosy patients with horribly deformed faces, feet, and hands. I was enraged by the stories of their rejection and discrimination, and full of romantic admiration for the heroism of Father Damien, who braved the prejudices of society and risked his life to serve. Despite my Catholic upbringing, I had no urge to become a missionary, but this solitary, repeated exposure to a forgotten disease, social injustice, and the mesmerizing trinkets of faraway cultures quickened in me a desire to help the poor and to explore the world.

That's really why I ultimately chose medicine—though my initial choice for university studies was engineering because I loved mathematics and solving practical problems, which I did for a few months in Ghent. Those were my two main desires: to work for greater social justice and to travel. Medicine dovetailed with my childhood passion for science; a medical degree was a passport to work anywhere in the world; and ill-health was surely the worst kind of injustice, so as a doctor, you could really be useful. But when, after seven years' study at the medical faculty in Ghent, I broached the idea of specializing in infectious diseases, the unanimous verdict of my professors was that I would be a fool to do it. There were still a few infectious illnesses around, of course, plus the occasional outbreak of a nasty new contagious disease in some distant, benighted place. (Although I had certainly never heard of them, Congo-Crimea fever was first identified in 1956, for example, and Lassa fever first appeared in 1969.) But in general, infectious diseases weren't considered interesting or cutting-edge in 1974. They had just about all been conquered by advances in antibiotics and vaccines.

My professor of social medicine grabbed my shoulder firmly, to make sure I was paying attention. "There's no future in infectious diseases," he stated flatly, in a tone that bore no argument. "They've all been solved."

But I wanted to go to Africa. I wanted to save lives. And it seemed to me that infectious disease might be just the ticket and full of unresolved scientific questions. So I ignored him.

I don't really know why I had developed this fascination for Africa. My parents were hardworking people. My father was an economist, a senior civil servant promoting export of Belgian agriculture in the nascent European Union, and my mother worked in her father's construction business. They came from village people, bloody-minded peasants, not the bankers or silversmiths and weavers of the Flemish guilds that made our region famous in the Middle Ages. In a region that has been churned up and snarled over by greater nations since time immemorial, we inhabited a tiny world of small, dim, villages and fields under a leaden sky. Just about every Sunday of my childhood, my parents took us to our grandparents' houses; until I was eight, we had all lived within four miles of each other. The women of our family were all great cooks, and on my father's side the men were all serious drinkers.

Nobody from my family had ever traveled to the Belgian Congo, the private kingdom of King Leopold II that was to become independent as Zaire. My parents and grandparents saw colonial settlers as lazy good-for-nothings who lived off other people's labor. "Rest is rust" was the motto of my great-grandpa's workers' bicycling team, the Downhill Riders of Wijgmaal, and its stiff old blazon, embroidered in 1905, hangs even now in my study at home.

GUIDO AND RENÉ picked out the one remaining test tube of blood from the thermos and set to work. We needed to look for antibodies against the yellow fever virus, and other causes of hemorrhagic or epidemic fever such as typhoid. To isolate any virus material, we injected small amounts of the blood samples into VERO cells, an easily replicable cell lineage that is used a lot in labs. We also injected some into the brains of adult mice and newborn baby mice. (I never liked this aspect of the work. Sometimes we needed to inject patient tissue into the testicles of rats, to isolate *Mycobacterium ulcerans*, the cause of Buruli ulcers, and it made me cringe.)

All this work was done with no more precautions than if we had been handling a routine case of salmonella or tuberculosis. It never occurred to us that something far more rare and much more powerful might have just entered our lives.

In the next few days, the antibody tests for yellow fever, Lassa fever, and several other candidates all came up negative, and it seemed likely that the samples had been fatally damaged by their transportation at a semithawed temperature. We bustled nervously around the mice and checked our cell cultures four times a day instead of two. On the weekend, each of us popped in to check the samples. All of us, I think, were hoping something would grow.

Then it happened. On Monday morning, October 4, we found that several adult mice had died. Three days later all the baby mice had also died—a sign that a pathogenic virus was probably present in the blood samples that we had used to inoculate them.

By this time our boss, Professor Stefaan Pattyn, had also gleaned a little more information about the epidemic in Zaire. It seemed to be centered on a village called Yambuku, where there was a mission outpost run by Flemish nuns—the Sisters of the Sacred Heart of Our Lady of s'Gravenwezel. (S'Gravenwezel is a small town north of Antwerp.) The epidemic had been raging for three weeks, since September 5, and at least 200 people had died. Although two Zairean doctors who had been to the region had diagnosed the malady yellow fever, the patients suffered violent hemorrhagic symptoms, including extensive bleeding from the anal passage, nose, and mouth as well as high fever, headache, and vomiting.

Hemorrhagic manifestations are quite unusual in yellow fever. But although Pattyn could be a bit of a bully, he was hardworking and knew his stuff. He had worked in Zaire for six or seven years, and exotic viral illnesses were right up his alley, though his specialty was mycobacteria—tuberculosis and leprosy. I recall him telling us that this had to be that strange and lethal phenomenon: a hemorrhagic fever.

I was just a recently graduated physician; none of the rare hemorrhagic fevers had ever crossed my path. Nor had they featured at all during my medical training. So I made a quick run to the institute's library to try to absorb as much as I could. It was a small but diverse group of viruses, from mosquito-borne dengue to exotic, recently discovered rodent-borne South American viruses with names like Junin and Machupo. All, by definition, caused high fevers and massive bleeding, and their fatality rate was often in excess of 30 percent.

Previously I had been excited about the work we were doing; now I was inflamed. If we were hunting for signs of a hemorrhagic virus, this was outbreak investigation of the most stirring variety. I truly loved the detective thrill of working in infectious disease. You came in and figured out what the problem was. And if you managed to figure it out quickly enough—before the patient died, basically—then you could almost always solve it, because, just like my medical school professor of social medicine had said, solutions had by this time been found for almost every kind of infectious illness.

In the early 1970s, when I was a student, infectious diseases didn't exist as a stand-alone specialty in Belgium; you had to study clinical microbiology, which meant cultivating and analyzing bacteria, viruses, fungi, and parasites—any kind of microorganism capable of causing disease. This was fine by me. I was very interested in microbes. And I didn't necessarily want to devote my life to caring for individual patients all the time. As a hospital intern, I had already concluded that too many people in Belgian doctors' waiting rooms were there with a small cough and big drama. The underlying cause of most of their problems seemed psychological—issues with their relationships, or at work. They didn't really need to see a doctor.

However, there's a huge area of medicine that is neglected, and that's making sure people, collectively and individually, *don't* get sick. I was interested in understanding the forces that make people sick— the microbes, which are usually relatively straightforward, and also the complex social forces that make people vulnerable to ill health. I wanted to combine a scientific career with clinical and public health work in a developing country, where there was real medical need and I could truly make a difference.

While clinical microbiology excited my scientific curiosity, epidemiology promised the thrills of investigation and discovery. And thanks to our often blood-soaked, century-long colonial occupation of Africa, in Belgium's medical history there was a rich tradition of both. The Prince Leopold Institute of Tropical Medicine in Antwerp was founded in the early 1900s to train medical personnel for the colonies and conduct research on exotic diseases—mostly parasitic infections such as sleeping sickness and malaria, which were major killers of colonized and colonizers alike. Even in the 1970s, it was dominated by professors who had worked in the former Belgian Congo, and who had a political outlook that was ultraconservative and steeped in racial condescension—much to the dismay of their students, who like me were primarily inspired by dreams of social justice and third world liberation. The director, Professor P. G. Janssen, and my boss were two of the exceptions.

That's why, when I graduated, I applied for a job as a junior researcher in Pattyn's lab with the aim to obtain a doctorate. His attitude to all new arrivals was that you began in the kitchen. In those days, there was almost no plastic in a scientific laboratory: plastic was expensive. All the equipment was glass and was recycled, even the pipettes. And all the bacteriological and virological media, which today any self-respecting lab would order from a catalogue, were prepared in-house, by hand. So for the first three months I sterilized pipettes and prepared gels and broths. It was very much like starting out in a restaurant kitchen by working as a sous-chef, chopping onions; or like learning to become a medieval artist by first grinding pigments as an apprentice. If the basic media are not properly prepared the entire experiment is invalidated, and so I needed to understand all the ingredients and all the processes of microbiology, from the ground up.

I liked it. I had always liked doing things with my hands. I started learning how to identify bacteria—a shigella, a salmonella—under a microscope and using biochemical tests. My first real assignment was to grow *Mycobacterium leprae*, the cause of leprosy, in mice footpads. This was part of clinical trials to test the effectiveness of a combination therapy that would ultimately cure the disease, as demonstrated by several research groups. Pattyn's microbiology lab was located at the Institute of Tropical Medicine, but he worked with the University Hospital and also, incidentally, with the Antwerp zoo. When someone (or some animal) fell ill, a sample of stool, or urine, or blood, or a throat swab, came to us for analysis. I cultivated it and then stared at it—not focusing intently but trying to detect something unusual, something striking.

It took about a year to master that routine work. Our techniques would be considered laughably ancient today. For salmonella, you took the person's stool, diluted it, put it on a plate spread with agar and a culture medium, and placed it in an incubator. You waited and watched what grew. You needed an eye to pick out which colony of bacteria looked like a possibility. Ah, *this* one might be a candidate. You picked it up, put it on another plate, grew that, so there'd be a sizable amount, and then you began doing biochemical tests, checking perhaps five or six different chemical combinations. Then you knew it was salmonella. But which serotype? A *typhi* bacteria, which causes typhoid, or something banal that merely gives you the runs?

I found a lot of weird anomalies staring down the familiar funnel of the microscope in Pattyn's lab. I isolated a number of bacteria for the first time—specific subtypes of salmonella, things like that—from people, seals, elephants, flamingos, and shrimp. These weren't world-class discoveries, but they validated my feeling that I was where I needed to be—that I had that particular, slightly obsessional, very meticulous skill that microbiology requires, an approach that crucially involves *not* throwing away things that don't fit into your preconceived scheme of ideas.

After about a year, Pattyn let me begin working on viruses. In the days before PCRs and DNA probes, the viral detection techniques were very difficult and precise. As we say in Dutch, you had to be even more of an ant-fucker than with parasites or bacteria—really obsessed with detail. First you had to isolate the virus—say, polio. You took the patient's stool, diluted it, and then, instead of placing it on agar you injected it onto cells. Most of these cell lines, such as VERO, were derived from cancer cells, because they replicated easily; but in those days you couldn't just buy them, you had to prepare them. You placed a sample of the stool on them, and then twice a day you observed the cells under a microscope. Certain viruses kill the cells; they detach from the side of the glass container, creating a pattern of holes as they fall away. When you saw that, you took a sample and put it on another cell layer to be certain that it stemmed from an infectious virus. And then to identify herpes virus, for example, you brought it in contact with antiserum treated with a fluorescent dye or looked at it under an electron microscope, where you could really see the virus.

It was a tiny, detailed job, and it wasn't exotic, and it didn't involve traveling. But I was content, even thrilled, to do it. I knew I needed to arm myself with this knowledge and these skills before I could go to Africa and work there, to discover new diseases and new solutions that would save lives.

ON SEPTEMBER 30, the Flemish nun who was the source of the original blood samples died in Dr. Courteille's clinic in Kinshasa. He sent us some fragments of her liver to us for pathologic examination. (Again, the samples were flown to Belgium on a *passenger* aircraft.) To add to the diagnostic confusion, microscopic examination of the samples showed swollen "Councilman bodies"—lesions considered typical of yellow fever. However, as Pattyn knew, they may also feature in Lassa virus, an African hemorrhagic fever whose transmission is mainly from rodents shedding virus in their urine and feces. So although Pattyn's hypothesis that the samples from Kinshasa contained a hemorrhagic virus was not confirmed, it was not disproven either.

By this point for him to keep us working on those samples was sheer folly; he knew we were not equipped to do the work in safety. In 1974 there were only three labs outside the Soviet Union that could handle hemorrhagic viruses: Fort Detrick, a military lab in Maryland that did high-security work on anthrax and other highly lethal diseases; the Army High Security Laboratory in Porton Down, in England; and the so-called hot lab at the Centers for Disease Control, in Atlanta.

Nonetheless, we continued to bustle around like amateurs in our cotton lab coats and latex gloves, checking our VERO cell lines. The cells began detaching from the glass sides of their containers: it was either a toxic effect or an infection, but either way, cytotoxicity had kicked in. That meant we might be close to isolating a virus, and we began extracting cells to cultivate them in a second line of VERO cells. And Pattyn had been told we should expect more samples from Zaire in the next few days.

But just as we were beginning to cultivate the second VERO cell line, Pattyn intervened. He had received instructions from the World Health Organization's Viral Diseases Unit to ship all samples and biological material from the new mystery epidemic to Porton Down in Britain. (In fact, a few days later Porton Down sent them on to the Center for Disease Control in Atlanta, which was the world's reference lab for hemorrhagic viruses.)

Pattyn was furious, and I too was upset. It looked as though our outbreak investigation was over before it had even begun. Glumly, we prepared to pack everything in tightly sealed containers: the patient serum, the inoculated cell lines, and the autopsied mouse brains and samples. But then Pattyn told us to keep some of the material back. He claimed that we needed a few more days to ready it for transport. So we kept a few tubes of VERO cells, as well as some of the new-born mice, which were dying. Perhaps it was a stubborn rebellion against the whole Belgian history of constantly being forced to grovel to greater powers. That material was just too valuable, too glorious to let it go. It was new, it was exciting—just too exciting to hand it over to the Brits or, in particular, to the Americans.

Pattyn was a colorful character, with a razor-sharp brain. He didn't have the smug, colonial attitude of so many men of his generation; he wore funky eyeglasses and collected contemporary art. And although he could be contemptuous I never felt his scorn was connected to skin color or social class—only to stupidity. But he certainly had an outsized ego.

There was a rack of secondary tubes in the lab, which we had inoculated after the first VERO cell line was killed. We knew there was something in there—something that was trouble—but still, we had taken out the rack so we could examine the tubes under the microscope. Doing that kind of work wasn't Pattyn's job. He was a micromanager but he wasn't a technician, and in fact he could be rather clumsy. But impulsively he reached for one of the precious tubes, to check it out himself under the scope, and as he did so it slipped from his hand and crashed on the floor.

Little René Delgadillo was the one who got his shoes splashed. They were good, solid leather shoes but René bleated, "Madre de Dios" (Mother of God!) while Pattyn swore, "Godverdomme" (Goddamn!)—and there was a moment, just a beat, of blank fear. Immediately we whisked into action: the floor was disinfected and the shoes removed. It was just a small incident. But it struck me only then how lethal this thing really might be and the huge risks we had been taking in handling it so cavalierly.

ON OCTOBER 12, our semiclandestine secondary cell line was ready for analysis. Guido took a sample and treated it so an ultrathin slice could be examined under an electron microscope. Then we took it over to Pattyn's friend Wim Jacob, who handled electron microscopy in the university hospital lab. A few hours later he came over to our lab with the photographs.

"What the hell is this?" said Pattyn.

There was a long pause as he glared at the photographs, at us, at the walls of the corridor. I peered over his shoulder and saw what were by virus standards very large, long, wormlike structures: nothing like yellow fever. Pattyn's excitement, or irritation, was rising.

"This looks like Marburg!" he exploded.

I didn't know much about Marburg.

Everyone else in the lab seemed to know about Marburg, and today of course all you'd need to do to find out would be to check the Internet. But back then I needed an atlas of infectious diseases. So I went to the institute's library and sure enough our virus *did* look like Marburg.

In those days Marburg was the only known virus that was this long—up to 14,000 nanometers, or 0.000014 millimeters. Huge. (In comparison, polio is up to 50 nanometers.) It had been identified just nine years before, in Germany, when a number of pharmaceutical workers became infected by a batch of monkeys imported from Uganda. It appeared to be extremely virulent and swiftly lethal. Seven of the 25 people infected by direct contact with the monkeys died with hemorrhagic fever, and six more individuals fell ill following contact with those primary infections.

Marburg was clearly a very scary illness, and as we did not have Marburg virus–specific antibodies, we could not definitely conclude whether our isolate was Marburg. Perhaps it was a different virus with similar morphology.

Pattyn was not suicidal. Once he had established that "our" virus was—at the very least—closely related to the terrifying Marburg, he had the sense to shelve all further work on it and sent the remaining samples directly to the high-security lab at the CDC.

I was still very excited. It felt as though my childhood fantasy of exploration was almost within my reach. I kept arguing that we had to follow up our work, go to Zaire and check out the epidemic. I felt strongly that we shouldn't hand this world-class discovery over to some other team. *We* had identified this virus, after all, so *we* should be the ones to establish its lethality and its real effects on the ground.

Pattyn was not immune to this line of argument himself, but our lab had no budget to pay for anything so bold and unscripted as an expedition to Zaire. He went to the Ministerial Department for Development Aid, and was told they funded programs to help poor people, not programs to assist medical research. It was my first encounter with the sobering reality of fund-raising: how crucial it is and how difficult it can be to raise money when you wait until the crisis arises. It was also the first of a long series of confrontations with bureaucracies, a major lifelong source of irritation.

Even if safety demanded that all the research had to be done in an expensively equipped, high-security lab, why *should* we leave it to the Americans and WHO to do the epidemiological work on the ground, where the epidemic was certainly still underway? How often does a small research institute in Belgium have the opportunity to make medical history? It's not often that a twenty-seven-year-old comes within reach of the discovery of a new virus, and it looked as though the virus we cultivated had a fighting chance of being just that.

On Thursday October 14, the answer came by telex: it was indeed a new virus. Karl Johnson, chief of Special Pathogens at the CDC, reported that his team had isolated a similar virus from other samples of blood from the same Flemish nun in Kinshasa. Pushing our information one step further, he added that this virus did not react with Marburg antibodies. Therefore it was different from Marburg, though we did not know how different it was.

I learned two things. One was that my institute (and indeed my country) had very limited means. The other was that there was a worldwide network of scientists who could solve almost any problem in no time. Back then we didn't even have fax machines—only the phone and the telex—but this network seemed all-knowing, and most of it was implanted in America. That's when I began to tell myself that I wanted to go to America, to plug into that network and learn how we could become world class too.

As for my impossible dream of taking our outbreak investigation to Zaire, I figured it was over. It was time to go back to looking for salmonella in the stool samples of patients with a nonspecific belly-ache. I was crestfallen.

But Pattyn was not a bad guy. I think he saw how despondent I was, and on Friday, October 15, he sent me to Paris for the weekend with my then wife, Greta Kimzeke. (We met when I was in medical school and she was a psychology student. At this point we'd been married for just six months.) Pattyn had been invited to a conference organized by Beecham, the pharmaceutical company, about some new antibiotic they were bringing out. He hated that stuff, and he was kind enough to let his young assistants make trips that pharmaceutical companies constantly offered him.

However, when I walked into the conference room at the Hotel Nikko on that Friday afternoon, my name was on a screen, with a message: I should urgently contact a phone number in Brussels. What the heck?

Before doing anything, I called Pattyn, who was still at the lab. He said the Department for Development Aid and the Ministry for Foreign Affairs had been ringing his phone off the hook: we had to get to Kinshasa. The Americans were going there to take a look at the epidemic, and there was some kind of French delegation already in place; even a South African was on his way. Also, Belgian expatriates in Kinshasa had begun panicking, sending their children to Europe because of the epidemic.

"The Belgian government is under pressure to do something," he told me. I thought, surely that "something" can't be just me, a recent graduate from medical school? But I kept my mouth shut.

"This is now a political priority!" Pattyn continued, and I thought: So, that's how it goes. Unless something is a *political* priority, figuring out how to save lives is not a big issue.

"It's *our* Congo, you know," he said, and I had no idea whether he meant it ironically or straight up, no ice.

So I phoned a Dr. Kivits at the Department of Development Aid. There was minimal discussion. He said I should leave the next day on a 10-day mission. I asked if it would be OK if I waited until Sunday, and Dr. Kivits said fine. So I said yes. I didn't think about it for a second but asked Greta, who was three months' pregnant and immediately agreed.

In a sense, it would be a voyage of self-discovery as much as discovery. In that classic way of the Grand Tour, I was leaving my home, at the age of twenty-seven, to discover myself. Leaving the plain, hardheaded Flemish world of no bullshit—head down, nose clean, hard work, low profile—and heading to a place of big, apocalyptic emotions: despair and exuberance and tragedy and fear. A place that was really coming apart at the seams; a slow-moving disaster scene that had just once again hit a new catastrophe. It was my dream: I was going to the heart of Africa—Zaire—to explore the outbreak of a new virus.

CHAPTER 2

Adventure at Last

GRETA AND I cut short our Paris weekend and quickly returned to Antwerp, where Pattyn and Guido met me in the lab, together with Dr. Kivits, head of the health section of the Department of Development Aid in Brussels. We spent a few hours hunting down protective gloves and masks and some basic lab equipment. I tried to familiarize myself with the procedures for maximal protection from hazardous viruses, both in the lab and in the field. It basically means protecting your eyes, mouth, nose, and hands, and avoiding needle pricks. Guido gave me some motorbike goggles, which turned out to be extremely useful.

I was also quickly trained in hematology lab procedures and blood tests. Because this was a hemorrhagic-fever epidemic—which included, by definition, symptoms of bleeding—I would need to monitor all kinds of blood parameters: the degree of disseminated intravascular coagulation, which causes uncontrollable bleeding; the number of platelets and hematocrits; and so on.

But Pattyn was mostly interested in teaching me how to capture bats. For some reason he was convinced that they would prove to be the virus reservoir (the place or animal where the virus normally hides). To be honest this was the only thing that scared me about the trip. I am poor at catching flying objects at the best of times, even when they don't have claws and teeth. I nodded while he explained, but I decided on the spot that I wouldn't catch a single bat (and didn't).

Meanwhile, WHO had just released the news of an outbreak of a hemorrhagic fever in southern Sudan. Nzara was 450 miles east of Yambuku, where "our" Zairean epidemic seemed focused. And analysis at Porton Down "had revealed a new virus, morphologically similar to Marburg, but antigenically different," WHO said. This meant that by October 15, three laboratories—ours, the CDC, and Porton Down—had independently identified what seemed like it could be the *same* new virus, which was the probable cause of *two*, simultaneous, deadly epidemics.

The telex from WHO was the first we heard of the Sudan outbreak, and this startled us. There was something very sinister about a virus suddenly unleashing in two such isolated places. Where would it strike next?

I went back to the library. Pattyn had told me that the American team from the CDC included Karl Johnson, the man who had discovered Machupo fever in Bolivia. I tried to photocopy everything he'd written.

I raced home and packed enough for 10 days. Pattyn insisted I take a suit and tie, as I would "represent the Belgian government" and meet with Zairean government officials—something I had absolutely no interest in then, but would have to do hundreds of times two decades later as head of UNAIDS. Luckily I did own a suit; I had bought one for my wedding.

Then I hunted down my passport, no easy feat. It had long since expired. (I didn't need one to go to Paris, since I was a European Community national.) I had even cut out my passport photograph to use for some urgently required sports-club membership card. And of course this defunct and defaced excuse for a passport didn't have any kind of visa for Zaire in it. I knew that Pattyn had decided to come with me to Kinshasa, just for the week—but I had no idea if they would even let me get on the plane. That night I couldn't sleep for nerves and excitement.

Dr. Kivits reassured me that he would get me on the airplane, even with my shredded and useless identity document. Indeed, when Pattyn's wife Renée drove us to Brussels airport on Sunday evening—while her husband ranted nonstop about various bat species, the viruses that nestled in their organs, and the need to keep our guard up with those confounded Americans and French—Kivits was there in the departure lounge, a mild smile on his face.

At check-in, when the police officer at immigration wordlessly gestured me to one side with a hostile glare, Kivits stepped in and exhibited some kind of official supercard that magically gave me passage through immigration and out of my own country. So far so good, but without a passport, how would I manage to get into Zaire?

It appeared that Dr. Kivits had several such tricks up his sleeve. He told me, "Find a passenger called Paul Lelievre-Damit in first class. He knows you're on the plane. When you get to Kinshasa, just follow his instructions. Do exactly what he says and you'll be fine."

I felt like Tintin, the boy hero, in some sort of comic-strip thriller. I wanted to laugh out loud. It was absolutely nothing like real life.

On board the aircraft, I still couldn't sleep. When our DC-10 stopped off in Athens at about 4 A.M. to refuel, only four people left the plane to stretch their legs. All of us were men and all of us headed to the airport bar, where we introduced ourselves. One was Paul Lelievre-Damit, the very man I was supposed to meet.

Lelievre-Damit was chief of the Belgian Development Cooperation in Zaire, and one of the most powerful foreigners in Kinshasa. He was probably mightier than the Belgian ambassador, since Lelievre-Damit sat on the money sack. When he figured out who *I* was, he interrupted my halting story about an epidemic outbreak and started swearing.

"Goddamn! It's always the same with these bloody bureaucrats in Brussels! We're facing a terrible epidemic, and all they could find is you? How old are you? *Twenty-seven?* You're a totally green trainee, barely even a doctor. You've never seen Africa in your life . . ."

I winced at his robust and graphic outburst of Flemish epithets. It was undeniable. I had no expertise; few skills; I could no more save the African heartland from a mystery virus than a comic-strip boy could have done. But after a couple of glasses of ouzo it emerged that Lelievre-Damit had played cards with my dad when they were both penniless students in Leuven, and that helped a lot.

"When we arrive in Kinshasa, just stick to me," he said. "Don't look left or right or turn around. The airport is pandemonium, the police are worse than the criminals, and you're as clueless as a puppy—you'll be eaten alive. When we land, follow me as close as possible. Don't look left or right, don't reply to any question, and above all, don't hand your piece-of-shit passport to anybody but me. We'll go straight to the VIP room, and I'll make sure you'll get into the country. OK?"

I nodded, speechless.

The next morning the pilot smoothly navigated our DC-10 into Ndjili airport in Kinshasa, where we parked near several wreckages of less fortunate airplanes. Out of the windows I could see hundreds of people on the terrace of the airport building, waiting for family or hoping for business, and when the doors of the plane opened, a steaming sauna of air rushed into my face. I pushed to the front of the plane to find Lelievre-Damit, and as instructed, I glued myself to him when descending the DC-10 stairs, as tightly as a baby monkey clings to his mother.

To be honest, I wasn't just bewildered and hungover: I was slightly afraid. The light was very bright—it must have been 10 A.M.—and the tarmac was full of women swathed in cloth and men in *abakos* (an acronym for *à bas le costume*, "down with the suit," a Mao-style jacket that Zaire's longtime dictator, Mobutu Sésé Seko, had made compulsory after a visit to China). They cried out and waved and grabbed at the passengers.

With practiced, fluid movements Lelievre-Damit and Pattyn glided me into the VIP room, where a very respectful official smiled and accompanied us to Lelievre-Damit's diplomatic car. There was no mention of anything so vulgar as an identity document.

THE ROADS OF Kinshasa were unbelievable, with people and animals wandering randomly across them, not to mention the vehicles, which hurtled from every direction. It looked to me like the most unbridled chaos. We drove straight to the headquarters of the Fométro, the *Fonds Médical Tropical*, a nongovernmental organization that operated much of Belgium's vast program for medical aid in Central Africa. We were told that an important meeting of the *Commission Internationale pour le Contrôle de la Fièvre Hemorragique au Zaire*, chaired by the minister of health, was already underway.

We found a large number of men, and one woman, seated around a table in an intense fog of cigar and cigarette smoke. When we entered the room all of them had just stopped speaking, and as their heads swiveled almost all seemed to be glaring at us. Pattyn's reputation had clearly preceded him, and hackles were rising in anticipation of a turf battle.

Everybody introduced themselves. The Zairean health minister, Professor Nguete, was a sharp-minded, obese man, about sixty years old, with a half-chewed cigar screwed tightly into his mouth: I rarely saw him without it. The American Karl Johnson—head of Special Pathogens at the CDC—had a thin beard and small, sharp eyes; he smoked a pipe. His right arm, Joel Breman, was taller, burlier, with an amiable smile and was speaking French with a funny accent; I liked him immediately. Pattyn curtly shook their outstretched hands and then stiffened when the lone Frenchman, Pierre Sureau, introduced himself as the representative of the World Health Organization and the French Institut Pasteur. A lean man with silver, curly hair, Sureau was a true *Pasteurien*, a veteran of exotic epidemics from Vietnam to Madagascar, and he was to become something of a mentor to me.

Margaretha Isaacson was the only woman among us; her eyes glinted behind metal-rimmed glasses and her dark brown hair remained helmetlike as she acknowledged our presence. Born in Holland, she escaped the Holocaust and emigrated to Israel, where in her youth she was a fighter pilot. Now she was a South African national, thus a most improbable presence in Zaire, a country that, at least theoretically, observed the ban on travel for citizens of the apartheid regime. But in 1974 in a hospital in Johannesburg, Isaacson had treated a couple of Australian backpackers who had come down with Marburg and infected one of their nurses. The male Australian died, but the two women survived. Thus Isaacson brought with her, from forbidden Johannesburg, the world's entire, tiny supply of serum from Marburg convalescents.

Although we knew our mystery virus wasn't Marburg, we all hoped that it would prove to be a close enough relative that we could use the Marburg antiserum from South Africa to treat patients from this epidemic. Even if not proven clinically, the hypothesis was that high levels of serum antibodies would inactivate the virus in the patient's blood.

There were others present, too: Jean-Jacques Muyembe, a sleek and brilliant young Zairean professor of microbiology for whom I later came to develop profound respect: Gérard Raffier, head of the French Medical Mission in Zaire, and his equivalents at the Belgian Fométro, Jean-François Ruppol and Jean Burke; and André Koth, a slim, bespectacled young doctor from the Kinshasa Medical Service who looked extremely intimidated. Except for Koth, I was by far the youngest of the lot.

Karl Johnson rapped us to attention—it was clearly his meeting—and summarized the situation in a few words. We were dealing with a virus that was completely new to science. Its potential for transmission—particularly to medical teams and caregivers—appeared to be extraordinarily dangerous. Reports claimed that more than 80 percent of people infected were dying. We had only one possible treatment option in the form of serum from convalescents who had very high levels of antibodies, but we needed to track down such individuals, test their blood to be sure it didn't contain live virus, and then treat it to be able to inject antibodies into people currently sick. These tests required very specialized material and highly qualified researchers working in extremely safe environments. In the meantime—here he nodded at Margaretha—we would attempt to use the Marburg serum. Furthermore, since the immediate cause of death was severe hemorrhage, and given the probable role of coagulation in the development of uncontrollable hemorrhaging, we would endeavor to treat patients with heparin, an anticoagulant medication.

He went on: the worst scenario we faced was the specter of a full-blown epidemic in Kinshasa, an unruly megacity with poor infrastructure, an unreliable administration, and 3 million citizens accustomed to defying arbitrary government controls. Barely a fort-night before, three people from the Belgian mission in Yambuku—two nuns and a priest—had been brought to the capital for treatment. All were now dead, and they had infected at least one nurse, Mayinga N'Seka, now hospitalized in critical condition. Efforts were being made to track down all her contacts in the city to quarantine them. They included—here Johnson paused for a second—personnel of the US Embassy, where the nurse had recently finalized arrangements for a student visa to the United States.

Was this the beginning of an outbreak in Kinshasa? Once a virus this lethal is introduced into an environment this chaotic, it is almost impossible to control it. It is also an explosive political situation for the government, and it was clear from the health minister's agitation that news about the epidemic was out and panic was already setting in. At that time we had no real indication of how contagious the dis-ease was, only that it seemed highly lethal.

Karl spoke no French, though by necessity that was the language of our meeting, so Pierre Sureau and I translated for him, back and forth. This is a role I've often picked up and it's useful, because trans-lators have a lot of power and connections. It also keeps your mind from wandering, which is crucial, because when I heard the phrase *"probably the most serious risk to public health in the past 25 years,"* some-thing inside me went oddly quiet.

The top priority, then, was Kinshasa, and it was decided that most of the international team would remain there temporarily, while a small contingent would travel to Equateur province for a three- or four-day scouting trip to do the logistical groundwork and sketch out a plan for a full-blown investigation.

Karl asked for volunteers. I was the first to raise my hand. The others were Pierre Sureau, the Frenchman; Ruppol, a jovial man with a leathery tan; and Joel Breman, the younger American. André Koth was later deputized to join us, to represent Zaire.

With an airy wave of his hand, Pattyn then also volunteered me to visit the infected Kinshasa nurse with Sureau—"my young colleague will accompany you."

We were driven to the Clinique Ngaliema in a Fométro four-wheel-drive car. It suddenly began to rain heavily; I was not yet used to tropical storms. The Clinique Ngaliema was actually a hospital for the wealthy. It was near the Congo River, in Gombe, one of the nicer parts of town, which in colonial times had been a neighborhood reserved for whites. But still, the roads were gashed with deep potholes and the earth beneath was red. Even something as ordinary as the ground you walked on was different here, more vivid and alive.

There was a very fearful atmosphere in the corridors of the clinic. Dr. Courteille, the director of Internal Medicine, who received us, briefed us first about safety precautions. After the deaths of the two Belgian nuns—and their infection of nurse Mayinga—their mattresses were burned, and their rooms locked up and fumigated with formaldehyde vapor on four successive days. Disposal of bodies was carried out by wrapping them in cotton sheets impregnated with a phenolic disinfectant, and the fully wrapped bodies were sealed inside two large, heavy-duty plastic bags before being placed in their coffins.

Courteille, who was taking care of the nuns and of Mayinga, was careful not to accompany us to the sick nurse's bedside, and it seemed that all the personnel kept a guarded distance from their former colleague. But Sureau had already visited Mayinga and he seemed at ease. Despite our cumbersome protective garments—balaclava-style bonnet, surgical robe, gloves, overshoes, and goggles—he had obviously struck up a rapport with the young woman. She was very sick, and completely desperate, and convinced she was going to die.

Mayinga had been hospitalized on Friday, October 15, with a high fever and a severe headache. Now, on Monday the 18th, she began bleeding; there were black, sticky stains around her nose, ears, and mouth and blotches under her skin where blood was pooling. She had uncontrollable diarrhea and vomiting. She clung to Pierre, who soothed her, telling her about the serum that Margaretha Isaacson would administer, which contained antibodies that might strengthen her immune system to fight the virus. Sadly the serum didn't work and Mayinga died a few days later.

We drew blood to perform a number of blood tests that would guide the decision to prescribe supportive treatment for intravascular coagulation, which we thought might be the cause of death in hemorrhagic fever. We took the vials of blood over to the hospital lab to look at them under the microscope—Mayinga was lucky to have been hospitalized in her place of work, because Ngaliema was a private clinic for privileged people, and it did have some basic equipment. But none of the technicians or personnel was willing to handle Mayinga's samples for some good reasons, as the hospital lab did not have a containment facility.

I examined her blood, and it was a catastrophe. The platelet count was terrifyingly low. As green and unimaginative as I was, the real lethality of this virus began to sink in, and my hands shook a little as I handled her blood. Who knew how this virus was transmitted—by insects, or body fluids, or dust.

We also visited Pavilion 5, the isolation ward. Clinique Ngaliema was constructed in the colonial manner, with separate pavilions connected by covered walkways to maximize the potential for isolating contagious patients and to keep as much air as possible circulating around. About 50 people were quarantined at that point, either because they had cared for the two Belgian nuns from the Yambuku mission or because they had had close contact with Mayinga. They included a fourteen-year-old girl who had eaten from the same plate as Mayinga the day she developed a fever; there was even a pregnant woman, quite visibly only days away from giving birth.

We checked them out briefly; although clearly frightened, and perhaps depressed, they seemed physically normal. They remained in isolation for nearly one month, but none became ill.

We returned to the Fométro for a quick shower before the International Commission's second meeting of the day. Once again we all filed into the large meeting room, to discuss details of the trip that Sureau, Breman, Koth, and I would take. I noted that an obviously important white man was already seated at one of the chairs along the wall. Broad-faced, with a trim gray moustache, he wasn't taking notes—didn't even look as though he was paying much attention—and I swiftly forgot about him. But at the end of meeting, he took over.

"So we'll need a C-130 transport plane," he began to dictate, speaking French with an extreme American accent. "We'll need a

Land Rover, with supplies of gas . . . " and he listed an improbable amount of equipment and supplies.

At some unseen command, an assistant holding a wooden box entered the room. Inside the box was the coolest contraption I had ever seen. It was a mobile phone—the kind of thing you saw only in movies in those days. Bill Close picked up the handset and said in his funny accent, "I want to speak to General Bumba"—the commander in chief of the Zairean Air Force, who had the same last name as the town where we were headed.

"Mon vieux," he drawled. "I'll need a C-130 tomorrow morning at 4 A.M. sharp to drop a team in Bumba, OK? Merci!"

And then without really waiting for a reply, he put down the handset and his assistant closed the box. We all just gaped at them.

Bill Close (incidentally, the father of the actress Glenn Close) had come to Congo just before Independence as a missionary worker, though he was a trained physician. Somehow he became President Mobutu's personal physician as well as director of the biggest hospital in the country, Mama Yemo Hospital in Kinshasa (it was named for Mobutu's mother). But this didn't fully explain the extent of his power and influence in Zaire. He was a mysterious man, thoroughly likable, with an unmatched knowledge of Zaire and connections at all levels in society. A year later, he left Zaire, disillusioned by the Mobutu regime. We stayed in touch until his death in Wyoming in 2009.

AFTER THE MEETING broke up, it was suddenly nightfall, the abrupt equatorial sundown another new and surprising experience for me. I hadn't had lunch and I was ravenous, so a few expatriate Belgians took me out for a night on the town. They filled me up with stories of the epidemic—how pilots were refusing to fly to Bumba because birds that caught the mystery disease were falling out of the sky; how Zaireans believed the virus was caused by witchcraft and was impossible to escape.

In sum, these expats were eager to tell the greenhorn all about the realities of "Darkest Africa." Although there were of course exceptions, I didn't much like what they said—a lot of disrespectful, sneering stories about those Zaireans.

But I immediately loved Kinshasa's night scene. The music was terrific—a very elegant, intricate rumba-type sound—and the dancing was fascinating: in Zaire people moved their hips, not their feet, swaying in a minimal space, creating a wave that was subtle, suggestive, complex. In Belgium at the time, we discoed, jerking around. This was beautiful.

It was a different planet, and yet I felt part of the scene—completely natural, not scared or threatened in any way. That slight beat of panic at the foreign and unknowable nature of this country fell away, and it came to me that everything would be absolutely fine.

CHAPTER 3

The Mission in Yambuku

I N THE 4 A.M. darkness, with a pulsing hangover, I watched our
military pilots striding angrily back and forth on the tarmac.
They were clearly bursting with resentment at the prospect of
flying to the epidemic zone. They refused to help us load the aircraft.
Finally they agreed to fly us to Bumba as instructed, but they told us
they wouldn't stop there—just drop us off and fly on.

A Land Rover was driven on board and secured. We loaded in
some gasoline, a few crates of protective gear and medicine, and some
supplies for the Belgian mission. We settled into the military-style
seats along the walls and braced for a rocky ride to Bumba, the capital
of the subdistrict.

As the sun rose the pilots loosened up a little. They let us move,
one by one, into the cockpit, where we could take in the incredible
vision of the tropical rain forest that flowed beneath us like a vast,
heaving green sea punctuated now and then with a hamlet of frag-
ile huts. The plane was basically following the Congo River—huge,
nine miles wide in places, the other bank often barely visible. Again
I heard the story of pilots watching birds fall dead over the forest

around Yambuku, struck midair by the mystery virus, but there was a new twist: dead human bodies lining the roads.

We landed in Bumba, a riverside town of then perhaps 10,000 people and the administrative and trading capital of the district—a territory half the size of Belgium, with mostly dense forest interspersed with coffee, cocoa, rice, and palm plantations, almost all owned by Unilever corporation. For about two weeks the entire zone had been in quarantine and under martial law, cut off from the rest of the country. And this had occurred during the crucial rice and coffee harvest, the area's main (if not only) source of cash. The timing could not have been worse for the population and for the few businesses struggling to survive in this forgotten corner of the globe.

As soon as the C-130 came to a standstill, I moved to the hatch at the back, impatient to get to work. What I saw through the open loading dock is permanently imprinted in my memory: hundreds of people—the whole town it seemed—were standing on the red-earth airstrip in the burning sun, first staring at us and then yelling, "Oyé! *Oyé!*"

When Ruppol drove the Land Rover out of the huge plane, the crowd cheered and a steady murmur of comment began. The crowd was yelling because they were expecting supplies of food and basic goods—this was the first plane to land in several weeks. When they realized we were not delivering foodstuffs, the more desperate pushed forward, hoping to board the plane, but the military police beat them back.

As soon as the last box was unloaded, the pilots shouted, *"Bonne chance"* (Good luck!), with a look of pity and, if I'm not mistaken, scorn, before gunning the engines and taking off. We too were now part of a quarantined population. As soon as the noise of the engines died away, Ruppol, who had grown up in Zaire, addressed the crowd in Lingala, with the natural authority of a man born to rule.

"Good morning men and women of Bumba. We know that you are suffering from the terrible epidemic of Yambuku fever. We know that you all suffer from the quarantine. We have been instructed by President Mobutu Sésé Seko to come and help you, to stop the epidemic so that the quarantine can be lifted and the harvest can be shipped to Kinshasa. We ask for your cooperation in respecting the quarantine, isolating any person who falls ill, and reporting them to the authorities."

The crowd responded with approving calls of "Eh" and "Oyé."

A determined Flemish man appeared, perhaps 10 years older than I, wearing dark glasses and a local shirt made of African *wax* material. He introduced himself to us: Father Carlos, from the Order of Scheut, thus a colleague of the Catholic missionary priests who had died of the virus in Yambuku. I was startled—priests, to me, were old and wore vestments—but Carlos drove us to his mission, where a photo of Mobutu adorned the fluorescent green wall alongside the smaller wooden crucifix. (This bright green was, I soon discovered, the color of Mobutu's "Party of the Revolution.") We were plied with steak and French fries (from the mission's cows and potatoes) and whisky and beer and cigars (at noon!).

Though very committed to the well-being of his flock, Father Carlos was also a very practical man, and he briefed us about the epidemic. It had all started in Yambuku in the first week of September, when the headmaster of the mission school, who had been traveling through the north on vacation, returned and fell ill. After his death, crowds attended his funeral, and within days the mission hospital began filling with other sufferers, including the headmaster's wife. They suffered high fever, headache, hallucinations, and usually bled to death. One after another, his caregivers at the Yambuku mission hospital fell ill, along with members of his family, other patients, and dozens of other, apparently unrelated, people. Father Carlos listed their names, emphasizing—perhaps naturally—the Belgian nuns and priests who had succumbed to the epidemic: Sister Beata, who acted as midwife; Sisters Myriam and Edmunda, who had been transported to Kinshasa and died there; Father August, Sister Romana, Father Germain. With the Zaireans every patient was preceded by a kind of rough genealogy—"the son of"—so I grabbed a notebook.

Nobody knew how many people had died, but all those who fell ill died within eight days. The few nuns still alive at the Yambuku mission were convinced they too would die soon. Only one person was known to have recovered from the virus. As for current cases, there were some in Bumba, and several people who had traveled to Bumba from Yambuku and were being kept in quarantine.

After lunch Pierre and I strolled down to the river, 16 miles wide at Bumba—almost half the entire coastline of Belgium!—and choked with blue floating-hyacinth flowers. The entire town of Bumba had to come here to get water to drink and wash with: though the colonial administration had installed pipes to bring running water to some of the houses, the system had already, 15 years after Independence, fallen into disrepair. There was also no electricity in the town apart from a few privately owned generators.

We circled back to the Portuguese grocery store, Noguera. The shelves were bare—a bit of powdered milk, salt, matches, white flour, cooking oil, cylinders of gas. There were, however, some cans of pilchards and blue workers' overalls: both Pierre and I liked the idea, and bought them. They seemed more practical than the few clothes I had packed, and better adapted to the unbearable humid heat.

It was time to pay our respects to the *Commissaire de Zone* (District Commissioner). *Citoyen* Ipoya Olonga was almighty in the region, second only to the military commander and the chief of the feared state security service. Citoyen Olonga also represented the omnipresent MPR—the *Mouvement Populaire de la Révolution*—Zaire's sole political party, of which every newborn automatically became a member. After President Mobutu visited China, Zaire was completely organized into the propaganda terminology of Maoism and riddled with official corruption, the country quite openly structured into a sort of fiscal feudalism, in which each level of tax collector took a cut of the tax he'd collected and sent the rest up the hierarchy, until President Mobutu placed a great portion of his citizens' earnings into his own bottomless pockets.

I found myself enduringly fascinated by this totalitarian, nearly Orwellian, type of organization, which gave a creepy, fascistic overlay to so many kinds of interactions that would otherwise have amounted to simple gangsterism. Everyone complied with the command to call each other *citoyen*, betraying a very pervasive fear; in every type of relationship in Zaire you could smell this corruption and abuse of power.

Our meeting with Citoyen Olonga was pointless but necessary, the first of many empty protocol visits I would have to endure in my life. We were kept waiting for the obligatory hour, so that we would be impressed with the Commissaire's power. Fortunately we had a chance meeting with the director and doctor of the Unilever plantation in Ebonda, 10 kilometers from Bumba and the main employer in the region. The epidemic was an economic disaster for PLZ (the Lever plantations in Zaire), because they couldn't transport their harvest and many of their workers had fled. Together with the missions, they provided the only logistical support that we could count on in Zaire. They had come to ask advice on how to handle funerals of patients dying with hemorrhagic fever; they had seen several deaths and feared for the lives of two sick children aged three and five years old. We agreed to see them the next morning, on our way to the Yambuku mission.

At last we were permitted to enter the office, where we had to endure the ritual of tea and coffee and a pretense of polite conversation. Finally Ruppol, who was easily the most familiar with this sort of proceeding, broached the need to provide our short expedition—and the full team's much longer one—with backup assistance, including transportation. It was all done with few words and some highly scripted gestures.

"How can the poor region of Bumba provide you with all this logistical help? I have no budget for this kind of assistance! We're all suffering here, and I can't even go to Kinshasa to join my family" (a kind of shuffling of papers, a highly telegraphic frown of worry, a terribly regretful shaking of the head).

More empathetic smiles from Ruppol, whose face must have been aching. "Ah, but we have considered that. And what we have here will help you to do it." Suddenly a shiny, medium-sized suitcase materialized in Ruppol's hands.

Ruppol had come with a *suitcase* full of local currency. I had never seen such wads and wads of money. Officially, one Zaire was worth one US dollar; in reality the currency was worth a fraction of that. Still, when he opened his suitcase to display its contents to the Commissaire de Zone it was like a drug deal in a movie. There was no receipt, no detailed estimate, no pretense that we were hiring so many people for such-and-such a length of time. Indeed, whatever we had to do afterward we had to pay for separately.

But the suitcase had broken the ice. Citoyen Olonga told us about the very real worry of food provision in town; no boats or trucks had been allowed to enter the zone for more than three weeks, he said. The military camp in Bumba had been without food for several days.

Back at the mission, I slept like the dead. I had missed three nights of sleep—in Antwerp, on the flight to Zaire, and in the bars of Kinshasa.

The next morning we visited the small Bumba hospital, where a dozen people traveling from Yambuku were quarantined, along with one or two other patients suspected of possible hemorrhagic fever. The Clinique Ngaliema in Kinshasa was a little dirty from a European perspective, but still, relatively decent. Here I saw real deprivation, conditions that were truly shameful. The few suspected fever patients were clearly ill, but their symptoms were not spectacular: they had high fever and chest and abdominal pain, but a cursory exam gave no indication that they had hemorrhagic fever. They lay on beds without any mattress—just the bare metal springs, covered by a cloth if they had one. There were no medicines. The walls and floors were really dirty and had literally fallen away in parts. All this was apparently "normal." These vulgar conditions had no connection to the sudden health crisis—things were always this way.

All around the hospital were women with shaved heads, some screaming and crying, others preparing food with a lack of hygiene that made me blanch. The patients themselves were in a condition little short of horrific, blood oozing from their mouths.

Dr. N'goy Mushola, the doctor in charge, was a fairly young man, accustomed to performing surgery and C-sections in conditions that would cause a European medic to faint. But he was clearly overwhelmed and terrified by the hemorrhagic fever. Several people had died in his care, and he described their violent, uncontrollable bleeding to us in apocalyptic tones.

I drew blood from all of N'goy's patients for further examination in Kinshasa. Together with Masamba Matondo, the chief medical officer of nearby Lisala—coincidentally the birthplace of President Mobutu, the man whose photo was on every wall—N'goy gave us a quick, clear overview of the epidemic situation based on his visit to Yambuku. Again there was the litany of names: X got it, and her husband Y, and also her sister Z, and she was cared for by her aunt Z from the village of Something—so that it became quite difficult for me to follow and I grabbed my notebook and raced to get it all down. At least 44 villages in a radius of 60 miles around Yambuku were affected. Most of the first people to be affected had apparently visited Yambuku hospital but, Masamba said, many secondary cases had occurred—in other words people who had not been in Yambuku. Virtually everyone who had been infected with the fever had died within a week.

N'goy nodded: everybody died. He had heard of only one survivor, perhaps two, but none of his patients had lived.

By the time we left for Yambuku we had heard of well over a hundred fatalities. My natural skepticism began to fall away, replaced by doom. The stories of Father Carlos and Dr. N'goy, the reports at the Bumba hospital, the evident fear of the pilots and the townspeople of Bumba and their desperate attempts to flee the town . . . the apparent virulence of this disease, the high mortality—put together with the poverty and poor organization that characterized Zaire and the potential for contagion in Kinshasa—added up to a picture that Joel Breman summarized as "potentially the most deadly epidemic of the century."

We left in two Land Rovers—one of them lent to us by Father Carlos—and drove in silence through the overpowering, unstoppable, exuberant force of uncut equatorial jungle, well over 30 feet high. All kinds of green pressed in on us, high walls of leaves and muscular lianas like something out of a Tarzan movie. I had never experienced how powerful and all-invading nature can be, and somehow it compounded my sense that we were making our way to something horrible and uncontrolled.

We stopped off at the Unilever plantation in Ebonda. The personnel were frantic. They had incredibly high expectations for our visit, and our brief stay clearly disappointed and further upset them. Women were chanting and shouting in mourning around the small clinic; a number of deaths had recently occurred. We met with three frightened Peace Corps volunteers who had holed up at the plantation—blonde American girls, about twenty years old, who were completely hysterical with fear, in floods of tears. My guess was that even without a mysterious, lethal epidemic, the stress they went through on a daily basis, trying to teach English in Ebonda, must have been really quite something. But I had no idea how to handle them. Joel took over, and promised to get them out, and home, on the first available form of transport.

I had a photocopy of the image of the virus that we had seen under our electron microscope in Antwerp, and for some reason it occurred to me to pull it out and show it. This had a fascinating placebo effect on the crowd. I suppose it made the virus seem more real—less supernatural, and perhaps less potent.

Beyond Ebonda the road became almost impassable, barely more than a sinkhole of mud and water, with entire sections washed away by the torrential equatorial rains. We drove through small villages of not more than 10 to 25 huts, snuggling like nests at the foot of the towering tropical trees. About half of the villages had erected barriers to control people's movements in this time of quarantine. The elders explained that they had done this without any official instructions, just as their elders had done in the time of smallpox epidemics. We asked if anyone in those villages was currently ill; all shook their heads no. There was no way to check whether this was true, but we told them that if anyone fell ill, they should isolate the person as much as possible and seek to get a message to us at the Yambuku mission.

Suddenly after four hours the dirt road opened out into cleared land, with a few dozen huts and some brick houses that bore remnants of paint and red tiled roofs. That was Yandongi, the administrative capital of the subdistrict, a sleepy town of perhaps a thousand people with a few brick houses from colonial times and a few shops with hardly any goods. Oddly, Yandongi was almost the only village in the Belgian Congo to appear in any work of Flemish literature: in the 1960s Jef Geraerts, a colonial official, had written about the more or less soft-porn adventures of an assistant regional administrator in this sad little place, which he bewilderingly described as seething with ecstatic naked dancing and a primal, wild, rich energy.

Then the thick green curtain around the road closed in again, and we advanced with great difficulty until first the coffee plantations and then the church and red roofs of the Yambuku mission appeared, like mirages, in the blinding sunlight. Surrounded by a neatly swept courtyard lined with royal palm trees and immaculate lawns, they seemed surreal. It was difficult to believe that this clean, orderly, even idyllic place was really Yambuku, the heart of the mysterious killer virus.

To the right of the small church lay the building where the fathers lived; to the left lay the convent where the nuns slept, and the school; and behind them was the clinic. In between was the guesthouse, where three nuns, all aged between forty and fifty-five, and an old, white-bearded priest stood outside the door as if they had been waiting all day.

As our group walked up, Sister Marcella, the mother superior, shouted, "Don't come any nearer! Stay outside the barrier or you will die just like us!"

Although she was speaking French, I could hear from her accent not only that she was Flemish, but also the region that she was from, near Antwerp. (This doesn't make me a linguist; Flemish dialects are very distinct, and this was particularly the case for the sisters' accents.) I jumped over the line of gauze bandage that had been strung up to warn away visitors and shook her hand. In Flemish, I said, "Good day, I'm Dr. Peter Piot from the Tropical Institute in Antwerp. We're here to help you and stop the epidemic. You'll be all right."

There was a very emotional scene as the three nuns, Sisters Marcella, Genoveva and Mariette, broke down, clinging to my arm, holding each other and crying helplessly as they all began talking at once. Watching their colleagues die one by one had been an appalling experience. They talked and talked in a rush of relief. They felt, I think, that we had come to save them and, specifically, that they could count on me. I felt so glad that I could speak these women's language, both in terms of their dialect and their mentality, the attitudes that they came from.

All these women were younger than my parents, but they seemed antiquated. Their voices reminded me of my father's grandmother, a big, round-faced woman who was known for miles around as Moe Dolf—Mother Dolf. (Her husband, who died in 1921, was named Adolf, so she was Mother of Adolf's children.) Moe Dolf grew up on a farm near Wijgmaal, a village near Leuven, and she had never been to school. Still, she could count, and she was sharp; she had a hard head and she was a great cook. She owned a tavern in Wijgmaal that doubled and tripled as a dancing hall, inn, restaurant, village shop, and social club for the men from the Rémy factory down the road, which manufactured starch and where one of my great-grandfathers worked as a machinist, and everyone in the neighborhood celebrated births and marriages, and mourned deaths, with a party at Moe Dolf's place. Her seven children and many descendants—including my father and his mother—all grew up serving beer and waiting tables, and tending to the pig, the chickens, and the vegetable patch out in back.

Sister Marcella, a short but determined woman, appeared to be in charge. She looked and sounded a little like my great-grandmother and she had the same capable hands and broad cheekbones, but she didn't have that hard-edged scrutiny in her eye or the same sense of brisk energy. Perhaps it was only to be expected, after weeks of fearful isolation, that she seem so drained of life. In any case it was clear that to her I represented a young but valiant rescuer, someone who had come from home to restore things to their proper place. Though I was the youngest, most junior, and quite possibly the most inept among us, we were bound together through the links of language and shared tradition.

Later the sisters told us that they had read that in case of an epidemic, a *cordon sanitaire* had to be established to contain the spread of the disease. They had interpreted this literally, with an actual cord that they strung around the guesthouse where they had taken refuge. They had also nailed to a nearby palm tree a sign in Lingala, warning *"Anybody who passes this fence will die."* It instructed visitors to ring a bell and leave messages at the foot of the tree. It was scary and sad and spoke volumes about the fear that they had endured.

As Sister Mariette prepared dinner for us, Sister Marcella showed us the notebooks where she had recorded all the deaths of hemorrhagic fever patients, and any data she felt was relevant to their illness, such as recent travel. Nine out of 17 hospital staff had died, as had 39 other people among the 60 families living at the mission, and four sisters and two fathers. She broke down several times as she described their symptoms and the agony of their deaths, particularly those of her fellow nuns. This small group of women, all from the same area northeast of Antwerp, all of whom had been in Zaire for more than six years, had naturally developed a profound bond in this small outpost of Flanders in the equatorial forest.

"We prepared ourselves to die," she said simply. "We spent our days in prayer." I knew that to her this was a simple, factual description, but these modest words conjured a suffocating sense of doom, the sense of an invisible disease closing in on a dwindling number of women.

Sister Marcella continued reading out from her neatly kept records as I scribbled down more precious pieces of information. She listed the names of villages where deaths had occurred. She wondered whether the illness might be linked to eating fresh monkey meat: the villagers often foraged for food in the forest and the headmaster who was, tentatively, our "Patient Zero" had returned from his travels with several monkey and antelope carcasses. She noted a high number of deaths among newborn children born at the mission clinic, and observed too a sudden spike in stillbirths among their herd of pigs. Three months ago, she said, there was an epidemic among goats in the region of Yandongi.

These were all good lines of inquiry. (Later I took blood from the pigs through their tail veins, a new experience for me.) None of them panned out exactly, but another of Sister Marcella's hypotheses proved to be exactly right. "Something strange must be happening at the funerals," she told us. "Again and again we've seen that the funerals have been followed a week later by a batch of new cases among the mourners."

She was clearly pleading with us for answers, but there was nothing we could say. Our first job was just to ask questions. To break the ice I showed the electron microscope photos of the new virus, as I later did in every village we visited. The sisters too were fascinated by the wormlike structures that had caused so much pain and devastation in their community.

Joel handed over the supplies we had brought with us—essentials such as petrol, but also comfort items: Gouda cheese, beer, some correspondence, and Flemish newspapers. Although we had no authority to do so, we told the nuns again and again that we would not leave them until the outbreak was over. Although we might be going back and forth we would not abandon them.

Pierre suggested that starting the next day we split up into three teams, one per vehicle. Each team would systematically visit as many villages as possible for a preliminary epidemiologic survey, to identify active cases of hemorrhagic fever, to provide whatever basic care we could muster, and to make sure that the patients were kept isolated and, if necessary, buried without the normal rituals, to prevent further spread.

We then briefly visited the hospital, which was made of a few small, square pavilions with red metal roofs, connected by covered walkways, much like the Clinique Ngaliema. Everything was empty: most of the patients had fled, fearing they would be contaminated by the fever, and finally after several of the nursing sisters died the decision was made to close it down completely. The rooms were clean, the blood stains barely visible, but as a medical center it was very rudimentary and the surgical theater was the most basic kind imaginable: a high bed with a plastic-covered mattress. I didn't see any anesthesia equipment. *How do you do surgery without anesthesia?*

With the diesel oil we brought, the nuns started up the mission's generator so we had some light in the black tropical night. As a feast, they prepared *Carbonnades à la Flamande*, a traditional Flemish winter stew with beer that we settled down to consume in the steaming tropical heat. To me the effect was slightly comic, but I could also see that to the sisters it was almost magically comforting. We had brought beer and wine, and taciturn Father Léon emptied half a bottle of the Johnny Walker whisky that Jean-François Ruppol had brought him. The sisters sipped a few tots of Dubonnet fortified wine, their carefully rationed evening tipple: they seemed to be allowing themselves to relax for the first time since the death of Sister Beata on September 20, exactly one month earlier. They spoke almost endlessly about their families, their religious order, and Flanders.

As we had no clue how the virus was transmitted, and whether the virus could somehow survive on materials such as mattresses and linen, we decided to sleep on the floor of a classroom in the girls' boarding school, which we first fumigated with formaldehyde and mopped with bleach. I was exhausted, but once again could not sleep. There were too many impressions and questions racing through my head. We had no idea whether the epidemic was still spreading or how fast, but we clearly were approaching the heart of it: soon it would be staring us in the face. I wondered too what on earth happens at a Zairean funeral, and what could motivate a Flemish woman to spend her life in the middle of a faraway jungle, totally disconnected from her world, without the most basic infrastructure and communication. How could you run a 100-bed hospital without even one physician? How did people survive in these villages? How could I be most useful here?

The night was bursting with the caws and cries of animals. I went outside in the blackest of nights, where stars shining uninhibited by city light seemed so close above my head that I might almost reach them, and I listened to the distinct and ominous sound of drumming. Perhaps, in the ancient manner, our arrival was being announced.

CHAPTER 4

Ebola

T HERE'S A KIND of excitement that takes over when real discovery is at hand—almost like light drunkenness, but with
tingles. Laying on the floor in the Spartan comfort of the
girls' dormitory in a village thousands of miles from anywhere any
member of my family had ever reached, I knew that this was a defining moment in my life—scientifically, geographically, in terms of
every kind of emotional and physical horizon. I was facing a total
unknown: a new virus, a new continent. Even the insects were mon-
strously unfamiliar, the cockroaches as long and fat as my finger. But
I had no room for fear or worry. I felt *alive*.

The next morning—Thursday, October 21—the nuns introduced
us to the only two known survivors of the mystery fever. One was
the wife of the deceased headmaster of the mission, our Patient Zero.
"Mbuzu ex-Sophie" was a small young woman with hunched shoulders. (President Mobutu banned Christian names, forcing everyone
in Zaire to take an African name; those who continued to use their
previous identities were obliged to camouflage them behind the pre-
fix "ex.") Her head was shaven (I learned in Bumba that mourners in
this region commonly shaved their heads) but she was quite robust,

and though she had clearly been ill she reported only a high fever, headache, fatigue, vomiting, and diarrhea, no bleeding or other signs of internal hemorrhage. Sukato, a male nurse at the hospital, reported a similar set of symptoms, and although he was extremely thin there was no way of telling whether that was due to his illness.

It was a real relief to find two healthy convalescents so quickly. If we could confirm that they really had been infected with the mystery virus—and if we could persuade them to act as donors—these two former patients could provide the precious plasma that seemed to be our only hope to treat other victims of the disease. The problem, however, was that our plasmapheresis equipment was still in Kinshasa. We would also need to test their plasma before using it, to be sure that it didn't contain live virus, and these tests would require specialized material operated by highly qualified researchers working in an extremely safe environment—a virus lab like the one at the CDC in Atlanta. It would not be easy to transport potentially highly lethal substances to Atlanta from Kinshasa; from Yambuku, or even Bumba, it just could not be done. In other words, we would have to persuade these two villagers to travel back to Kinshasa with us when we left. We broached the subject: Sophie, who had lost two of her eight children to the virus, as well as her husband, rejected the option immediately. She initially didn't even want to give blood, though she wanted to help.

We needed to get out on the road before the midday heat and afternoon storms made travel very hard. Leading out from Yandongi, there were four roads we could follow (though they were not "roads" in any Belgian sense), and we had four cars: one that we had brought from Kinshasa by plane, one that Father Carlos had given us from the mission in Bumba, and two that belonged to the Yambuku mission. This meant we could split up. Our objectives were pretty basic. We needed to know whether the epidemic was still active, and if so how active it was and how extensive its geographic spread. The only way to learn these things was to go out and look for clues. We also needed to nail down a preliminary sketch of possible risk factors and, of course, the mode of transmission. And we also needed to take blood samples from the sick—as many as possible—because so far we only had one sample of the virus and we needed to confirm it.

I was to travel with Pierre Sureau and Sister Marcella, the mother superior, in her ancient Land Rover. We would take the road west. We were also planning to act as "firemen," on call for the other teams, though we had no communication equipment whatsoever with us. To reduce the number of people exposed to the risk of contamination, Pierre and I would be the only ones to take blood from acutely ill patients.

The forest erupted with noise like a living thing as we hurtled and lurched our way along the well-trodden paths. At several points we came across barricades—huge branches and bamboo sticks slung across the roads. Although the whole zone was supposed to be under official quarantine, Sister Marcella said that the village elders had received no orders from the medical or military authorities to build these obstacles; they were prompted by old knowledge, ancestral memories of experience with smallpox epidemics that had periodically devastated the region before being eradicated in 1979. These barriers were mostly manned by small children and the elderly; many of the older men and women were smoking pipes that smelled strongly of marijuana. Seeing Sister Marcella they acquiesced and let us pass.

The villages were closely nestled hamlets of mud huts with banana leaf roofs. Outside them, wispy cooking fires burned all day under their dried-leaf awnings. We were quickly surrounded by villagers. There was no doubt that every person we saw, in every village that we went to, had heard about the killer epidemic. Just about every village had suffered at least one death. We took down as much information as possible about those cases and how they were cared for, noting that in almost every case the corpse was buried right behind his or her hut. In addition, there seemed to be no quarantine or precautions other than the barricades, and those were clearly less than total: people spoke freely of family members traveling to other villages to care for their loved ones.

Still, in the first few hamlets the chiefs reported no active cases. I was suspicious but felt that surely they would have no reason to hide a dying patient.

Then after perhaps five or six villages, we were brought to a hut where two patients lay: man and wife. We were told they had been sick for several days. Standing outside the small hut, we robed in our protective gear, with gloves and gown and motorcycle goggles and paper surgical masks. We had been equipped with full-face respirators that provided airtight isolation, and thus better protection from airborne virus particles, but they were suffocatingly impossible to wear in the midday heat. It was the first time I had ever entered an African village home, and in this astronaut gear I was certainly as much of a shock to its inhabitants as they were to me.

The sick couple lay on raffia mats, piled on top of a low platform made of branches. Flies settled insistently on the black crusted blood around their mouths, noses, and ears. Both had dark blotches on their torsos and their eyes were darkly bloodshot. They had barely the strength to move. The husband began vomiting blood, painfully and spottily. Both had a look in their eyes that I later became familiar with in AIDS patients but had never seen before. It is an empty look, a ghostly deadness that some people describe as "glassy-eyed."

With easy, skillful gestures of care, Pierre Sureau slipped over to the bed. He nodded an attempt at reassurance and slipped a syringe into the woman's arm. I merely watched; I had no idea how to be useful, for I knew we had no possible treatment to offer these people. We had supplies of tetracycline, a broad-spectrum antibiotic, and loperamide, a strong antidiarrheal, but neither of these was going to help.

As Pierre drew the blood out of the wife's arm, her husband gave one last strangled choke and then stopped breathing.

I had seen dead people; in medical school I had *cut* dead people. And occasionally patients had died in various hospital wards where I had worked as an intern, as well as violent deaths during my work in the emergency room in Ghent in Belgium. So I had thought I was inured to dying. But most of those had been *sedated* deaths—unfortunate, sure, but sanitized, predicable. Watching someone die in front of me was new.

Both Pierre and I froze: How would the other villagers react? Would they assume that in our nightmarish outfits we had killed this young man? I glanced at Pierre and saw that he, too, was shaken, and the same thought flashed through both of us: if the man had died while Pierre was taking his blood, we would quite possibly be killed. We explained what had happened and left as soon as possible, giving instructions that the bodies should be buried immediately, without any cleansing or ritual, and should only be touched with gloves (we left several pairs in the village).

That morning we saw eight sick people, though none as obviously close to death as the first couple. All had the glassy look in their bloodshot eyes, severe abdominal pain, and bleeding from various orifices. We also saw a number of people who reported that they had suffered what seemed to be an attenuated version of the disease, with swollen face, severe headache, high fever, and chest and abdominal pains, but no hemorrhage. We asked them to allow us to take blood for antibody testing. This was difficult: they seemed convinced that witchcraft of some sort was involved, and it fell to Sister Marcella to persuade them.

Although they seemed reluctant to discuss this in front of Sister Marcella, most of these people attributed their recovery to the intervention of the *nganga kisi*, the herbalist or sorcerer. Pierre and I both noted this, and later discussed the obvious difficulties of asking people for information while using as a translator a person who for religious and medical reasons was so obviously likely to disapprove of certain answers.

We returned, stunned, to the mission in torrential rain, churning with difficulty through the sodden jungle paths. A midafternoon meal was waiting for us. I don't remember exactly what it was, but the sisters ate largely African food: *foufou* porridge; local rice; goat or chicken or game from the forest. Once we even ate monkey—a dish of *carbonnades*, a quintessentially Flemish stew made with fresh monkey meat, probably from a vervet, *Cercopithecus aethiops*, as we were informed when the meal was over. Since we considered monkey a possible vector of the disease, this was perhaps not the most prudent of choices. But we found it hard to be rude to our hosts, and I reasoned with myself that the meat was so extremely overcooked that surely no virus would remain active.

Later that first afternoon, Sister Marcella called the order's mission in Lisala on the crackly old ham radio that was Yambuku's only connection to the outside world. Her colleague in Lisala passed on a message to us from Karl in Kinshasa: Mayinga, the young nurse whom we had visited at the Clinique Ngaliema, was dead. In other words, the Marburg plasma that Margaretha Isaacson had brought with her from South Africa did *not* deliver protection from our epidemic.

That evening there was a new sense among us of the gravity of the situation. A real camaraderie had sprung up among us. Joel Breman from the CDC was our leader—an experienced field epidemiologist, a veteran of smallpox, with a great sense of humor. Pierre Sureau, too, was a real inspiration to me. A chain-smoking fifty-year-old who had more experience in his left elbow than I had in my entire body, he nonetheless was never snide or scornful, indeed treated everyone with the same gentle courtesy. Dr. Masamba, the regional director of public health, who joined us in Bumba, was an excellent organizer, and he seemed impervious to fear. The Belgian Jean-François Ruppol took care of logistics. He spoke Lingala and Kikongo, having grown up in Zaire on his parents' cattle ranch, and he was a good man in a pinch.

Sitting around our lamplit dorm that evening, it struck me that the scene was a little like in those jokes where a Belgian, an American, a Frenchman, and a Zairean might all walk into a bar.

FOR THE NEXT two days we toured villages every morning, taking blood where we could, jotting down every potentially telling detail and piece of data we could muster. We saw patients with blood crusting around their mouths or oozing from their swollen gums. They bled from their ears and nose and from their rectum and vagina; they were intensely lethargic, drained of force.

In every village we organized a meeting with the chief and elders. After the ritual passing of a plastic cup of roughly distilled *arak*—banana alcohol, which Pierre had the courage (or perhaps the common sense) to refuse—we asked them to describe their experience of the new illness, the number of cases and deaths, the dates, whether they had knowledge of any people currently sick. We questioned every villager we came across about day-to-day practices—unusual contact with animals, new areas of forest cleared, food and drink, travel, contact with traders.

We heard of entire families who had been wiped out by the swift-moving virus. In one case, a woman in Yambuku had died days after giving birth, swiftly followed by her newborn. Her thirteen-year-old daughter, who had traveled to Yambuku to take charge of the child, fell ill once she returned to her home village and died days later; followed by her uncle's wife, who had cared for her; then her uncle; and then another female relative who had come to care for him. This extremely virulent interhuman transmission was frightening.

We were all familiar with our terms of mission: we were here just for three or four days, to act as scouts in preparation for the arrival of a larger team that would try to set up systems to control the epidemic and break ground for further research. Our job was to document what was going on, sketch out some basic epidemiology, take samples from acutely sick patients, and, if possible, find recovering convalescents who might provide plasma to help cure future sufferers.

And we were doing that job—harvesting samples, collecting data, and cataloging the basic logistical equipment that the larger team would need to bring. But we knew that from a human point of view this simply wasn't enough. We needed to stop the virus from infecting and killing people.

The mystery fever's epidemic curve was starting to take shape. The classical epidemiological curve is pretty simple; it plots the number of new cases of an infection against time. In the simplest type of outbreak the number of people infected rises gradually, then picks up pace, reaching a peak at the midpoint of the graph. Once the virus has exhausted its stock of easy victims (the weak or easily accessible), the rate of new infections begins to wane until the epidemic fades to a whisper.

All of us were aware of the many exceptions to this in real life— the unexpected outliers, the blips and lags, the complications of propagated epidemics with secondary and tertiary infections. But night by night, as we jotted down data and sketched out a picture from our interviews and notes, it appeared that although people were still dying (and dying horribly), the peak number of new infections around the Yambuku mission might be, at least provisionally, behind us.

This was a huge relief. But another conclusion also began to take shape, and it was a great deal more uncomfortable to deal with. Two elements linked almost every victim of the mystery epidemic. One factor was funerals: many of the dead had been present at the funeral of a sick person or had close contact with someone who had. The other factor was presence at the Yambuku Mission Hospital. Just about every early victim of the virus had attended the outpatient clinic a few days before falling ill.

We developed near-certitude about the mode of transmission one evening, when Joel and I were drawing curves showing the number of cases by location, age, and gender. (Working with Joel was a real education, like a terrific crash course in epidemiology.) It seemed likely by this point that aerosol contact was not enough to transmit the disease. But particularly in the eighteen- to twenty-five-year age group, at least twice as many women had died as men. We knew that there was something fishy about the hospital, and about funerals, but this was the real clue. What's different in men and women at that age?

Being a bunch of men, it took us a little time to figure out the answer. Women get pregnant. And indeed, almost all of the women who had died *had* been pregnant, particularly in that age-group, and they had attended the antenatal clinic at the Yambuku mission.

Masamba and Ruppol were the first to figure out the picture. Vitamin shots. They were usually completely pointless, but many African villagers considered them vital: to them the act of injection with a syringe was emblematic of Western medicine. Thus there were two words for Western medicine in the region. Anything you ingested orally was *aspirin*, and it was hopelessly weak. An injection was *dawa*, proper medicine—something strong and effective.

We needed to take another tour of the Yambuku hospital.

Knowing what we now did, the empty rooms and bare metal bed frames of the mission hospital seemed more disturbing—grim killers of the joyful young mothers who had come there to be cared for but left with a lethal disease. When we reached the stockroom, we hunted through the large multidose jars of antibiotics and other medications.

Their rubber bungs had been perforated multiple times by syringes. In some cases the bung had been removed and was stuck down with a simple bandage. Nearby were a few large glass syringes, five or six.

We politely interviewed the nuns. Sister Genoveva told us quite freely that the few glass syringes were reused for every patient; every morning, she told us, they were quickly (and far too summarily) boiled, like the obstetric instruments employed in the maternity room. Then all day long they were employed and re-employed; they were simply rinsed out with sterile water.

She confirmed that the nuns dosed all the pregnant women in their care with injections of vitamin B and calcium gluconate. Calcium gluconate is a salt of calcium and gluconic acid; it has basically no medical value in pregnancy, but it delivers a shot of energy, and this temporary "high" made it very popular among patients.

In other words, the nurses were systematically injecting a useless product to every woman in antenatal care, as well as to many of the other patients who came to them for help. To do so, they used unsterilized syringes that freely passed on infection. Thus, almost certainly, they had unwittingly killed large numbers of people. It looked as though the only obstacle to the epidemic had been the natural intelligence of the villagers, who saw that many of the sick came from the hospital, and thus fled it; who knew to set up at least some barriers to travel, thus creating a semblance of quarantine.

The nuns were totally committed women. They were brave. They faced an incredibly difficult environment and they dealt with it as best they could. They meant well. We had shared their table and their lives for what seemed like far longer than four days, and every evening, as they sipped their little tots of vermouth, they had told us about the villages of their childhoods. Every evening the discussion had ended up circling around and around the same subject—the epidemic. Who had fallen ill first, when it had happened and how. The dread of infection, the horrible deaths of their patients and colleagues. They had been trying to map out the frightening terrain until, I suppose, it would seem more manageable, less horrific. It was a narrative in which they had felt like heroes of a sort, and certainly martyrs.

Now it appeared that they were in some sense villains as well. It was very hard to formulate the words that would inform the sisters that the virus had in all likelihood been amplified and spread by their own practices and lack of proper training. In the end I think we were far too polite about it: I'm not certain at all that it really sank in when we told them our preliminary conclusions.

OUR THERMOSES WERE full of blood samples that we needed to deliver to a lab for detailed analysis. After great persuasion, the two survivors, Sophie and Sukato, agreed to come with us to Kinshasa for further testing and, assuming that their blood did indeed have antibodies to the virus, plasmapheresis. It was time to head back to Bumba for our rendezvous with the pilots who had agreed to return us to Kinshasa.

Pierre Sureau and I argued that there was no need for *all* of us to leave. We felt that a continued presence could be useful, if only as a placebo—a totem that could relieve the sisters (and to some extent, also the villagers) of their fear of being alone with the epidemic. There were still some active cases of the virus around Yambuku, and no way of knowing whether the epidemic would flare up again to full strength. However, although Pierre radioed Karl Johnson his most strenuous recommendation, our orders were to return.

But when we got to Bumba no plane came. A day went by and an airplane engine rumbled the sky, but when we scrambled out to the airfield it circled overhead and flew off without landing. Another day went by, and another. We were told there was no fuel for the airplane. Then it was a national holiday. Then the weather was not good. Meanwhile we were running out of carbon dioxide canisters to manufacture the dry ice that we had packed around our blood samples. We had to drive over to Ebonda from the mission in Bumba, where we were staying, to persuade the Unilever plantation officials to accept these small potential bombs of contagion into their freezer and then hope against hope that their generator wouldn't fail.

You learn to wait for things in Africa. Initially you are overcome by a swell of irritation, but after a few days it wears off, as most things do. You learn to sit on a veranda or under a tree and talk, or nod in silence, knowing that when the plane comes, you will hear it. It's a good life lesson.

I spent quite a lot of time with our convalescent Sukato, who spoke some French and could translate, too, for Sophie, who was already missing the children she had left behind in Yambuku. Neither of them had ever been to Bumba. Sophie in particular was a deeply modest and devout Christian, and to both of them this ramshackle townlet seemed to represent the fearful temptations and corruptions of the big city. They felt humiliated by the knowing sneers of the locals, who looked down at them as primitive forest folk, and Pierre and I bought them clothes from Noguera so they would feel more at ease. I was a bit anxious when I thought of how they would react to the truly chaotic metropolis of Kinshasa.

I also spent time with Father Carlos, who really was a most curious character. (He still lives in Bumba, and we correspond, now by e-mail!) He must have been in his early thirties—slightly older than I—but though he drank beer and wore Jesus sandals and colorful short-sleeved shirts made of local cloth, he seemed from an entirely different generation. He had inherited money from his family in West Flanders (I gathered that his father had been a banker) and he spread it around Bumba, paying for projects, helping people out. He was totally acclimatized to his environment, preaching in what seemed like fluent Lingala, deploying skills of diplomacy and negotiation that were truly admirable; he was a figure of authority almost equal to the local Commissaire.

With Carlos, as with the sisters of Yambuku, I perceived aspects of my own Belgian culture far more clearly than when I was actually living it. The dialect they spoke; the heavy, traditional winter food they enjoyed despite the sweltering heat: all of it seemed so confined, so tightly wound, and redolent of the 1950s. Every day, once work was over, they ate together, prayed, and then they sat, sipping old Flemish liqueurs such as Elixir d'Anvers, and talked, conjuring up a fantasy of an old Flemish village. For them the motherland was frozen in time that was situated somewhere between their own childhoods and those of their parents. I knew this country was partly imaginary, but it was also partly where I came from too. This was how my people used to think and see the world.

I saw then that I had left my tribe. I had far less in common with the sisters than I did with the piebald, random team of scientists that chance had cobbled together to fight a virus that none of us yet understood.

WHEN THE PLANE finally came to pick us up after four days of waiting, the pilots refused to load our two convalescents or our samples of virus. They had arrived with a load of construction material for a villa that General Bumba was building in a nearby hamlet, and they planned to take off with a load of local produce, breaking the quarantine embargo. Thankfully it seemed there was no logistical problem that Jean-François Ruppol could not solve. The aircraft finally took off, in pouring rain with all of us on board as it lurched and hiccupped perilously across the tree line.

We arrived in Kinshasa and escorted Sophie and Sukato to the Clinique Ngaliema. None of the people quarantined there had developed symptoms. But that also meant that so far, no antibodies had been found in any blood samples. The blood Sophie and Sukato would give—like the vials we had brought with us—was crucially important.

There was still a high degree of panic among the medical staff at Ngaliema. Perhaps intensifying the sense of gloom, a negative-pressure isolation bed, one of only two or three in the world, had arrived from Johannesburg. It is a kind of hermetic tent that basically prevents viruses from leaving the space because of the negative pressure in it. It stood grimly in a special room in Ngaliema, to be used in case one of the international team fell ill. Basically, if one of us caught the virus, we would be entombed inside this contraption for the duration of our treatment, or our few remaining days alive. The ultrasophisticated material demanded experienced and specialized personnel, and it was far from clear that it would ever really work as planned.

Staring at this apparatus, I recalled a potent image from my early

childhood: the iron lung. In 1958, when I was nine, Belgium hosted
the World Fair. My father, who worked at the National Agency for
the Promotion of Belgian Agriculture and Horticulture, oversaw one
of the displays, and my parents took us there every Sunday afternoon
from April to October. It was far and away the most exciting thing
that ever happened in my childhood. My younger brothers and sisters
were too young to roam about, but I was allowed to roam freely across
that one square mile of futuristic exhibits.

There were colorful glassed-in cable cars, like something out of a
Jetsons cartoon. A gleaming monument, the Atomium, dramatized
the chemistry of molecules; it loomed high above the cantilevered
pavilions, all angles and glass and curved steel. A huge fairground
was open every day until 4 A.M. Rockets, on one ride, carried you
across a city of the future, where houses showed off fantastical gadgets; then you flew past the Milky Way and around Mars before
returning to Earth. Robots distributed bars of chocolate. There was
a machine that manufactured and bottled Coke; a mine shaft complete with trolleys; a model of an oil refinery. There were people
with strange skin colors and extraordinary looking eyes. There
were pavilions for plastics, for explosives, for chemistry, for photog-
raphy, for glass, and for every imaginable country and international
organization.

But there were just two objects that drew me back, again and
again. The Russian pavilion contained a Sputnik, a small silver sphere
that was suspended just beneath a massive, frowning statue of Lenin.
It was barely a year after the first Russian space flight, and here was
a real representative from that new world of discovery, outer space.

And in the United States' pavilion, just next door, there was an
iron lung—a terrible, sealed glass container that breathed for you.
In a way, I think that ugly, cylindrical cage had a profound impact
on my life. Everyone was terrified of polio in those days; the oral
vaccine wasn't licensed until 1962. If you caught the virus, you could
become paralyzed and may not be able to breathe without the support
of an iron lung, perhaps your only hope for long-term survival. The
nightmarish vision of being caged for life was I think something that
motivated me to care for the sick. I pondered it intensely. Surely there

must be some better alternative? Turning away from the negative-pressure isolation bed, I felt uneasy.

NOW THAT IT was clear that our virus was not a subspecies of Marburg, but was in fact a new (and possibly far more virulent) hemorrhagic fever, more international personnel began flying in to join the team. My friend Guido Van Der Groen arrived with enough equipment to install a field virology lab at Clinique Ngaliema. For several days he had been working there in a plastic isolator—a small laboratory bench under a plastic tent, accessed via two plastic built-in sleeves, the low internal air pressure maintained with a small electrical pump. With a grin, he handed me a good-bye note penned by our boss, Stefan Pattyn, who had returned to Belgium to pursue his hospital and teaching work. His note urged me yet *again* to catch as many bats as humanly possible, and warned me to beware of traps that would be laid for me by our American and French team members.

Another new arrival was Joe McCormick, a bespectacled young CDC staffer with a Paul McCartney fringe who had broken off his work on Lassa fever in Sierra Leone and was planning to travel from Isiro in northeastern Zaire to southern Sudan, where the mysterious twin epidemic to our own was still advancing.

We made a full report to the International Commission about our preliminary conclusions and our sketch of a hypothetical epidemiological curve. There was a strong possibility that the epidemic had peaked, but there were still at least a dozen people around Yambuku who were critically ill, with almost no provision for quarantine, so a strong potential for flare-ups or another big wave of infection remained. In addition, even if we were right about the scope of the epidemic in Yambuku, if just a few isolated cases reached Kinshasa or any other major city the epidemic would certainly explode. And the logistics situation at Yambuku was extremely dicey. Everything had to be brought in by plane and helicopter.

Karl was ordering radio and laboratory equipment, and he began working on plans to install a special medical center at a distance from Yambuku and other significant villages, so that patients could be separated from their families. It would have to include a highly secure inpatient ward; a highly secure field lab equipped with a centrifuge and other equipment for hematological analysis; a separate quarantine center to isolate suspected cases; and an outpatient ward where serum donations could be obtained and the sick could be brought for diagnosis. Naturally the very ill would need to be transported from their villages, and that meant a helicopter would have to be available on a daily basis.

I could see that setting up a treatment center like this was going to take weeks at the earliest. Meanwhile, we were spending our lives in meetings, which I detested. (Little did I know that meetings would *become* my life.) At every endless meeting Pierre and I argued for our swift return to Yambuku. We had promised the sisters that we would be back, as well as the people in Bumba, and our only contact with them was the haphazard link provided by the radio operator at the Order of Scheut's Kinshasa headquarters, which passed on messages via the mission in Lisala. There was no direct communication at all, but every message ended with a plea for us to return.

This went on for several days. All of us were still camping out at the Fométro offices, not the easiest setup for a competitive pack of men. (Only Margaretha Isaacson had her own room.) Late one night we were drinking Karl's Kentucky bourbon—it was one of those half-gallon bottles with a handle—discussing what our new virus should be named. Pierre argued for Yambuku virus, which had the advantage of simplicity; it was what most of us were already calling the disease. But Joel reminded us that naming killer viruses after specific places can be very stigmatizing; with Lassa virus, discovered in 1969 in a small Nigerian town of that name, it had caused no end of problems to the people from the locality. Karl Johnson liked to call his viruses after rivers: he felt that took some of the sting out of the geographical finger-pointing. It was what he had done when he'd discovered Machupo virus in Bolivia in 1959, and it was clear that night that he had every intention of doing the same in Zaire.

But we couldn't call our virus after the majestic Congo River: a Congo-Crim virus already existed. Were there any other rivers near Yambuku? We charged en masse to a not-very-large map of Zaire that was pinned up in the Fométro corridor. At that scale, it looked as though the closest river to Yambuku was called Ebola—"Black River," in Lingala. It seemed suitably ominous.

Actually there's no connection between the hemorrhagic fever and the Ebola River. Indeed, the Ebola River isn't even the closest river to the Yambuku mission. But in our entirely fatigued state, that's what we ended up calling the virus: Ebola.

CHAPTER 5

A Pseudo Outbreak
and a Helicopter

T HERE'S A STRAIGHTFORWARD formula that's crucial to the
life and death of epidemics. (And thus, of course, also crucial
to the life and death of humans.) I would study it later in the
classic work of Robert May and Roy Anderson, who 30 years after the
epidemic attracted me to Imperial College in London where he was
then rector. The components of this equation are β, virulence (how
contagious the virus is—the probability of transmission in a contact
between an infected individual and a susceptible one); c, contacts
(the number of contacts, on average, per infected person per day);
and D, duration, the number of days you are infectious. Combine
those three factors and you come to a number—the Basic Reproductive Rate, R°—that determines how fast the epidemic will spread,
and whether it will simply die out of its own accord or develop into a
long-term pandemic.

$$R^\circ = \beta\, c\, D$$

If R° is less than 1, the outbreak of disease will peter out. If R°
equals 1, the disease will become endemic. If R° exceeds 1, a full-

blown epidemic will break loose. The question was which calculation fit Ebola.

In the first 21 villages we looked at, we found evidence of 148 fatal cases of Ebola, and 12 cases where people showed antibodies—in other words, 12 people were confirmed as survivors. This suggested the astronomical fatality rate of 92.5 percent, though in the absence of a serological survey in the population we could not yet exclude that a lot of people were asymptomatically infected, as is the case for many viral infections. And we suspected that Ebola was highly contagious in at least some households. We didn't know exactly how or exactly how much. But its incubation period was very short, and it killed people so quickly—within 14 days of initial contact—that they probably weren't infectious for long.

So although β, virulence, was playing against us, D, the quick kill rate, was, paradoxically, an advantage from an epidemiological point of view. People simply didn't stay infectious for very long, because they died so rapidly. While we would, of course, seek to improve patient survival, we also needed to cut down on c, the number of infective contacts per sick person.

In that respect, we were extremely lucky that Ebola still had not flared up in the sprawling, intensely interconnected megacity of Kinshasa, where contact patterns were almost uncontrollable. Because Ebola was still isolated in the remote Yambuku region, and because the village elders had of their own accord set up a measure of quarantine, we could just about hope that it would die down on its own.

Meanwhile, I was stuck in Kinshasa, at Karl's orders. I liked the city. It was huge—far larger than Brussels—and it flashed with a terrific energy, generosity, and joy. When there weren't any evening activities at work (on most days), Guido and I went out in the evening and ate grilled "Capitaine," a white river-fish, and huge *cossa-cossa* shrimp with some of the hottest *pili pili* spices in Africa. Then we took a taxi to some bar in Matonge and submerged ourselves in the rich atmosphere of this crazed metropolis and the intricate cadences of Congolese *suka suka*. We drank locally brewed *Primus* and *Skoll* beer while discussing local and international politics with Zaireans and foreigners, and I learned to dance with my hips in the huge mirrors that were often a feature of the dance halls, from a series of grinning women who took pity on a poor foreigner with jerky sticks for limbs.

But I wasn't in Zaire to learn to dance.

I spent a lot of time in Kinshasa's three main hospitals: Mama Yemo Hospital, named after Mobutu's mother (I noted later how much dictators seem to revere their mothers); Clinique Ngaliema; and the University Hospital, up the hill. In spite of its name, the latter was the worst off in terms of infrastructure and equipment, but it had very competent physicians. In the past week I had seen more cases of hemorrhagic fever than anybody else in Kinshasa except for Pierre Sureau, and was thus what might pass in the dark for a world "expert" on the subject! It was also an opportunity to soak up more knowledge about medicine in Central Africa, and to learn from my resourceful Zairean colleagues, many of whom were intellectually brilliant but had to hold down several jobs and run side businesses to feed their extended families and put their children through decent schools.

I became friends with the head of the clinical lab at Ngaliema, a young Flemish lab technician named Frieda Behets who had trained in our lab in Antwerp. She was one of the most practical and energetic people I met during my work in Africa and helped me out numerous times with both logistics and political advice. (She later played a major role in AIDS research in Africa and elsewhere and is now a professor at the University of North Carolina.) Her then husband was a veterinarian who introduced me to two important places: the Bralima (Heineken) brewery and the presidential farm in Nsele. The brewery was not only a welcome source of cold beer but more importantly a generous source of CO_2 to produce dry ice, necessary for transporting virus samples. And the farm was a source of an even more precious commodity: liquid nitrogen, used to preserve semen for artificial insemination of cows, and the best medium to store viruses at $-170°C$. I also helped him later with some microbiological research on diseases of Mobutu's chickens and pigs.

Meanwhile, at the Fométro office Margaretha Isaacson was driving me nuts. She was constantly at us to report our body temperature three times a day, to detect early signs of viral infection. Although she was right, I was still enough of an adolescent that this annoyed me to an unreasonable degree.

There were also discussions and tensions between Karl and Pierre Sureau. Pierre and I wanted to return to Yambuku immediately, while Karl argued that it was far more important to secure Kinshasa and to wait for the crates of equipment that were on their way from the United States. I was bursting with frustration.

It was around this time that I came down with diarrhea and fever. I felt dizzy, and my head began to ache as though it was circled by a metal vise. As one of the few members of the team to have actually seen an Ebola victim, I was perhaps hyperaware that these were invariably the first symptoms of the disease. In any case, we were all under the strictest instructions to report any kind of incipient infection. But I knew that if I did I would be put in a plastic-wrapped isolation bed under the care of Margaretha Isaacson, and that as soon as my condition stabilized I would be sent to South Africa for weeks of quarantine.

So, unforgivably, I decided not to tell anyone. I tried to isolate myself as much as possible. I was so frightened that I could barely admit to myself what I was risking, and the kind of risk to which I was exposing my colleagues. When the fever dissipated after less than 48 hours—it had probably been some random intestinal bug—I was a little less arrogant; I recognized the kind of fear that the sisters and the other inhabitants of Yambuku endured, night after night, fever after fever, death after death, for over two months.

Then a report came in that the hemorrhagic fever had hit a prison in the town of Kikwit, about 250 miles away from Kinshasa. Three people were dead and another three were said to be sick. I volunteered to accompany Jean-François Ruppol, the seasoned Zaire hand. And I will never forget traveling there in a little Fokker aircraft from Air Zaire. We were the only two passengers and the pilot told us to sit on either side of the plane to maintain the aircraft's balance. Suddenly, as I was looking out at the rain forest, the Fokker swung sideways and as I watched, one of the engines literally broke off in front of my eyes and fell off the plane. I thought this was the end but, unbelievably, the pilot landed us safely.

Kikwit was another sad and shabby town, with a few decaying old colonial buildings and shacks no cleaner or more orderly than those of Bumba. As in Bumba, there was no electricity and little sanitation: the infrastructure had collapsed since Independence.

The hospital surprisingly was one of the cleanest and best managed I saw in all my decades in Zaire. It was run by Paul Janseghers and his colleagues from the Belgian development agency, and had reasonable supplies and competent, active staff. (Sadly, Belgium later withdrew support from the hospital as part of policy changes in development aid stressing that local institutions should not be managed by Belgians, and Mobutu's concept of authority did not include investment in local services for his citizens. One dramatic result of the predictable breakdown in basic infrastructure and management were hospital-based epidemics, such as the Ebola outbreak that Kikwit did indeed witness in 1995, which killed over 200 people.)

Within an hour we established that there was no outbreak of Ebola in the dilapidated prison. In reality, the prisoners had acute hepatitis, with massive liver necrosis, and this, combined with rumors of a mystery killer disease afoot in the country, set off panic. The local medical authorities had already done liver biopsies but the results (and the samples) hadn't gotten to Kinshasa, because of the haphazard nature of transport links. (In those days it was said that there were only 600 miles of paved road in Zaire, a country half the size of the entire United States. There are probably even fewer now.)

We drove back to Kinshasa in a car lent to us by Kikwit hospital, and stayed there for another day or two; finally Karl gave Pierre and me the go-ahead to return to Yambuku. We left in the first week of November, with a heavy load of food supplies—cans and C-rations that had arrived from the US Army, to counteract the damaging effects of the quarantine. (You're obviously not going to solve a systemic problem of hunger by handing out a few cans of corned beef, and, in any case, there was no famine whatsoever in either Bumba or Yambuku. But these food supplies had arrived in Kinshasa, so we took them with us.)

In retrospect, it was all very amateurish. I have since, for my sins, become a professional of humanitarian assistance, and this sort of individual charity solution violates all the rules. In fact, the money I had with me, to hire people and set up teams was far more useful to the region than the cans of meat.

I was in charge of logistics, again in preparation for the arrival of a far larger international team, with a lab. Inwardly I quavered, because although I did have some claim to a little knowledge of viruses, I really could have no pretense of any ability to organize a long-term expedition to the jungle beyond 10 years of Boy Scout training and my high school summer jobs working for a professional travel outfit in Turkey and Morocco.

Before we left Kinshasa I made one phone call to Greta. This was a very complex production. Even the powerful Fométro office had no international phone line, and the local lines had been out of operation for years. But the Fométro administrators knew a man at the telephone company, where you went to book a long-distance call. If you asked the proper person (and if all other factors in the telephonic constellations were correctly aligned at the time), the Fométro phone miraculously came to life at the appointed hour. You were patched through by the operator and after an unpredictable few minutes the line went dead; subsequently, the special phone guy to whom you owed this extraordinary service came to the office for his *matabiche*, his tip.

Greta was worried. Ebola was making some minor news in Belgium, and all travelers from Zaire had to submit to medical exams. She was alarmed to learn that I was about to go back to Yambuku and that I would be staying in Zaire for considerably more than 10 days. I felt strangely disembodied. I was sorry that she was anxious, and I was relieved that her pregnancy was advancing without problems, but my life in Belgium now seemed very far away.

Again we took the president's C-130 airplane to Bumba, and again the pilots kept the engines running as we unloaded. As soon as we disembarked, they took off. As we watched the plane take off from the red dirt airstrip I wondered when, how, and even whether we would see it again. We had set no date for them to return, and there was no other way to get out of quarantined Bumba. I had an empty feeling as we headed over to Father Carlos's mission.

With the help of Dr. N'goy Mushola, I hired and trained a few men to create a surveillance network around the town. These men sought out cases of Ebola and brought symptomatic patients to the hospital in Bumba or the clinic at the Unilever plantation in Ebonda. We drew blood to test later for Ebola antibodies. (Patricia Web's lab at the CDC in Atlanta was frantically developing the antibody test that Guido later deployed in Kinshasa and Yambuku.)

We also needed medical staff. N'goy told us that none of the local nurses or medics had received their pay for months. These were government employees, so the money for their salaries had to come from Kinshasa. The doctors and nurses in Bumba were at the bottom of a huge pyramid, and as the money percolated down, at every level—regional, local—a portion of their wages was sliced off by corruption, and the slices had become so vast and shameless that there was often nothing left.

N'goy suggested that we simply agree to pay their normal, full salaries for a while. For us it was hardly any money at all, but for them it was a gift: to be actually paid, in predictable fashion, a fair, agreed-on wage for your work.

All the people we hired for the mobile surveillance networks were men. In those days it didn't occur to me that there was a specific need to hire women. I knew, but at the time didn't *perceive*, the fact that whenever we went to villages we saw only men, partly because women traditionally worked the fields and did all the heavy work. If we asked to talk to women—or to a specific woman—a man would say, "Why? I can tell you what you need to know."

We established our main logistics base at the Ebonda plantation, which we had visited during our first trip, because they had direct radio contact with the Unilever office in Kinshasa. So Karl Johnson and the others could drive over to the Unilever HQ and talk with us directly: a small matter, but a huge improvement over the sisters' patchy hookup in Lisala.

Then we drove up to the Yambuku mission, now lashed on a daily basis by torrential storms. We brought a lot of stuff for the sisters, including mail, which we had picked up at the *Procure*, the logistics base of most of the Flemish missionary orders in Kinshasa. (I had also purchased a most unexpected little artifact: a Flemish-Lingala dictionary and grammar book. I studied this for an hour every day and picked up quite rapidly enough words to hold a very basic conversation.)

A few days later, a Puma helicopter—another of President Mobu-tu's personal aircraft—arrived to serve us. Accompanying it were two pilots and a mechanic. The mechanic was a *Kibangiste*, a member of a Christian church founded by a Zairean prophet, Simon Kibanga, who died in a Belgian colonial prison in 1951. Because of this, he didn't drink or smoke or sleep around, whereas the two pilots did very little else. Accustomed to accompanying President Mobutu about the country, in high luxury and low supervision, they were deeply resent-ful of their assignment to our service: there was no champagne, no fun, and little opportunity for profit. They spent some of the next six weeks using the big Puma helicopter to fly from one bar to another, impressing women, and I, in my tightly wound Flemish way, resented this greatly, for I was paying them a per diem for their expenses, as well as buying all the fuel.

We needed the Puma because we planned surveillance visits to areas that couldn't be reached by four-wheel drive, particularly in the rainy season. Many villages were now completely inaccessible by land, and the rivers were so swollen they could no longer be forded. We planned to head north up the Ubangi River, a trip which, though it represented only 60 miles on the map, would have taken a day or more of almost impossibly hard labor by road.

We also made a second tour around every village in the Yambuku area. Yahombo, Yapama, Yambonzo, Yaongo, Yandondi, Yaekanga, Yalitaku, Yamisako, Yalikombi, Yaundu, Yanguma, to the west. Yalikondi, Yamoleka, Yamonzwa, Yaliselenge, Yasoku, Yamotili, to the east. Little strings of villages, like tiny beads lost along the muddy paths that meandered through the thick forest.

When we arrived in a village we settled ourselves under an awning or largish tree and were rapidly surrounded by people—chil-dren with bright eyes and prominent bellies, young girls with high round breasts, women in their forties with breasts hanging to their knees, and old men and women smoking marijuana. (We endeavored to arrive early in the morning, before work in the fields began.)

Later on I visited a few distilleries hidden in the forest to safeguard from theft. Many villages had a basic distillery: Bananas were left to ferment in a hollowed-out tree trunk and then flavored, by local specialty, with leaves or bark. This mixture was cooked, slowly, in an enamel pot covered with leaves. The vapor was caught and cooled in a hollow bamboo stick, with a carefully shaped piece of bicycle tire creating a bend and guiding the now-condensed liquid down again. Congolese moonshine. My favorite had a small Perrier bottle to capture the distillate (only God knew how that bottle arrived there).

I always sipped from the *arak*, out of politeness, though it was presented in a single, collectively used cup. I also occasionally sampled the communal cannabis pipe. However, I didn't partake of the plates of caterpillars or flying termites fried in palm oil, or the villagers' *boucané* monkey meat. Game (whether squirrels or monkeys) was the most common source of protein, and the villagers smoked it and hung it until it was blackened and half-rotten; the smell was so vile that it caught in throat and made you choke.

Family by family, Pierre and I slowly questioned everyone who seemed to have any relationship with the hemorrhagic fever, scribbling the details into a notebook. In only one village did we find a cluster of women and children who had died from Ebola without a clear narrative beginning with a hospital or funeral. This cluster remained something of a mystery until, on a second visit there, I met with one woman who had survived her illness and noted the scarifications across her forehead. I asked if they were recent and what they meant, and she said, "We had headache, so the *nganga kisi* [traditional healer] came to do this."

What had happened was that one young woman had gone to the antenatal clinic in Yambuku. When she returned with Ebola symptoms, including the typical searing headache, the *nganga* treated her with scarification, slicing her skin lightly with a knife. And just to be on the safe side, he performed the scarification on a series of other women in the village as a preventive measure—using the same knife.

Later, I met this particular herbal healer. He was a polite man, who received us in a room not very different from any other village hut. There were no fetishes or masks in evidence, though a series of liquids were macerating in gourds along the beaten-earth floor. We asked how he treated people who had Ebola, and how he protected himself, and he politely showed us: household bleach. He bought it at Noguera's shop in Bumba, and though he presented it to the villagers as traditional medicine, this bleach was apparently the main element in the potions and poultices he used to disinfect wounds and heal people.

There was a certain lack of poetry in this, but at the same time a welcome dose of common sense. Whether or not this *nganga kisi* also used traditional magic that he chose not to discuss with us, his use of bleach had probably saved a number of lives—though sadly he had not thought to use it to keep his knife clean.

THE LAST EBOLA victim in the Yambuku region died on November 5, two months after the beginning of the epidemic. Pierre left Yambuku on November 9 to return to Paris. The heroic phase of the epidemic was over: it was clear that the outbreak was coming to an end. But epidemics can rebound and rear up unpredictably. My job was to keep an alert watch for new cases; we didn't want to take risks.

The international team still planned to arrive with a generator and lab equipment for plasmapheresis, and we planned a solid epidemiological investigation to find out exactly how Ebola was transmitted. We knew blood was involved, but what about mother-to-child and sexual transmission? We also needed to learn about the natural animal reservoir of the virus: was it bat, bee, rodent, or smoked, dried monkey. Finally, Karl was also planning a serum survey, because although we had identified people who had been very sick, or who had died, it was entirely possible that Ebola had infected half the population and only some had fallen ill.

Pierre's departure left me alone with Father Léon and the sisters of the Holy Order of Our Lady. We spoke mostly about work and about Flanders. Despite all the trauma, they seemed to have gone back to hard work and their daily routine—no posttraumatic stress here (that came later). It was hard to have a more personal conversation as our worlds were too far apart, even if we all told about our family backgrounds. Only with Sister Genoveva, a humorous woman of about forty-five, could I have something of a discussion. At one point she made a comment—something like "God will protect us"—and, weary of courtesy, I said, "Do you really believe this?" She admitted to doubts, and that was something I cherished, for it made her seem more human, and in a way more tragic—doubts as later also expressed in the letters of Mother Teresa.

If Sister Genoveva was my favorite nun, my favorite village was Yamotili Moké—*Little Yamotili*, in Lingala, meaning its inhabitants had split off from the village of Yamotili. There was nothing really special about it, but the people seemed more open, and their agenda of needs (for food, supplies, cash) was perhaps a little less intense than in other villages. Also, it was close to Yambuku. I started going there nearly every evening, bringing some beer, or tins of sardines, or a little cloth to offer as a gift. If people had a medical problem they came to me, and I gave them an aspirin or an antimalarial—never a shot, but whatever I had. (I suspected that most of their fevers and so on were malaria and certainly everyone had parasites. We did a little lab work at a later stage; filarial and amoebas and all sorts of things showed up in their blood and feces.)

But for some reason I felt comfortable; I didn't feel I had to play the Big White Doctor who investigates disease and saves the world. Mostly I sat with the elderly men: they smoked their pipe and talked among themselves, not even in Lingala but in Buja, the language of their tribe, and I felt I was accepted by them. There was an older man whose name I forget (perhaps he was only forty-five but he had hardly any teeth) and like most men in Zaire he knew far more about Belgian soccer than I did, thanks to the magic of transistor radios. The goalkeeper of the Belgian national team at that time was Christian Piot, who shared my name, so that made for some comment and a funny sort of bond. But most of the time our companionship was a silent one.

No women ever participated: they were sweeping, cooking, pounding or grating manioc (cassava) roots, their staple food. Sitting with the Yamotili men was basically an alternative to sitting with my own tribe at the Yambuku mission.

I was answering those questions that had occurred to me when I first arrived in Yambuku. These people were living closer to the Middle Ages than to the year 2000. How did they manage to survive? Weren't they scared? To me they seemed so vulnerable, both to the invasive forces of nature—animal, viral, climate—and to soldiers. They told stories of insane cruelty culled from the multiple rebellions that had already crisscrossed the region. It was still only 16 years since Lumumba's speech at Independence and already there had been many wars, much killing and looting and rape. Even in times of peace, Mobutu's soldiers stole their meager possessions and raped girls and women. Even now, thinking about how vulnerable the villagers were gives me pain; their stories, and many subsequent experiences in Zaire, made me appreciate our well-functioning states where the rule of law is intended to protect its citizens, not scavenge off them.

In addition, though, by just hanging out with people, drinking arak and chatting about soccer I put together the very beginning picture of a whole culture. I'm a strong believer in what I later learned is called *qualitative* research. You do need the standardized epidemiological questionnaires, of course, for quantitative analysis, but you may also sometimes need to develop a kind of feel that's a lot less systematic, but may reach out to places that are deeper and more unexpected.

So, for example, that was how I put together a picture of what happened during funerals. As in so many cultures, funerals were a major event for the Buja, stretching across several days and could easily cost a full year's income. What made those funerals so lethal, apart from this prolonged and intense contact, was the preparation of the cadaver. The body was thoroughly cleaned, and the process often involved several family members, working bare-handed. Since the bodies were usually covered in blood, feces, and vomit, exposure to Ebola virus was enormous—particularly since the usual custom was to clean all the orifices: mouth, eyes, nose, vagina, anus.

People don't tell you this sort of thing. You get at it obliquely. You're talking about washing the body, and you say, "So, of course you're cleaning the anus?" Some people say, "Sure," and another says "No," and for a long while you don't know what to believe. One woman said that the body was licked. But nobody else agreed with that, and we were talking about the body of her very young, almost newborn child, so perhaps that had been a special case, not the norm. Then the body was wrapped in a cloth and buried in the ground right outside the door of the person's hut: (I often saw a row of mounds just outside a house—the burial ground of family members.)

The nuns were one source of information, but while people reported that their behavior was Christian, they had a separate, extra religion that they hid.

I became immersed in this place. I developed genuine respect for these people. I was growing up and answering my own questions, I guess. I wasn't thinking of Belgium, but of course I worried about my pregnant wife, particularly at night, in my austere cell with its crucifix on the brick wall. But what could I do?

Perhaps I was also finding that there was more to me than I had thought. I wasn't a boy with a great deal of self-confidence; that wasn't part of a Flemish education in those days (fortunately my own children are quite different). You learned humility and silence, to work hard and never think you're better than anybody else. This has its advantages: it protects you from snobbery and the corruptions of power. But it also means you aim small.

Now I was "director of operations" for the International Commission. A C-130 full of food and equipment arrived and I had to organize distribution. I was hiring people, paying them, negotiating with the Commissaire de Zone (who badly wanted the Puma for his own use), making sure the money didn't disappear, organizing the collection of specimens, and building a system so that 25 people could arrive from Kinshasa and operate in a clinic and a lab.

A SECOND HELICOPTER arrived, this time an Alouette donated by French President Giscard d'Estaing to Mobutu in return for God knows what favor. It lent an almost comic flavor to my life. I did not request it or need it, but Bill Close sent it to me, and by this time I was starting to find all this normal. Need a helicopter? Here are two! People in the humanitarian field are often like this: it's a mentality that's somehow not very grown-up, part cowboy and part Boy Scout.

Actually both the Puma and the Alouette were an enormous hassle to manage. The pilots constantly demanded money and caused havoc all over the region, blowing the roofs off huts and sleeping with an apparently endless loop of girls, dirt poor and in need of some cash. The sexual appetite of some pilots was apparently unslakable and the village men were not happy. Even the children were fascinated by the helicopters, and started producing toy helicopters made of wire—one of them is still in my office.

One afternoon the pilots flew the Alouette up to Yambuku from Bumba to tell me that Karl wanted me to fly back to Bumba with them to meet with the US ambassador and the head of the Kinshasa office of USAID, who had flown in from Kinshasa and wanted to be briefed on the epidemic.

Then the pilots disappeared. They always did a lot of business, buying stuff in the villages and selling it in Bumba, where people were still short of supplies because of the quarantine.

Sitting on the verandah of the Yambuku mission, I threw a kind of tantrum. If these big shots wanted to know about the epidemic, I thought, they should damn well come to Yambuku where the epidemic was. When the pilots returned, they asked me for a beer. I could smell beer on their breath already.

The sky was becoming dark, as it did every afternoon as the storms formed. I don't love flying; to be honest, in these helicopters that I was supposed to be ordering about, I was actually kind of scared. I also knew that the Puma pilots refused to fly in this kind of weather, so why fly in a much smaller Alouette, with pilots who had clearly been drinking?

So I said to myself, "The hell with it, I'm not going to go."

As I told the pilots to return to Bumba without me, a middle-aged man who was sweeping the courtyard spoke up. "*Patron*," he begged—"Boss" (I had long ago stopped asking people not to call me this)—"I have family in Bumba. I have never been in a *hélico*—can I go?"

"Sure," I told him. "Have fun." And they left. Soon afterward the sky broke into torrential equatorial rain and I felt glad for a moment that I had avoided being shaken up in the helicopter; then I went back to work.

The next morning I turned on the army radio that had come with the Alouette, for my daily contact with Kinshasa, and Karl was at full volume.

"You sonofabitch, where the hell are you? Where the hell is the Goddamn helicopter? You kept the ambassador waiting for hours! And the USAID guy! That's where all our money comes from!"

I said, "The helicopter left last night and the next time your ambassador comes he can bloody well come to Yambuku"—we were both angry—but then we both realized that the helicopter and the people in it were missing, and we fell silent. I had a sinking feeling that it had crashed somewhere in the storm.

All around me there was so much death, with people dying because they had cared for a sick person or asked for a shot of vitamins or helped bury a relative. And although I pretended that it didn't affect me, I think I must have been a little too close to breakdown by this time. In terms of contact with patients and the crazy parameters of operating in Zaire, I had been taking risks that were calculated, but still very real, and although I faked a great confidence about all this, deep down I knew how dangerous it was. Now I had survived two brushes with my own mortality—the frightening fever in Kinshasa and the Alouette crash. I was cut off from my normal support system and literally from the rest of the world, and knowledge of my vulnerability, which I had suppressed, flooded in. Thinking of the young sweeper who had probably perished in my place I was petrified, overwhelmed.

I cut off the radio transmission, went to my room, and laid down on the metal bed. I missed Greta. Our first child could have been born fatherless. I felt a wave of self-pity, then righted myself: sentimentality wasn't going to help anyone. I reached for those traditional Flemish coping mechanisms, repression and work. Sweep everything tightly under a rug. Above all, get the job done. But, at the same time, I realized that my newfound lack of respect for authority and on-the-fly risk assessment had literally saved my life. A cherished lesson to trust my own instinct.

Two days later, the Puma helicopter arrived from Bumba with orders that I return to see the Commissaire de Zone. The pilots were extremely unpleasant. They were, of course, colleagues of the downed Alouette pilots. Now, flying to Bumba in their care, I was really scared. The Puma is a combat aircraft, and it can fly with the doors open so you can shoot out; only a patch of webbing holds you to your seat.

Citoyen Olonga was menacing. In essence, he accused me of knowing in advance about the crash, perhaps even causing it; that was why I had not taken the trip myself. In Zaire, in this population, nothing could happen by coincidence; if there was an accident, or an illness, then someone had caused it to happen, by hex or by potion. He announced that a hunter had found the crashed helicopter in the forest, and that since I was responsible, I must go there to collect the bodies, as well as pay compensation to the families of the dead young man and the pilots.

I went to see Father Carlos and said, "Now I really have a problem." I needed three coffins by early next morning, and by now it was late in the afternoon. We bought some planks, some disinfectant, and a fumigator spray full of insecticide at Noguera, because after three days in the heat, these bodies weren't going to be that nice. (I also brought an aspirator mask with me from Yambuku—not just a surgical, paper mask, but a gas-mask type of thing.)

As we drove this load back to the mission, we passed a group of prisoners working on the side of the road, and an idea hit me. I asked the prison commander to let me have six prisoners for 24 hours. I didn't bribe him—I never paid a bribe in Zaire—but he agreed to my request. (Although when everything was over I did pay them a little money for their pains, and the prison commander probably figured that out and took it from them.) That night we banged the coffins together in the courtyard of the mission. It was almost a relief to be working at something manual—all of us together, shirtless, in the evening heat.

The next morning the Puma pilots flew me and the six prisoners to another Unilever plantation deep in the forest. A huge crowd of people had gathered there: I had no idea how so many people had come to be present in such a remote area, but I suppose the noise of the helicopter engine had called them to the scene. The pilots loped off for a beer—they didn't bother to come with us to recover their colleagues' corpses—and the hunter, the six prisoners, and I marched into the forest. The prisoners slung the coffins with lianas onto big sticks that they balanced on their shoulders. The hunter was in front, slashing the undergrowth with his machete. I stumbled behind, in my blue workers' overalls, with socks rolled over my legs to protect myself from the snakes, spiders, giant centipedes, and other insects that teem in the Central African rainforest, which I cringed to even think about.

It was absolutely virgin forest, thicker than any kind of vegetation I had seen around Yambuku, and I was sweating with resentment and anger, in addition to the already suffocating equatorial temperature. I knew that we were being followed at a distance by possibly a hundred villagers. I couldn't see or hear them but I could feel them; it's dark in the Zairean rain forest, but I knew that they were there.

After well over an hour of marching through the virgin jungle, which was a very tiring experience, given that I had spent the night hammering coffins and had barely slept, I suddenly smelled something unmistakable. So I put on the mask, and when we saw the smashed helicopter the prisoners dropped their coffins and ran away. They didn't go too far, I guess, but what the hell was I going to do now? The hunter merely gazed at me with curiosity. We shared no language.

I went up to the helicopter, which was lying on its side; it hadn't burned or exploded. The pilot and copilot were still in their seats, totally swollen, and although I pushed a bit, I couldn't extract them. It felt like a scene from some B movie, and I took pictures of the horror scene with a disposable Kodak camera I had bought in Kinshasa. Then, to give myself some more time to think, I began to fumigate the corpses, spraying great gusts of insecticide. I tried to remove the mask, because it was so hot I was almost suffocating, but then I almost fainted from the cadaver smell.

Nobody else was there, so if I didn't manage to do this, it wasn't going to get done. And if anything bad happened to me while I was out here, nobody was going to notice. In a situation like that, you can have self-pity, you can snivel and quaver, but it doesn't make any difference: you're alone.

One of the pilots' legs was stuck out of the door at a sick-looking angle, and I noticed he had smooth new Italian boots on. A rather unpleasant idea came to me, and I yelled out, "The first one who helps me drag out this man gets these boots." I said it in French, and to the best of my ability, in Lingala. So then a few of the young people who were watching from nearby stepped up, and the prisoners emerged from the undergrowth, since basically they had nowhere to go but home with us to Bumba; this was not the region where they belonged. And in the end, after some really hideous maneuvers that I would prefer not to remember, we got the corpses out and jammed them into the coffins, which we had lined with plastic tarps. The bodies were so swollen we had to jump down the coffin lids as if closing overstuffed suitcases. It was a really ugly scene.

Then we wound the coffins shut with lianas and back we went, marching for nearly two hours through the impenetrable rain forest, the prisoners staggering under the weight of their loads and the immensity of the stench. As we left the scene the hidden villagers moved in and began to deconstruct the helicopter for parts. (Years later huts were still decorated with bits of the Alouette!)

We loaded the coffins into the Puma, and I then joined the pilots for a lukewarm beer. No words were exchanged. I stared at the beer coasters, which exhibited the logo of Mobutu's incredibly corrupt Mouvement Populaire de la Révolution with the utterly hypocritical slogan "Servir oui. Se Servir non." (To serve: yes. To serve oneself: no). I swept the coasters into my pocket as a souvenir, paid for the beers, and then told the pilots I was done: they could drop me off in Yambuku. But they wouldn't do it, they had orders to bring me back to Bumba for another dressing down.

Meanwhile, I had made a mistake: in my stress I had forgotten to dilute the disinfectant. In other words, I had poured pure Dettol (a powerful disinfectant on the basis of chloroxylenol) on the corpses. It was fortunate the helicopter doors were open, but even so our eyes were totally bloodshot by the time we landed. And I didn't go to the Commissaire de Zone. I went straight to the mission, to Carlos, and said, "I need to get drunk." I had never felt anything like it in my life, and indeed I have never had that urge again.

I suppose I was waking up to the fact that I wasn't living in a comic strip. I wasn't Tintin, and in fact there was nobody *drawing* this comic strip, nobody but me. I had put myself in a situation where I was alone, far away, and wholly reliant on complete strangers, who could drop me out of the sky as easily as not and who had no real reason to help me in any way. In African terms, I was really still a child, because I had never truly understood before that life does *not* go on forever, and I too will die.

Carlos drew himself up and I actually saw him slip into his professional role of pastor. As I recall, he actually called me "My son" and said something about the bitterness of life and the hereafter.

I said, "Carlos, I don't need this," and went to one of the little shebeen bars in what passed for downtown Bumba. And after I'd had a few beers a white man walked in speaking Lingala. It was Simon Van Nieuwenhove, a sandy-haired young Flemish man with broad shoulders and eyes that constantly moved, scanning the room. He had just arrived in Bumba from the Sudanese border. Joe McCormick, the American whom I'd met in Kinshasa, had flown back to the Zairean capital with his blood samples, but Simon, who had accompanied him on his tour through southern Sudan to establish a link with the other Ebola epidemic, had continued by road, to meet up with me.

Simon was perhaps thirty-four years old, a physician, and he worked for the Belgian Development Cooperation agency in Isiro. He had been living in Zaire for several years and spoke a few local languages. He was a real bon vivant who knew far better than I did how to carry himself in a Zairean bar, where both men and women were quite naturally working on me for beer money and ready cash. He appeared at so precisely the perfect moment that it was almost hard to believe in the coincidence.

Everything bubbled up, the emotions and the alcohol. We talked about Ebola, of course, and he briefed me about the epidemic in Sudan, and we bought drinks for everyone in the bar—that was the mood I was in, I wanted great gestures and high drama—and in that instant of profound brotherhood we became friends for life.

CHAPTER 6

The Big Team

E VERYTHING CHANGED WHEN the big team came to Yambuku, at the end of November, because until then I had been the chief. Now trucks from the Ebonda plantation unloaded generator, a liquid-nitrogen tank to be kept at $-170°$, lab equipment, radio equipment, even video equipment. Two young physicians from the University of Kinshasa joined the team, Dr. Miatudila and Dr. Mbuyi as well as Mike White, a CDC epidemiologist from Atlanta, and two Frenchmen—a hematologist, to organize plasmapheresis from Ebola survivors to obtain hyperimmune plasma, and an entomologist, who planned to investigate possible Ebola reservoirs or vectors in the local insect population. (However, the hypothesis of an insect *vector* already seemed unlikely: Ebola's main mode of transmission was pretty clear.) Finally, a young Englishwoman who worked at the British Embassy in Kinshasa came along to organize the administration. There were even two Zairean electricians, whose job was to install an additional power supply for the generator and rewire the Yambuku hospital.

All this increased considerably the burden on the mission in terms of everything from catering to toilets. With all of this to manage, and lots of large personalities on display, I kind of withdrew into my shell. These people wanted to start all over again investigating the epidemiology on the basis of highly structured questionnaires. Karl and Joel rightly argued that it was important to gather as much information about Ebola as soon as possible. This was a very scary virus, and it's always better to do the work when an epidemic is fresh in memory: months later, people do not remember.

Thus we repeated the work that Pierre and I had already done. But this time we did it more thoroughly, as a more structured case-control study that retrospectively compared the sick and the healthy, to identify contributing factors. Basically we collected information on a case and compared it to that of two or three people who didn't get the disease, to try to eke out all the differences.

In addition, we mapped every house in the villages around Yandongi and Yambuku, and organized a vast survey of several thousand randomly selected people whom we tested for Ebola antibodies. The point of this was to assess the extent of Ebola infection in the area and to establish whether some people had already contracted the infection but had either manifested no symptoms or survived them. (We did find the occasional person with an old infection, but the main conclusion of this work was that survival of Ebola—and asymptomatic Ebola infection—is very rare.) It wasn't until 10 years later in 1986 that I fully appreciated the value of this precise and disciplined approach to a random population survey: because of the records we kept, and the CDC's excellent specimen storage, we used these same blood samples to take a look at the prehistory of HIV.

Joel Bremen was my mentor. After the theoretical courses I had studied in Antwerp, I was finally learning epidemiology in practice. Joel taught me the Zen of a robust case-control study, hammering into my head that precise case definition and careful selection of controls creates or destroys the value of research. A walking encyclopedia with experience of health in Africa, Joel had the patience of a monk, a heart of gold, and a sharp and comic delivery of Jewish jokes in both English and French.

We were constantly following up false rumors and dead ends. One Sunday Joel, Mike White, Guido, and I took a trip upriver to a village that was only accessible by dugout canoe. Those are some pretty unstable boats—two-person dugouts, with one man rowing with a stick. We were seated a few inches from the water line, and God only knew what parasites and crocodiles were in the water. A separate dugout transported the drummer, who gave the beat.

Every so often the rowers stopped, and someone climbed a tree to fetch down a stash of fermented palm wine. (There are palm trees whose trunks you can cut, much like a rubber tree. The sap is collected in hollowed-out calabash gourd, where it ferments in the heat to create an insect/moonshine stew of varying degrees of alcohol.) It tasted foul, but the rowers were clearly getting high. On the riverbanks there were all kinds of monkeys and birds, and the village too was like something out of *National Geographic*. When we arrived, all the inhabitants were at the landing stage, drumming and dancing and chanting. Many of the men were in loincloths, and the women bare-breasted.

Again, it quickly emerged that nobody was particularly sick, and the rumor of Ebola had been just that, so we paid for a huge meal and everyone laughed a lot and then we poled as best as possible our zigzaggy way back to Yambuku. (Guido's boat overturned, to everyone's joy but his own.) That was the only relaxing day I remember.

Guido had set up a very sophisticated portable lab, complete with enclosed working cabinets, fluorescent microscope, laminar flow facilities, electronic blood-testing apparatus, and a refrigerated centrifuge. This meant that as well as testing for antibodies in people, we also had the resources to begin investigating any Ebola antibodies in domestic animals and rodents. Since I had experience dealing with pigs and goats, the sampling fell to me: seizing these skinny, half-wild pigs and slicing off a tiny piece of their tail to the total hilarity of every child.

We were becoming a close-knit community. Guido began fooling with the video equipment that had been delivered, entertaining the team and villagers with funny clips that he shot—"YBC News from the Yambuku Broadcasting Company." None of the local people had ever seen television, so what to us was merely amusing was to them deeply powerful and fascinating.

All this sounds relatively lighthearted, but we all knew that the stakes were deadly serious. Before the big team had left Kinshasa, they were informed that Geoff Platt, a virology technician at the high-security Porton Down facility in Britain, had come down with symptoms of Ebola after pricking himself while attempting to inject some of our blood samples into a rodent. He was placed in an isolator in intensive care, his family and other contacts were quarantined, and a sample of serum from Sukato, the Yambuku nurse who had recovered from the infection, was rushed to Britain. When the team arrived in Yambuku, Platt was still very seriously ill. (He did ultimately spontaneously recover.)

Because Ebola virus had been detected in Platt's semen, as well as his blood, it was resolved that we should collect some sperm from the local men, particularly those who had survived infection with Ebola. Actually I had begun trying to do this before the Kinshasa team arrived, but it was a little delicate to communicate. Obviously this was not something I could ask a nun to translate, and the word *masturbation* was not in my Flemish-Lingala dictionary. After a couple of conversations in which I waved my forearm a lot and felt extremely foolish, it really did seem to me that masturbation didn't figure at all in the local culture. Nobody seemed to acknowledge what I meant.

So I asked Joel and Karl to bring a gross of condoms with them from Kinshasa. There was a long silence on the other side of the radio, and then a guffaw of laughter; what kind of superlover did I think I was, asking for a *gross* of condoms? But I had thought to use them to collect sperm. And indeed, this was easier to communicate. I explained, with a stick, how to roll a condom on a penis; the men went off to find their wives and girlfriends; and they emerged later with my trophies—used condoms, full and warm. It made me wonder whether I would have acquiesced if some African scientist had asked me, in Belgium, for such a thing. Clearly I was just as strange to the people of Yambuku as they were to me, and quite possibly more so.

As our camaraderie deepened, I began to develop great admiration for the power of American science, management, and entrepreneurship. I essentially shed the primitive anti-Americanism that I had developed, in common with so many Europeans at the time, and told myself that we Europeans should stop complaining about the United States, learn the best from them, and get our act together. I also decided I wanted to go to the United States for further firsthand experience of American science. I was determined to spend the rest of my life working on health in Africa; I felt that I would be marked for life by what I had seen of the degrading conditions of extreme poverty, and the intolerable suffering and disease to which it exposes people. But to do this as well as possible, I needed more training, more knowledge, and more skill.

In early December, Del Conn—a Peace Corps volunteer who had joined us from Kinshasa to provide precious logistic support—came down with fever and rash. Del was less lucky than I had been when I had my two days of bad diarrhea in Kinshasa: he was put in a plastic isolator and flown to Johannesburg with Margaretha Isaacson. Fortunately he did not have hemorrhagic fever—I don't know what he actually had—but he must have felt extremely lonely and scared in his plastic tent, with Margaretha as his caregiver.

Sometime after Del's departure, Stefaan Pattyn visited us, out of the blue. I now felt empowered enough to have a normal relationship with him.

On December 22, we finally flew out of the epidemic zone, to be replaced by David Heymann, a young American from the CDC who would be doing post-outbreak surveillance for two months. I had to hand it to him: it was nearly Christmas, but David was not only prepared to miss out on the usual holiday celebrations, he was also prepared to ensure the less than glorious work of postepidemic surveillance. This means ensuring that there is no recurrence of the epidemic and continuing the basic epidemiological surveys, while comforting the nuns and providing assistance to the hospital. He had lost his eyeglasses en route, and there was no optician for a thousand miles in any direction; I wholeheartedly wished him good luck. (As with so many members of the original Ebola team, our friendship developed further in subsequent years, as our paths crossed time and again—most recently when he became assistant director-general of WHO in Geneva and, again, in London, where we currently work together at the London School of Hygiene & Tropical Medicine.)

When the plane arrived to pick us up there was another big fight with the pilots of the Buffalo plane because General Bumba had demanded they bring a stock of rattan furniture back to Kinshasa, and a number of other people had bribed them to be allowed on board, so there was no place for our samples or lab equipment. (The quarantine had been lifted but no boats had yet arrived in town.) I argued and swore and joked around and cajoled.

Nonetheless, they ultimately conceded our right to board the plane, and allowed us to load our Land Rover, boxes, and nitrogen-gas canisters on board. Yet another storm was beginning. As we took off, the plane—overloaded and badly loaded at that—lurched and hit the trees. I could feel it straining against the wind to pull up and take flight. We had no seat belts, so we were flung about, and several of us were hit by heavy flying crates. There was quite a bit of blood and some shouting, and I thought, This time, this is it.

But weirdly I wasn't thinking about myself anymore. I looked over at the crate that held the liquid-nitrogen canister with all those precious samples of sera for further analysis and thought, Shit, all this work for nothing.

But then we pulled up, and out, back to Kinshasa.

I WAS HOME just in time for Christmas, after more than two months of absence, instead of the 10 days as originally planned—a quite transformed person. It took me a while to get used to the family and work routine again, to the absurd range of choices in supermarkets, and to the fact that, after all, Belgium is a well-functioning society. (Whenever I heard people say that we didn't need government, I reminded them what it is to live and do business in a country without a functional government and without the rule of law.)

I was grateful to be alive, and had learned that anything can happen, good and bad, in life. But also that more is in me than I assumed. Ebola showed dramatically that, in contrast to prevailing medical opinion in the 1960s and '70s, the world would experience a seemingly never-ending series of new infectious disease epidemics in humans and animals. This first-known outbreak of Ebola hemorrhagic fever was probably also the first example of highly integrated international collaboration to tackle an outbreak—a collaboration that was informal and ad hoc, driven by a very diverse group of scientists with a passion for solving problems in the field, and committed to working as a group (for example, we decided early on to publish our findings as an international commission, rather than as individuals, thereby avoiding the so-common conflicts among researchers about authorship). It was one of the last major disease outbreaks without global media attention, as neither CNN nor Internet-based social media existed in 1976. As so eloquently reported by Laurie Garrett, when Ebola hit Kikwit in 1995, 19 years after the false alert we investigated, there were nearly as many journalists as epidemiologists and doctors on site, which was a mixed blessing for those working in Kikwit, but certainly raised the world's understanding that we are under constant threat of new pathogens. Since then, there have been about 20 outbreaks of Ebola infection, nearly all concentrated around hospitals in Africa, and with very high mortality. In general it is an infection that causes epidemics only if basic hospital hygiene is not respected, and is really a disease of poverty and neglect of health systems. The heroic and well-meaning sisters in Yambuku had dramatically shown that doing good is not enough, and can actually be dangerous if it is not bedded in technical competence and sound evidence. Health, economic, and social development are unmistakably intertwined.

Finally, 35 years later, it seems more and more likely that my boss at the time was right: fruit bats are probably the reservoir where Ebola virus hides in between epidemics in humans and apes. If only I had listened to good old Pattyn, who died in 2008.

• PART TWO •

CHAPTER 7

From Ebola to Sex and the Transmission of Infection

WHEN WE RETURNED to Europe, Guido and I paid a visit to the convent of the congregation of the Sacred Heart of Our Lady to give the sisters a full report. S'Gravenwezel is a small town north of Antwerp, and the huge convent was an extraordinary place, very formal and grim; it felt like another era. We arrived at the appointed time one dark, almost-snowing afternoon in January. We rang a large bell and the heavy convent door slowly opened. A sister walked us through a series of freezing cold corridors to a waiting room. Finally we were called on to speak before the mother superior and all the assembled nuns.

I almost expected candlelight. I once again marveled at the series of historical events that had projected these women into a tiny village in Central Africa. You could hear a pin drop when we reminded them how the four sisters had died, and they asked too many questions to which we had no answer. We discussed also how we could raise money to refurbish the hospital, and they were very keen to recruit a doctor for Yambuku. Even after our presentation I'm not sure that the implications, in terms of their responsibility for the epidemic, had really sunk in. They profusely thanked us and said that they would pray for us, and then we focused on raising money for Yambuku.

This made me feel we hadn't done our job, frankly. Guido insisted that we shouldn't underscore their guilt: he saw their heroism and goodwill, their dedication, and loved them for it. But I thought it could have been an important lesson. Goodwill is not enough. You need to be competent, you need to know what you're doing, or you may do more harm than good. To be fair, it was true that they had had very little funding, extremely poor training, and they had not been able to pay for any doctors in the Yambuku hospital. Thus we promised to help them ask for government money so they could pay for a doctor at the mission. But I couldn't help wondering how many more mission hospitals in Africa were as underequipped and poorly run as Yambuku, and what earthly difference one doctor could make.

I was feeling sobered about the whole experience of traveling to Zaire. Maybe it was a kind of postcombat depression. I saw how irresponsible we had been throughout the whole assignment. No insurance, as traveling to an epidemic zone was an "extraordinary risk," against which the institute had not insured employees. No evacuation plan: the Americans had one, and all we did was rely on their probable help. Post hoc, I felt scared and angry at the scale of the risk.

I was also furious, because Pattyn without intending to do so, tried to deprive me of my reward. I was one of fewer than ten doctors who saw a case of Ebola; I participated in isolating the virus. One afternoon I walked into his office and saw on his desk the manuscript of the article he was writing to report the discovery of the virus. Neither my name nor Guido's was on it.

In a sense, this was how things often had worked in science in Europe until the 1970s: the young people did the work, and their bosses took the credit. Pattyn wasn't doing anything unusual, but it really made me mad. I grabbed the paper, went to find Pattyn, and calmly told him, "I am going to be an author of this article and Guido is going to be an author of this article!" Pattyn simply dissolved. He blinked a little bit and mumbled something about it being just a draft, after all, and wrote our names in right there while I was watching.

It felt like a small victory, however. Work at the lab seemed routine. My life—despite the comfort and friendliness and safety of it—paled in comparison with the drama of Ebola. A number of us must have felt the same way, for when the World Health Organization (WHO) convened a meeting of the international commission that month of January 1977 at the London School of Hygiene & Tropical Medicine, there was a tense and scornful dispute between the Zaire team and the group from Sudan—one that seemed way too emotional for its supposed subject. This was my first formal international meeting, and despite all the rituals of each speaker taking the floor and formally thanking everyone, there was tension. Each team accused the other of poor statistics. Ebola had killed only about 50 percent of its victims in Sudan, whereas the figure in Zaire was far higher, more than 80 percent. Later on it turned out that the two strains of the virus were different: almost unbelievably, there had been two simultaneous but unrelated outbreaks of the same, previously unknown disease within a radius of 500 miles. Again, there was a lesson here: something that may appear to be completely unlikely—even ludicrous—can happen.

The London School was an imposing establishment near the British Museum, its building nearly a whole city block, lined with the names of famous physicians of tropical medicine, which seemed to radiate all the imperial power of the British empire. Little did I dream that I would much later be appointed to direct this august institution. Too intimidated to speak much, I listened as my colleagues agreed on a number of recommendations for WHO. The main proposal was that mechanisms should be developed to identify and react promptly to new outbreaks of hemorrhagic fever, with mandatory reports to WHO of all new suspected cases, a Disaster or Outbreak Fund, and a constantly updated list of experienced people ready to participate in a rapid deployment team. We also recommended training for people who would coordinate expeditions; specific operational plans for surveillance, epidemiological studies, lab support, logistics, communications and information to the public; lists of the kinds of specimens needed for differential diagnosis, and where to send them; and a special, detailed checklist of recommended supplies. Basically none of it was ever implemented.

A few weeks later in February Pattyn received a phone call. The Ebola epidemic had perhaps flared up again in Yambuku and this time it might have already spread—maybe even to Belgium. Days before, a patient at the Yambuku hospital—a farmer, with a small shop—had developed what the sisters identified as Ebola symptoms and died. The nuns panicked. Rather than endure more weeks of quarantine and a continuing drumroll of deaths, they bolted to Kinshasa and caught the first available flight to Belgium. They were currently at the convent, consumed with fear.

Pattyn and I went to s'Gravenwezel. The sisters began crying. They could see that in taking flight they had not only abandoned what they conceived as their duty, but they had also potentially endangered other people. (They seemed to have posttraumatic stress syndrome—not surprising given what they went through.)

Then he turned to me. Pattyn wanted me to go back to Yambuku. He said that "we" would do the job *without* the Americans this time. "We" would get in there and find Ebola's natural reservoir.

I flew into the zone with Jean-François Ruppol and Dr. Weyalo, a young Zairean internist from the Clinique Kinoise, a brave and good companion. We landed in Gbadolite, the home village of President Mobutu's mother. Here Mobutu was engaged in erecting a series of three palaces—actually an entire Versailles—in which he and his wife (whose name, amazingly, was Marie-Antoinette) could indulge in his favorite tipple, vintage pink champagne.

Seen from above, the fake lakes and curving balustrades of this Italian-marble confection were simply obscene, a megalomaniac Disneyland that was emblematic of Mobutu's theft of resources and his distance from his citizens' concerns. The airport—equipped for intercontinental jets—was huge and empty. Leading from it, a four-lane highway lined with European tulips led past a number of villas said to be under construction for various dignitaries of Mobutu's régime, all of them jostling for proximity to the *Président-Fondateur*. Colonialism surely wasn't much worse than this loathsome régime.

We drove to Yambuku. The whole region was in panic. The mission hospital was deserted, though Sukato, the nurse who had survived Ebola infection, was still there. We stayed for two weeks, from

February 7 to 20, trying to develop a clear picture of events. Everywhere we went it seemed much more like an outbreak of rumors than an outbreak of disease. Although the sisters were now using sterile needles for injections, we followed up every possible needle contact we could; none seemed to have an infection. At every village we went to, people said, "Here there have been no deaths"—they were absolutely certain of that—"but in such-and-such a village the fever is back." But when we went there to check it out, we found nothing.

It was in a way more difficult to investigate a nonevent than an event. You had to prove that something *hadn't* happened. We wondered if people were hiding the disease so as to avoid the crippling economic effects of a quarantine, but we reasoned that this would have been a lot to hide. And there were other clues too. I saw no women with shaved heads, and I knew that meant there had been no deaths. People would not give up customs that ran so deep just to fool a couple of doctors. In the meantime we held consultations, and even did some emergency surgery, since the hospital still had no doctor.

In the end it was up to Dr. Weyalo and me to decide whether to quarantine the whole region. And we concluded that there was no need to do it. A single man had died following rectal bleeding. Probably he had had colon cancer. But in a region still seething with fear and tension months after a murderous epidemic that was all it took to ignite a new, quite pointless wave of terror.

I RETURNED TO Antwerp, a tolerant city in these days, and my son Bram was born in April, a few weeks after my return. To my surprise I found that this completely predictable event suddenly shifted my whole view of the world. Before, I felt completely independent. Now someone was relying on me, and a certain insouciant self-indulgence had to give way; I felt responsible, even anxious, about my—*our*—future. During the long evenings in Yambuku, Joel Breman and I had talked about my plans. I wanted to do more training in the United States. In Yambuku I grasped just how far ahead American medical science truly was. I was particularly impressed by the synergy between several disciplines to tackle a problem, and by the highly critical review of every step in the research process. And there was a joke in Belgium that if you wanted to get anywhere in academia, you needed the BTA diploma—Been To America.

Joel said that he would get me a place at the CDC's famous field epidemiology program, the Epidemic Intelligence Service course, which in those days took very few foreigners. But I knew he couldn't bankroll that; I would have to find the money. Pattyn, meanwhile, urged me to finish my specialty training in clinical microbiology. So while I was applying for various fellowships and sponsorships I continued working at the institute.

But then that spring a new adventure presented itself. André Meheus, a professor of epidemiology at the University of Antwerp, contacted me: he needed someone who knew about lab techniques to accompany him to Swaziland on a mission for WHO. I knew Meheus from my days as a medical student in Ghent; I was then an intern in the Department of Social Medicine where he worked. He was an easygoing and likable man with a lot of contacts, and somehow he had persuaded WHO to fund a five-week mission to southern Africa so that he could eliminate sexually transmitted disease from Swaziland.

When I heard this absurd premise I choked. But André told me this kind of thing was almost routine. WHO made up terms that were deliriously unrealistic and to receive funding you had to promise to fulfill them. But nobody ever checked whether you had achieved the impossible results you'd promised, and so long as you did some work and pushed the buck a little further down the road, everyone was happy. (Incidentally, at today's WHO this particular attitude has greatly changed.)

It was cold in Swaziland in June—the Southern Hemisphere's winter. The country was very different from Zaire. There wasn't the same exuberance of nature—in all its greenness and wilderness—or the same vivid personal style in terms of the way people dressed and moved and spoke. Zaireans were desperately poor, but they looked colorful, elegant, with elaborate hairdos and joyful gestures when they spoke. In Swaziland people were also very poor and were dressed in dingy sweaters.

They also had a stiffness about them, and a sadness that I interpreted as the shadow of apartheid: people, particularly men, seemed
to have been somehow broken. Even men over sixty were routinely
hailed as "Boy." It was strange, miserable, ugly. But after a while,
I understood that these people were as warm as those in Central
Africa, just different. Swaziland was a monarchy with an absolute
king. South African police were said to be everywhere, supervising
everything, so that the exiled African National Congress liberation
movement couldn't use the country as a base of operations. But many
whites whom I met at the hotel seemed to be present for two things
only—to have sex and to gamble.

In those days I knew hardly anything about sexually transmitted diseases (STDs). But André and I went to clinics, estimated the
numbers and type of sexually transmitted infection, reviewed their
treatment guidelines (which were almost uniformly ineffective), and
saw—it was clear—that the STD problem in Swaziland was enormous. I noticed when I was going through the mission records in
Yambuku, and at the Mama Yemo Hospital in Kinshasa, that there
seemed to be a sexually transmitted disease problem in Zaire, too;
chancroid and salpingitis and urethritis and gonorrhea seemed to figure far more often than I would have expected in Belgium. But in
Swaziland, the scale was off the charts.

We were doing clinical examinations, of course. And the kinds
of complications and combinations of STDs that we were review-
ing were simply mind-blowing. Every clinic was like a museum of
genital disease, a cabinet of sexually transmitted curiosities. The
patients were all desperately poor. A man would walk in wearing his
skirt and you would see that his penis was dripping on the floor. He
would pick his skirt up, show me a truly monstrous chancroid, and I
would ask, "So when did you last have sex?" And he would say, "This
morning."

I was astonished, because if it were me I wouldn't be able to put it
in my pants, it would hurt so bad. Speaking as a doctor, I was really
taken aback, because under those conditions the disease would clearly
spread fast and wide. And finally, as a human being I was shocked,
frankly. Because it quite often emerged that the sex partner was a

much younger woman, and the man could hardly have ignored the fact that his chancroid was highly contagious. Having sex in these conditions was just abominable. So I was quite judgmental about that, and also, incidentally, about the Swazi King, who at the time was seventy-nine years old, and almost every year married yet another virgin.

Prostitution was everywhere I went in Swaziland. The day I arrived at my hotel, the man at reception gave me my room key and when I went up there was a woman there. So I went back downstairs and said, "I want my own room—there is a woman in that room."

The receptionist looked at me, sort of taken aback, and said, "Oh? Want a boy?"

That, apparently, was the only other option imaginable. At first I assumed that such activity was limited to this particular hotel. I didn't grasp yet the scale of prostitution in the city.

André and I had no hope of eliminating STDs from Swaziland, quite clearly, but we could do something to help. We arranged to convene a training session for Swazi nurses a few months later, which I would return to direct alone. In the meantime I designed a simple way to identify STDs without any lab tests, developing something called algorithms for treatment. Basically it was a simple flow chart—a tree structure with questions. Are there red bumps on the genitals? Are there also open sores? Are the sores dripping pus? If so, treat with antibiotic XYZ. I sketched this flow chart out quite literally on the back of an envelope, and oddly enough it turned out to be so useful that it's still being used all over the world after being endorsed by WHO years later. You can find these charts on the wall in many a clinic in Africa today.

When I got back to Antwerp I found a letter waiting for me from the Zairean ambassador to Belgium, Kengo wa Dondo. "The President and Founder has appointed you an Officer of the Order of the Leopard," it announced. I had no desire to receive any kind of decoration from Mobutu, but I saw no polite way out. So I phoned the embassy and on the appointed day I went there and was handed a star-shaped medal on a piece of bright green ribbon, with the motto PEACE, WORK, JUSTICE. Sure thing, I thought: *Justice.*

The ambassador explained that I would soon receive a special card, personally signed by Mobutu (who, by the way, had a signature that was just a stab of ink—one line, no curls or letters—which I guess is how a man of infinite power signifies his status). This bright green fold-over card, which looked a bit like a Belgian driver's license of the time, would give me total immunity and total respect throughout Zaire. I would be guaranteed safety and protection from every kind of harm.

I decided not to go and get the card. I didn't want to profit from Mobutu's regime. I felt that Zaire had twice been the private property of a single individual—first the Belgian monarch Leopold II and now Mobutu—and I wanted no part of any of this corruption.

A few months later I also met Mobutu, the man whom French humanitarian activist Bernard Kouchner called "a bank vault in a leopard-skin hat," who had changed his name to mean "the rooster who leaves no chicken unplucked" or "the all-powerful warrior who goes from conquest to conquest, leaving fire in his wake," depending on the translation. Mobutu was on a state visit to Belgium, and he came to Antwerp to thank us for having saved the country. He was wearing that famous leopard-skin hat of his, and he held his magic walking stick, with the head carved like an eagle, and I shook his bloodstained hand. He was very charming, as were so many other dictators I met later as head of UNAIDS.

By this time I had decided to do my doctoral work in sexually transmitted disease. In a way this was logical. Hemorrhagic fevers, like Ebola? They were simply too dangerous and costly for our lab ever to hope to work with. Diarrheal diseases? Sure, that research would be useful, but there was already a group in Brussels that was doing a lot of work in the field. Malaria? It was such a complex problem; I wasn't sure I would ever be able to master the immunology. But STDs, such as I had seen in Swaziland, here was an area where I could really help people. Except for herpes in those days, you could always cure these diseases, and that's very gratifying for a doctor.

If you're a psychiatrist or a geriatric specialist, you're looking at chronic, complex problems; the work may be frustrating. Infectious diseases, sexually transmitted diseases—these were not prestigious specialties; in fact, they were at the bottom of the ladder in terms of medical status. But I was drawn to them, because these were problems that had solutions; as a doctor, your impact could be strong and quick. It could also be vital to reproductive health, a crucial issue for many women, whose medical needs in this respect (as in so many others) had clearly been ignored for far too long. Also, chlamydia had just been discovered as a cause of genital infection. This was an intracellular bacteria that was difficult to detect, but highly damaging to fertility. I found the microbiology of chlamydia fascinating. So although opting for sexually transmitted diseases wasn't the smartest career move, it made sense to me from the point of view of scientific curiosity and human need.

BECAUSE OF THIS new interest in sexually transmitted infections, I began seeing more patients in addition to my job in Pattyn's lab. The clinic that I worked in was housed in the same nice old art deco building as the lab—the Institute for Tropical Medicine—and its full name (which nobody used) was "Clinic for Colonials and Seafarers." This clinic was known for its treatment of sexually transmitted diseases because in Antwerp STDs were considered a tropical disease—there's a big harbor and a lot of sailors, and they tended to catch sexual diseases in outlandish places. I arranged to work there two afternoons a week, to further my research.

I liked the work. I wasn't only dealing with sexually transmitted diseases: this was a consultation for vaccinations, for leprosy and malaria, and what have you. A lot of people began coming to me specifically because they heard that I didn't share the half-concealed disapproval of some of the other doctors. Also, STDs were rising in Antwerp in the late 1970s, just as they were everywhere else—especially in the gay population, which had really only just begun to come out of the closet in Belgium, and openly live out what proved for some to be a dangerous lifestyle.

Obviously I knew that many medical doctors see work with sexually transmitted disease as embarrassing. It's dirty, it's low-life. But I never felt like this. When you work with STDs, you need to be able to keep your mouth shut (as in any interaction with patients). Confidentiality, competence, a nonjudgmental approach: these are what count.

I knew that ideally, my career and my life were going to be about developing countries. I was still searching, but it seemed now that it would probably involve something literally below the belt. So at the clinic in Antwerp I took samples from patients and tried to work them out in the lab. That's how I came to isolate a new, penicillin-resistant gonococcus from the urethral pus of a sailor who had sex while on furlough in Ivory Coast. Up to then, penicillin resistance in gonorrhea seemed to occur through mutations in the bacteria's chromosome. This meant that as resistance built up, you needed a bit more penicillin, but once you attained the correct dose the bacteria would succumb. With the new type of resistance an increased dose wouldn't help, because the bacterial strain produced enzymes that could actually *destroy* penicillin. Worse yet, the genetic information for producing these enzymes was transmitted by plasmids—extrachromosomal molecules of DNA—that could be transferred among different bacteria, a potentially serious public health problem.

The first gonococci of this type were discovered in US soldiers and Marines stationed in the Philippines; another was isolated in a man from Ghana. So my strain was the second found in Africa. I published the discovery in 1977. It was just a letter to the editor of *The Lancet*, but to a young researcher from Belgium that was the big time. The next year, when working in the laboratory of Stanley Falkow at the University of Washington in Seattle, we characterized the plasmid and the mechanisms of resistance.

All this work piqued my interest in gonorrhea; I tried to learn as much as I could. But when I looked into the medical literature, it was like looking into the Dark Ages. And it was the same with chlamydia. There was a whole field here crying out for some serious science, but at that time the only person applying scientific methodology to the study of STDs seemed to be someone named Dr. King Holmes, from the University of Washington in Seattle. He had worked with the navy in Vietnam, to estimate the risk of acquiring gonorrhea; he had worked on resistant strains, finding new etiologies; and he had started working on chlamydia and pelvic inflammatory disease (PID).

That really caught my attention because I saw so much of it in the records at the Yambuku mission. Holmes was doing very basic work on PID—what caused it, what microorganisms are associated with it. Common wisdom said it was bacteria ascending into the vagina from the environment—basically the scenario where you catch something from a toilet seat—but Holmes and his team demonstrated that it was almost always linked to sexually transmitted disease. This may not have been a socially convenient explanation but at least it indicated the correct treatment.

I met King Holmes for the first time at a conference in Rotterdam. I was coorganizing this founding meeting of the International Society of STD research—a group of young "Turks," who aimed to transform the science of STDs. As I recall the talk was on the various possible causes of nongonococcal urethritis—chlamydia, herpes, or other organisms such as *Ureaplasma urealyticum*—and I found King to be an inspiring, charismatic, even humorous speaker. He could have made the phone book sing. After his talk, I went up to have a few words with him.

I'm not sure what I expected, but it was certainly not that King Holmes would take the time to ask me questions about my work, and appear to listen to the answers. I didn't know yet that in the United States there was a totally different kind of relationship in academia, much more open and egalitarian. King is an extraordinary scholar, with an unlimited curiosity for disciplines far beyond his own specialty of infectious diseases, and above all, with a great capacity to mentor young researchers to get the best out of them. Soon after our brief encounter, he became my mentor as well.

A few months later, in early 1978, I obtained two fellowships—from NATO and from the Belgian Science Foundation—to go to the United States. My plan was, first, to attend the CDC's Epidemic Intelligence Service training course that Joel and I had discussed. In those days, this program was unique in the world. It was created in the 1950s to develop a corps of epidemiologists to investigate epidemic outbreaks, with a structured method for how to investigate disease outbreaks of known or unknown origins and what to do about them.

I also wrote to King Holmes and told him that I had a fellowship, and that I planned to attend the CDC course and work for a few months at the CDC's Special Pathogens Lab. I asked Holmes if I could then also come and work at his lab in Seattle. Holmes answered Sure. I felt I knew what I was doing. Nothing was really fixed, but I was a grown-up now and that suited me fine.

CHAPTER 8

America and Back

I ARRIVED IN ATLANTA in June 1978. Karl Johnson, our team leader in Yambuku and head of "Special Pathogens" at the Centers for Disease Control, picked me up at the airport in his old Volkswagen station wagon and dropped me at the home of Stan Foster, a CDC epidemiologist and smallpox veteran, where I stayed for a few weeks, before moving to Karl's house in Snellville, a small town east of Atlanta.

This was my first time in the United States, and it was as great a culture shock as going to Zaire—more, in some ways, because I had expected it to be essentially the same as Europe. People in Snellville left their air-conditioners on all the time, even when their doors and windows were open. Everywhere I went I needed a credit card but I didn't own one—this was 1978, remember, and in Belgium credit cards were rare. There were guns. Huge cars. The stereotypes piled up. In Georgia people call you by your first name after seconds. All around me in Atlanta were black people who were very different from Africans, while the CDC was all white, barely a single dark face in the crowd.

As part of the CDC course, I had to do a survey on contraceptive practices in inner-city Atlanta. I went with a veterinarian who was a black American from Harvard, and he was a bit nervous to do it. But I said, "No problem, I've been to Zaire"—I was the explorer. We drove around neighborhoods of burned-out buildings that looked like Beirut, knocking on doors. We asked questions to people who could barely understand my English; I certainly could not understand theirs. This was daytime work, so most of the people who answered the door were single women and perfectly friendly. Then a guy opened the door to his apartment and he had a Colt in his belt.

I have no recollection at all of the results of the survey, but I met some very interesting people at the CDC, chief among them the director, Bill Foege, the forty-two-year-old father of smallpox containment. He insisted on meeting personally with each foreigner who attended the course; he questioned me at length about my experience in Africa, and I found that remarkable. Foege was a very impressive figure, and not only because of height. Working as a medical missionary in eastern Nigeria in the 1960s, just as the people of Biafra began to fight for independence, he had had the job of performing smallpox vaccinations, but he didn't have enough vaccine to cover everyone. When a three-year-old boy came down with smallpox, he devised a system for mapping its likely spread and vaccinated only people in market villages and places where the child's family habitually traveled. His surveillance and containment scheme stopped the outbreak in its tracks and inaugurated a new tactic in the fight against the disease. (Thirty years later our paths crossed again as senior fellows at the Bill & Melinda Gates Foundation in Seattle, and he was as inspiring as ever.)

The plan was for me to work for a while with Karl at the high-security Special Pathogens Lab. I had to suit up in a space suit that had its own air supply and obey an incredibly disciplined, very highly organized regime. Really I just couldn't handle the discipline. I forgot things, and then had to undress and shower before leaving the lab to go get them, and go through the whole ritual again on return. It was too cumbersome for me—

After a couple of weeks I decided to cut short my now two months' CDC experience and head to Seattle to work with King Holmes, because my scientific interest had really moved from hemorrhagic fevers to sexually transmitted diseases. Greta had joined me in Atlanta, with Bram; we had bought a Toyota station wagon, in anticipation of exploring the New World, so the most logical idea seemed to be to pile everything into the car and drive across the country. We took our time, and stayed at campsites.

I was surprised by the number of churches on our way, though even a small European town like Antwerp has plenty of old Catholic churches. I could feel the unexpected agricultural power as we drove past miles and miles of fields planted with corn and wheat. The natural beauty of America was stunning, but although people were friendly, they seemed suspicious of us—with our accented English, we were clearly foreigners—and I remained startled and frightened of the pickup trucks with gun racks.

Bram, who was fifteen months old, took to running around the campsites without pants or a diaper. He liked it, plus it cut down on heat rash, and to us it seemed like a perfectly normal thing for a small child to do. But people couldn't seem to deal with this infant nudity. The more polite ones would come up to us with a concerned look and say, "Your son has lost his pants." The less inhibited would berate us—"Why is your kid going around naked?"

When we got to Seattle—beautiful, the Olympic mountains capped by snow, the coastline jagged with clear blue fjords—I telephoned King Holmes, who had perhaps forgotten all about me. He said, "Well, you'd better come for lunch at my place." This astonished me, though actually it turned out to be a peanut butter sandwich in his kitchen. When we finished, Holmes asked me, "So, what would you like to do?" and again I was startled: in Europe, the professor *tells* you what you're going to do.

I had my penicillin-resistant gonococci with me in the car, and I told him I wanted to study the plasmid's molecular mechanism of resistance, learn about sexually transmitted diseases, and also work on vaginitis. I had many women patients with chronic vaginitis (an uncomfortable discharge now called bacterial vaginosis), and although this problem seemed to be extremely common its cause and treatment were not well understood.

King said, "OK, why don't you start tomorrow." It was that easy. My jaw dropped.

I loved Seattle, in particular the unspoiled nature surrounding it, and its friendly people, but we were a bit frustrated by the lack of good food and coffee. This was Seattle before Microsoft and Amazon.com and with only one Starbucks on Pike Place Market. We drove 13 miles from our home on Lake Samamish to buy bread at a German bakery. Good bread is important for Belgians! Today the city is as sophisticated as can be for good food and many other essentials in life.

I also loved working with King Holmes—loved the atmosphere of intellectual freedom and confidence in an American laboratory, where young people are encouraged to develop their ideas; I flourished in this outlandish environment. King introduced me to Dr. Stanley Falkow, who was chairman of the Department Microbiology at the University of Washington. We agreed that I would share my time between Falkow's microbiology lab and the clinical work and epidemiology on STDs I was doing with Holmes. From Stanley I learned a lot about modern microbiology, including how to do some of the analytical techniques that were just being developed, such as genetic sequencing of plasmids, the Western blot (which identifies specific proteins), and molecular cloning. (He also taught me how to swear in English.) He is a superb scientist, whose main interest is pathogenesis, the step-by-step explanation of exactly how bacteria cause disease. He taught me always to put myself inside the bacteria—to try to think things out from a bacterium's point of view. How would I penetrate an epithelial cell in the gut? Why would I jump from an animal to a human? He was a superb mentor. Stanley is now emeritus at Stanford, and whenever we can we get together for very stimulating discussions around a superb pinot noir.

Holmes and Falkow worked together very easily, though they headed different departments. This is not always the case in science: people tend to guard their turf. But Holmes worked with everybody—psychologists, chemists, microbiologists, clinicians. Within his department he had a real flair for team building, which is another rare and important skill. Holmes was constantly traveling, but somehow was able to guide and manage this very diverse group, and when you saw him you received clear attention and guidance. He had assembled a group of incredibly talented people, all working on some aspect of sexually transmitted diseases. Many are now in leading positions in Seattle and many other places worldwide. When I left Seattle, King agreed to continue to be my mentor, and has been so for over 30 years now. We are also united by our appreciation for good wine, and I have kept many a wine label from our dinners all over the world.

I was following up on vaginitis studies, concentrating on a family of bacteria found in the vagina that we thought probably caused the problem. I had a whole collection of it, which I was analyzing. (Ultimately this work didn't really pan out; although we know now that this bacterium, *Gardnerella vaginalis*, does play a role, it has to interact with other bacteria to do so.) Later in Antwerp I also studied how to treat the syndrome best, and I demonstrated that the preferred treatment at the time—a sulfonamide cream—actually didn't work at all, was in fact no better than a placebo. The treatment that did work was metronizodole, an antibiotic active against some parasites and anaerobic bacteria. These were the days when the current evidence base of sexually transmitted diseases was established. This work was small in a way, but useful, and I liked it. I liked the very free and entrepreneurial style of American science. There was a great deal of private money—something almost completely absent in Europe except for the Wellcome Trust in Britain—but above all there was a wide open mindset. If you had a good idea and you were competent, you were given a chance to make good.

During my stay in Seattle, I had two encounters that turned out to be defining a few years later. The first one was with Tom Quinn, who had just joined King's group to study anogenital chlamydial infections. Tom is a very jovial infectious disease specialist, always sparking with new ideas, and with a voice you can recognize at a hundred yards' distance. (Five years later we joined forces to investigate AIDS in Zaire.) The second one was with Bob Brunham, a fairly shy and very thoughtful Canadian infectious disease physician and immunologist with curly hair, who was working on a vaccine against genital chlamydial infections. A little bit because we were the two foreign fellows in King's group, but also because of some common interests in

Africa, we became quite close friends. Bob told me about an epidemic of chancroid in Native Americans in Winnipeg, where he was at the University of Manitoba in Canada. Following my experience with this supposedly tropical STD, I was immediately fascinated by this outbreak in the Canadian prairies. His mentor in Canada, Dr. Allan Ronald, head of Infectious Diseases at the University of Manitoba, invited me to Winnipeg to exchange experience on chancroid and its cause, *Haemophilus ducreyi*, as there had hardly been any scientific and therapeutic advances on chancroid for several decades. When I landed on May 1, 1979, it was snowing! (I thought, This must be a tough place to live!) We hit it off, and decided to work together in Kenya, where chancroid was a big problem.

While I enjoyed every minute of work and life in Seattle, I was often disturbed by the absence of a social safety net—such basics as universal health coverage—as well as the easy assumption of some people I met that poverty was basically your own fault. But I also noted that there was far more talk than in Europe about gender inequality and the lack of fairness for women in society. Seattle was a very open-minded place; we were circulating among people who were interesting and diverse.

I became quite a fan of many aspects of American society. I could see that Belgium, and indeed Europe, was becoming ossified, suffocating entrepreneurship in science but also in many other areas of society. I was still deeply Flemish—my genotype so profoundly rooted. But the way those genes were expressed—my phenotype, as it were—was shifting.

However, Greta had no legal right to work in the United States, and as our year there crept by this became a problem. As my fellowship funds began running out we gave more thought to the idea of whether to stay in Seattle. I concluded that if all European scientists who came to America decided to stay, then Europe would really have a problem. I was all charged up with energy and knowledge and I wanted to help change things in Belgium.

WHEN I RETURNED to Antwerp in September 1979, my priority was to finish my doctoral thesis on the etiology of vaginitis. (I finally completed it in the spring of 1980.) I needed clinical material and that meant the STD patients at the Clinic for Colonials and Seafarers. But after a while it became clear that my research—and their treatment—would be enormously facilitated if we could set up a separate clinic exclusively for sexually transmitted disease. Instead of hiding these people, tucking them away alongside people with bilharzia or dengue, we could focus on their specific problems with more professional protocols better adapted to their lifestyles. We would become the first and most important STD clinic in the country. We could associate that work with the kind of outreach that I had seen in Seattle—epidemiological surveys of communities prone to STDs, even community talks.

So at the end of 1979 I marched into the office of the director of the Institute for Tropical Medicine and said so. He was a very conservative man and the idea simply appalled him. He didn't want to draw any more attention than necessary to this unsavory clientele of mine, with their dirty diseases. Although ultimately he did agree to set up a separate STD operation, he put our clinic at the very back of the building, next door to the animal house—the room where the small rodents were kept. Access was through the back door of the institute; I worked with one nurse; and our opening hours were 5 to 7 P.M.

However, I was undisturbed. The rest of the day I continued to work in the lab, where I was still just number four in the pecking order. And in that little clinic what I saw was that, particularly in the gay community, very serious epidemics of STDs were developing. And (mostly in heterosexuals) we were also seeing a huge rise in chlamydia.

I began appearing on the radio, in newspapers, and on TV, to talk about it, because the only way to solve this kind of problem is to discuss the risks and the precautions that people need to take. And just as I discussed homosexuality or sex-related drug use with my patients, I also had no special embarrassment about talking about intercourse on TV.

One evening at the end of 1979, I received a phone call from the pathologist of the Institute of Tropical Medicine. He wanted me to help autopsy a cadaver. The patient had died of galloping meningitis.

He was Greek, but he had lived for decades as a commercial fisher-man on the banks of Lake Tanganyika in eastern Zaire, and when he had arrived at the hospital he was already in terrible shape, with tremendous weight loss and a fever of unknown origin.

When we opened up his body we saw that it was devastated. He was riddled with an atypical mycobacterial infection, a clear sign that his immune system had totally collapsed. We were so taken aback that we kept blood and tissue samples in −70°C freezers. I wasn't smart enough to see that it was a new syndrome, but I knew I had never seen anything like it before.

CHAPTER 9

Nairobi

B Y THE SPRING of 1980, I had finished my thesis "The Aeti-
ology and Epidemiology of Bacterial Vaginosis and *Garde-
nerella Vaginalis*" and I had another, far more exciting project
underway. I was going back to Africa, for a research project that I had
dreamed up with Allan Ronald, the Canadian physician I had met
while in Seattle.

Allan was an amiable man and we talked a lot about Africa. He had
established contact with the University of Nairobi in Kenya, where
genital ulcer disease, in particular, chancroid, had become epidemic.
He told me that he wanted to start a research project on chancroid
and proposed that we work on it together. I had a little experience; he
had some contacts. It was an opportunity to develop a research base
in a city where basic infrastructure like phones and electricity posed
no particular problem, and there was a good university. So we made
a planning visit to Nairobi in January 1980.

Inspired by what I had seen in the United States, I incorporated
a nonprofit group the Foundation for Infectious Disease Research,
upon my return to Antwerp, intending to fund the new research program in Nairobi. From time to time, when I gave workshop train-

ing sessions to general practitioners, or lectures on STDs, I had my emolument deposited into the foundation. It was not a lot—$300 here, $3000 there—so it didn't add up to much. Short of robbing a bank, I didn't know how on earth we would raise enough money to support the Nairobi project.

Then, at a conference on infectious disease, I ran into a new antibiotic that seemed to me a promising candidate to step in as a new chancroid treatment, a more effective alternative to erythro-mycin. The drug was produced by Schering, a company I thought I could convince to fund a trial on the treatment of chancroid, even if chancroid treatment did not represent even a minor future mar-ket for any pharmaceutical company. Where to set up such a trial? While in Swaziland, I had worked with a highly competent and pragmatic English microbiologist who lived in South Africa, Ron Ballard, who had told me there was a truly massive chancroid prob-lem in the South African gold mines, and had asked for our help. The town he mentioned—Carletonville—was the largest gold-mining complex in the world, close to Johannesburg, and with what he described as ideal medical backup in terms of hospitals and labs. On the one hand I wasn't keen to work in apartheid South Africa, but Ballard argued that there was no moral high-ground to aban-doning the poor and needy.

Ballard, Eddy Van Dyck from my lab, and I went to Leslie Wil-liams Memorial Hospital in Carletonville, which indeed was one of the better hospitals I saw in Africa. Clearly the company needed to keep their workforce healthy and productive, but they definitely had no idea how to handle the chancroid problem. Conditions in the gold mines, often over a mile underground, were not only high-risk but also extremely hot and humid; wounds just couldn't heal, and appall-ing chancroid ulcers were incapacitating the miners.

The miners were from all over—Swaziland, Botswana, Lesotho, Mozambique, Malawi, Zambia, Zimbabwe—and they were well paid compared to any worker in their home country. I was never allowed down the mines; I would have liked to see what they were like. But I visited the hostels they lived in, and the places they drank, and saw, lining the red soil paths, the wooden shacks with corrugated iron roofs and simple cloth doors—a prostitute in many of them. Every payday there were lines of men outside these places.

The men worked in shifts, six days a week, around the clock; they all hated and feared the work, but all of them had families back home, and they were doing it for them, trying to bring home enough money to give an education to their children, start a business, maybe set up a shop. I knew, though, that many of them were also taking home some truly infernal diseases, in addition to the high risk of work-related accidents and tuberculosis—the highest rate in the world. These men were at the same time victims of pure exploitation and a source of hope for their community to get out of poverty. I was revolted by their working conditions (and those of the sex workers . . .), was deeply touched by their loneliness and songs full of nostalgia of home, and to this day cannot see gold without thinking of them and what it takes to produce it.

Under apartheid the men were away from home for 11 months to work in the mines, and whereas some established a stable relationship in South Africa, sexual expression was often limited to occasional commercial sex. From the perspective of sexually transmitted agents, many sex partners (the miners) for few women (the sex workers) is ideal and gives rise to explosive epidemics, as we saw then for chancroid. (This perverse organization of labor in the mining industry in South Africa undoubtedly paved the way of what became the world's most severe AIDS epidemic 10 years later, with some of the world's highest HIV prevalence rates occurring in sex workers around Carletonville, of whom 78 percent were HIV-positive in 2001.) In spite of the huge STD problem, the apartheid government of the time did not support STD prevention programs, not even condom distribution.

Within five weeks we studied enough patients in the clinical trial to demonstrate that the antibiotic indeed worked remarkably well, as compared to the then recommended treatment of erythromycin. (Despite its success the new antibiotic was never marketed.) Because the study concluded much faster than anticipated and we were very economical on our expenses, I made enough money to seed our Nairobi project. Meanwhile, Allan, in Canada, had put together enough money to start working, so I joined him in Nairobi at the end of 1980.

Nairobi was a lively city, full of small and bigger business, an infrastructure to host both business clientele and tourists. The people were mostly much better off than those in Zaire. But what struck me most of all were the huge slum areas, particularly the Kibera and Mathari Valley shanty towns, the largest slums on the continent outside South Africa—one mass of undulating corrugated roofs where everyone lived on top of each other, in garbage and sewage, while the Kenyan élite and expatriates flourished in spacious villas in the hills. Conditions in Kibera were far worse, in those days, than anything I saw in Zaire.

We worked very closely with the chairman of the university's Department of Medical Microbiology, a refugee from Rwanda and Uganda named Herbert Nsanze, a handsome sophisticated man who was very personable and very smart. We occupied a little office at the medical school at Kenyatta National Hospital, with a clunky Commodore computer that we used for statistical analysis. There was no phone. It was a smart group of people, and we became a very well integrated little project—not so little, after a while. Several years later we were joined by King Holmes's group at the University of Washington, and Marleen Temmerman's team at the University of Ghent, and the project grew to become one of the most productive and long-standing research collaborations in Africa, forging a very large number of groundbreaking studies.

Allan arranged for us to work in the municipal STD clinic, popularly known as Casino Clinic, because it was next door to the Casino Cinema on River Road. This was a very lively but also quite rough area, kind of a skid row, as described in "Going Down River Road" by Meja Mwangi, one of Kenya's most popular writers. There were countless bars that had tiny rooms where the prostitutes and bar girls went with their clients. They were dirty, really depressing places visited by mostly poor people. I've seen so many rooms like these, in Bombay and Bangkok and Kathmandu, and I still honestly don't know how anyone can have sex in a place like that. The smell alone would make me impotent, besides other considerations of love and disease.

Unlike in Kinshasa, there was hardly any music in this kind of bar, just a lot of straightforward drinking. When the alcohol level was high enough the clients headed upstairs with the women who worked there. And then the next day, or next week, quite a few of the men and women queued up at the Casino Clinic. Literally every morning hundreds of people were waiting when the doors opened at 7 A.M.

It was worst for the women. Dr. Da Costa, who was a Kenyan-born Indian Catholic, railed against them—"You whore, you slut"—and told them they only got what they deserved. As a doctor he was actually pretty competent, which was fortunate, because he was the only doctor in the Casino Clinic and it was basically the only sexually transmitted disease clinic in the city, as well as being at the time the largest STD clinic in Africa. As an empathetic doctor, however, he was a nightmare. I remember the young women crying at his pronouncements that now they would never be able to have children, which is indeed one of the major complications from untreated gonorrhea and chlamydial infection. I noted, too, that many of them were probably not involved in commercial sex; many were actually the regular partners and wives of male clients. Whereas I admired him because basically no other physician wanted to do this unglamorous and stressful job, I had to wonder why he was working there, since he hated his clients so deeply.

I tried to find out where these women came from. Most of them appeared to be Kenyan, but in other neighborhoods, such as the Pumwani district, there were concentrations of young women from Muhaya villages in the Akagera region near Lake Victoria in Tanzania. Their situation was a little like that of the gold miners in Carletonville. They traditionally came to Nairobi for a year or two, accumulated some capital, went back home, got married, and started a business. Just about everyone in their villages knew pretty much what they did to earn a living, but they pretended they didn't know and that made everything all right.

I spent about a month in Nairobi, to get things going. To staff the project on a permanent basis, I recruited Lieve Fransen, whom I knew from medical school in Ghent; she had worked in Mozambique for the first government after Independence and was tough as nails. She later became the director of the European Union's AIDS Task Force and is now a director at the European Commission Communication department. Allan had sent in a Canadian fellow, Frank Plummer, who was the real pioneer of the project (with Allan as mentor and driving force). Frank, a tall teddy bear from the Canadian plains, was the eternal optimist, an entrepreneur with more new (and excellent) ideas than any of us could remember, and always ready to support our Kenyan colleagues. He is now director of the Canadian equivalent of the CDC. When Lieve Fransen returned to Belgium in 1984, she was succeeded by Marie Laga, who had worked for *Médecins Sans Frontières* in Burundi, an unflappable woman who had a gift for communicating with people and who became a leading figure in HIV prevention work in Africa. And then there was Elizabeth Ngugi, a tiny, but superenergetic Kenyan nurse and professor of community health, who brought a local public health perspective. She pushed us continuously to work more with communities of women and sex workers, looking beyond the medical and epidemiological issues we were trying to resolve, and also addressing the root causes of prostitution and assisting women in their struggle for a decent life free of coercion. (The project increasingly did so.) All this created the foundation of a long-term partnership between the universities of Nairobi, Manitoba, Washington, and later Ghent, and the Institute of Tropical Medicine, which over 30 years later is still active.

From the onset, we were committed to ensuring that the results of our research benefitted the people of Kenya. This was not so easy, as this kind of translation of science into policy and implementation involves many steps and many institutions (as I later learned the hard way as head of UNAIDS). Our main interlocutor was the Ministry of Health and, fortunately, over the years the Kenyan administration became more open and committed to our work. I wrote grant proposals for the European Union, which had just launched a new program to support research on health in developing countries. At the end of 1982 Herbert Nsanze and I were notified that what seemed like a massive grant was on its way to us—150,000 écus ($200,000, at today's exchange rate) to fund a study to determine the best way to treat chancroid and resistant gonorrhea in Africa. The penicillin-resistant gonococcus from Cote d'Ivoire that I had discovered in Antwerp was already marching across the continent, spreading far faster than in heterosexual communities in Europe or North America.

By this time I was going to Nairobi three or four times a year, whenever I managed to scrape together the budget. Gradually we began working on other pathologies. We were the first group in Africa to work on chlamydia, which turned out to be a lot less common in Nairobi than it was in New York or Brussels. (We wondered at first whether this was because of a very common eye infection, trachoma, which was also caused by a member of the chlamydia family; perhaps suffering that eye disease as a child provided protection against the genital infection. But following studies in two areas around Nairobi, that theory didn't hold.)

We also became very involved in sexually transmitted diseases during pregnancy—what they do to the pregnancy and, if it continues to term, to the newborn child. The previous medical literature talked about gonorrhea making African women infertile, but there hadn't been any proper research on these complications using modern clinical and microbiological techniques since the early 1960s. It seemed to me though that given the number of women that we were seeing at the Casino Clinic—and the kinds of complications that appeared to be common—the problems caused by STDs in pregnancy were probably much bigger than people thought.

So we went to Pumwani Maternity Hospital, the largest maternity hospital in East Africa. It was like a baby factory, with 25,000 births a year, in an atmosphere so filthy and neglected that I wondered how anybody merits to start life this way.

The contrast between the maternity hospital where my children were born (in the meantime blonde Sara was born in 1980) and the conditions these long-suffering Kenyan women had to give birth in were simply intolerable. The doctors at Pumwani were paid a pittance, and so they were often completely unavailable. They concentrated on their private practices and left the whole place to the nurses and midwives, strong women who worked with incredible dedication. And yet many of the health authorities of the country, who quite obviously knew about the situation, didn't act, usually mentioning budgetary problems whenever I brought it up. Of course they had a point—in those days a major part of the nation's health budget was absorbed by Kenyatta National Hospital, the university hospital on whose campus we had our office. But better management and incentives would have gone a long way to improve the situation at Pumwani Hospital.

At the university, the professors were smart and committed, maintaining high standards of medical education. But the sobering reality was also that medical services were deteriorating fast. Women routinely bled to death; the level of preventable neonatal deaths and infections was inexcusable; and the appalling conditions I saw in Pumwani really motivated me a lot to work on simple methods of at least preventing the worst kinds of postpartum infections.

Beginning in about 1900, it was established medical practice to administer silver nitrate eyedrops to all babies at birth to prevent them from acquiring gonococcal infection from the mother and possibly going blind. It was a triumph of public health in Europe. But Nairobi hospitals abandoned this practice after caustic concentrations of silver nitrate—a consequence of evaporation—caused severe eye damage. Damned if you do, damned if you don't.

So Marie Laga and her colleagues Pratibha Datta and Warren Namaara did a number of classic studies to look at new ways to prevent the transmission of gonococcal and chlamydial infection by using safer tetracycline ointment. At the same time, we began working on ways to treat babies who had already been infected. As it turned out, instead of the recommended penicillin treatment, which was longer term and required hospitalization, all it took was one shot of ceftriaxone, a fairly expensive cephalosporin. Follow up of the babies in the slums was a real challenge, because "regular" addresses often did not exist. Therefore mapping was essential, with information such as "Go to toilet number 7, then three streets to the left, and she lives on the first house on the right with a red roof." This work remains the basis for current international guidance for the prevention and treatment of neonatal conjunctivitis.

I thought perhaps this was my niche in science: figuring out the connections between sexually transmitted disease in pregnancy and complications in newborns, and then figuring out ways to solve those problems before they happened. It was the kind of work that made my heart lift: applying solid science to a complex problem in poor countries, and developing better ways to prevent and treat disease—in a sense, producing the goods that other clinicians use.

When we started the project we had no business plan, no specific goals, and hardly any money beyond one year of functioning. We were young, optimistic, and committed to solving the formidable problems of ill health Kenya was facing. The challenges were enormous, and none of us had firsthand experience in solving them—logistics, finances, publication rights, and day-to-day management.

Nowadays there are dozens of similar projects in Africa, but at the time we began, none focused on sexually transmitted diseases and on women's health. The few existing research programs were nearly all linked with the former colonial powers, whereas it was always important to us to strengthen the capabilities and infrastructure of our African partners. I am particularly proud of the large numbers of Africans, North Americans, and Europeans we trained in Nairobi. Many are now established clinicians, epidemiologists, and researchers in their own right.

Of the researchers whom I recruited for our Nairobi project, almost all were women. This was far from the traditional approach: men dominated research in Africa. But I knew it would make a difference, in terms of the degree of attention that they paid to the African women on whose behalf we were working. Many a time I examined a woman or talked about a case with a colleague and felt overwhelmed with anger. These infections were not just painful, they caused a great deal of permanent damage. Infertility is a drama for women anywhere in the world, but in Africa it can destroy you—your marriage, your value in society, your self-worth. I wanted to dispel the unspoken and cruel assumption that if African women had a fertility problem perhaps that was not a terrible thing.

IN MANY WAYS I loved living in Belgium. I felt the country was changing for the better—becoming more international, particularly thanks to Brussels' being the headquarters of the European

Community, NATO, and a growing number of corporations, with a thriving economy and growing skills in biotechnology and microchips. I loved the food, the artistic life, and the social culture, centered on neighborhood cafés. But there was a strange atmosphere in the country in the early 1980s. There were a number of scandals involving kickbacks to individuals and to political parties, and ultra-right-wing activism by secret groups. A gang of killers went around the country, shooting up stores and supermarkets. A parliamentary commission investigated these crimes, but they were never solved. The extremist Vlaams Blok party emerged; it was mixed up with Flemish nationalism, and xenophobia, and campaigning for the independence of Flanders.

One evening a week I volunteered at a free youth clinic in a battered old terraced house near the Antwerp central station, which mostly involved prescribing contraceptives. Many doctors in those days wouldn't prescribe the pill to unmarried girls and women, let alone help women find abortions if that was what they desperately wanted. I also saw many drug users, an extraordinarily difficult group to work with as a doctor and emotionally charged for me—I had lost a friend from medical school to an overdose. He was one of our most brilliant students, and I never came to grips with his addiction and death, which occurred when I was in Zaire during the Ebola outbreak.

Often when I left for Africa I felt I could be more useful: I could make a difference. I welcomed the sheer physical space; Belgium is one of the most densely populated countries in the world. There was also the joy that I perceived in so many African cultures. People were poor, but in their poverty they were creative and energetic. In Belgium, by contrast, people complained so much, from the weather to their aches and pains to the state of hospitals and schools, and this seemed to me a gigantic waste of time and energy: Belgium has some of the best education and health care in the world. As our Nairobi research program grew, I began to travel much more widely around Central and West Africa. I went several times to Burundi, where the Institute of Tropical Medicine had a program to train doctors who had received substandard medical education in the former Soviet Union. I also helped out with one of Pattyn's research projects, monitoring some of his research on the treatment of leprosy, in Burundi and Senegal.

There was something of a revolution underway in leprosy treatment. Up to then, one form of leprosy ("paucibacillary" or "tuberculoid") was fairly easily treatable, although the treatment was long. But in lepromatous leprosy—where leprosy bacilli appear all over the body—the patient's immune system was so damaged there was no real treatment. Pattyn's group helped show that if you used several drugs in combination, you could actually cure the disease. It was the basis of the near-elimination of leprosy today. The work brought me full circle, to Father Damien, my childhood local "saint," who tried to care for and treat lepers in Hawaii. While I was still searching my way through the fascinating worlds of academia, research, clinical care, and international development, I was accumulating highly diverse experience and getting ready for the next chapter.

◆ PART THREE ◆

CHAPTER 10

A New Epidemic

MEANWHILE, IN ANTWERP, I became the go-to doctor for people arriving from Africa with embarrassing tropical infections and gay men seeking discreet medical advice. Some of the time, men and women who consult a doctor regarding matters below the belt are actually expressing psychological difficulties—pain in relationships. So many of the patients I saw at my clinic in Antwerp were actually the worried well. But the gay men that I saw displayed a truly baroque variety of illnesses, and there appeared to be a real explosion in the homosexual community of syphilis and hepatitis B. If some kind of epidemic wave was underway, we definitely needed to do something about it; but first, it needed to be documented. So, just as I did in Nairobi, I took a few of my students and went out to do a survey at what was clearly the local ground zero: Antwerp's gay bars.

There were a lot of them. I had gathered, from conversations with gay friends and patients, that the homosexual community in Antwerp—like everywhere else in Europe—was pretty hypersexed. But I wasn't prepared for what that really meant. I remember the first leather bar we went to, where I faced the startling sight of a man with leather chaps strapped across his bare bottom. And I was particularly surprised by the anonymity of the sex.

In Belgium, the early 1980s were a time when gay men at last felt they could burst into the open. (It wasn't like Belgium today, when a man easily mentions that he went somewhere with his husband, now that same-sex marriage is legally and socially accepted.) There was still quite a lot of discrimination; it was difficult, for example, to be an openly gay schoolteacher. But Antwerp was then funkier than Brussels, more connected to havens of tolerance like Amsterdam, and far more relaxed about homosexuality than the rest of the country. It had a lively fashion and art scene, a port and a sense of openness to the world, which may have explained the kind of sexual acting-out that I was seeing.

We took blood in the bars, and estimated the prevalence of various STDs. Seven percent had syphilis, and 34 percent had had hepatitis B, figures that were indeed far higher than for other populations in Belgium. We organized a vaccination campaign for hepatitis B, with flyers and feedback sessions in the gay community. And of course this brought more gay patients to our clinic; indeed, that was the intention: to seek people out and treat them. They received state-of-the-art treatment and advice. I've also always, instinctively, felt it's important to touch patients—take a hand, hold a shoulder—to help establish a real connection. My first experience, long ago, was with a leprosy patient, when I first began working with Pattyn. It was a Belgian priest, and he recoiled and said, "No—don't touch me." He was convinced I would catch his disease, and when I told him I really would not catch it, he almost broke down. But I was never frightened of touching. I wouldn't obviously go with bare hands somewhere where there's blood, or into someone's mouth, but touching the skin? There's always soap.

IT HAD BEEN almost five years since Ebola, and I was still fascinated by the sudden epidemic, not the chronic problems of medicine, but the rush of adrenaline that comes with a mystery outbreak. Anyway, it meant that I paged through every issue of the CDC's *Morbid-*

ity and Mortality Weekly Report ("*MMWR*" for the initiated), which would report on outbreaks in the United States and often also in other countries. And on June 5, 1981, the *MMWR* ran an item on five young, white gay men in Los Angeles who'd contracted *Pneumocystis carinii* pneumonia, which up to then almost exclusively appeared in severely immunosuppressed patients and rarely so since being identified in orphanages in Europe after World War II. All five men also had aggressive infection with cytomegalovirus. Soon after that first publication, cases were reported from other parts of the United States, with some men having aggressive Kaposi's sarcoma, a rare skin disease usually seen in Central Africa, and occasionally in older white men of Mediterranean and Jewish descent.

Because this seemed to be a new syndrome—and it was occurring in gay men—I read the item with more attention than usual. It rang a little bell, though not necessarily the correct bell. This was something new, something exciting and also intellectually interesting—a mystery. Gay men. Symptoms of unknown origin. I didn't immediately think of Africa, or about the Greek fisherman whose body I helped autopsy in 1978, but I wondered whether this was also happening in our gay community in Antwerp, in particular after the subsequent reports of what still did not have a name.

Then in October 1981 I went to Chicago to attend the annual meeting of ICAAC (the Interscience Conference on Antibiotics and Antimicrobial Chemotherapy) and the Infectious Disease Society of America, of which I was a member. There were a number of talks there about this new "gay syndrome" (a syndrome is a group of symptoms and signs that collectively are characteristic of one or more diseases). The hallmarks were Kaposi's sarcoma and *Pneumocystis carinii* pneumonia, so again, I didn't make any links with African patients we started to see in Antwerp. But when I returned from Chicago, I talked about it over a beer with my friend Henri Taelman, who was the head clinician at the Institute of Tropical Medicine.

Henri was a Francophone from Brussels, not much older than I, but he had vast clinical experience in Africa, and his work was his life: he lived and breathed for clinical medicine to a degree that I could only marvel at. It was almost difficult to talk to him about anything else, though he had a great sense of humor. He was meticulous man, with great integrity and a powerful dedication to his patients. (He died far too young in Rwanda in 1999, where he had returned after the genocide to help rebuild the university hospital in Kigali.) He often called me in to talk over a patient's case—take a look at the samples and the context, puzzle it out. Now it was time for me to call him in to help.

Henri and I began going through the hospital files, trying to check whether there was anything new—any kind of syndrome we missed earlier.

This was where the Greek fisherman's case suddenly became obvious: an inexplicable death, his body eaten away by an unusual infection, obvious signs of a powerfully degraded immune system.

Slowly, one after another, other patients started walking in to the institute, nearly all of them with an African connection. They had chronic diarrhea, with startling weight loss, and infections that were unusual, highly aggressive, and suggestive of an extraordinary and mysterious immune collapse: cryptococcal meningitis, for example, or central-nervous-system toxoplasmosis, and dramatic herpes zoster infections. Our team was accustomed to all kinds of tropical complications—from malaria, sleeping sickness, sickle-cell anemia—and we knew that these were not the symptoms of any ordinary tropical disease. By the end of 1982 we had perhaps a dozen of these patients, and in those days that was a lot, because every single case of this so-called Gay-Related Immune Deficiency was worthy of publication in a medical journal and was reported to WHO.

Although there were pieces of the puzzle that seemed to fit, what we were seeing was a spectrum of opportunistic infections that were quite different from the *Pneumocystis carinii* pneumonia and Kaposi's sarcoma being described among gay men, and from 1982 also in people with hemophilia and some Haitian heterosexuals. None of our patients said they had had homosexual contact. And we also had a few women; in fact, women were almost half our caseload.

They were African women, the wives of wealthy men or high-ranking government or military officials. They came from Central Africa—mostly Zaire, but in a couple of cases Rwanda and Burundi—

and they were desperate, very thin, very worried, very sick, with a peculiar, glassy look in their eyes that seemed familiar. I realized only much later that it was the same look that I had seen in the eyes of Ebola patients. Their medical situation deteriorated with spectacular speed. We had no idea how to treat them.

The pace of arrivals picked up. Henri and I began phoning each other—"We admitted another one"—another well-off African, or occasionally Belgian, from Central Africa, basically on the verge of death, hoping to receive better medical care with us than they would at home. Henri and I talked with them, over and over, trying to work out the epidemiological picture, because we thought there *had* to be a gay connection. It wasn't easy, because most African cultures are pretty homophobic and even the simple suggestion could be perceived as a mortal insult.

I remember one Zairean high-ranking military official who arrived in 1982: about fifty years old, formerly obese, his clothes simply hanging off his body. I recognized the cockiness, the brutality, the sense of entitlement and power of a real Zairean boss-man, and I knew I had to have a conversation with him that wasn't going to be easy. Having spent quite a lot more time than I ever really wanted to with those helicopter pilots in Yambuku, I had a decent grasp on how to talk to a Zairean military official about sex. I just didn't know how to ask about gay sex.

"So," I began, "a man like yourself could be a real *sportif*"—a sexual athlete, the innuendo was clear.

Of course he was; Commander X was very proud of his sexual prowess and the many, many notches in his belt. He laughed with barely a trace of embarrassment and said, "Naturally I'm a real man. A real man needs women, many women."

"Wow, you're a real man," I said. "Yeah, and maybe, you know, you're a great athlete, so maybe, in between women, also a man from time to time?"

"What!" bellowed the general. "Never! How can you even think that? How filthy! How deranged!"—and his voice rang with sincerity and spontaneity.

Again and again I had this conversation with African male patients.

Sometimes they were totally upfront about their large number of female partners; sometimes they were a little embarrassed, as if they anticipated a white person's judgmental attitude to something that might be perceived as African animality. (I never looked at it that way as I knew European men and women with as many partners, but they couldn't know that.) Sometimes they simply led a fairly monogamous life. But although some admitted to having sex with dozens or even hundreds of women, they were adamant: every one of them affirmed loud and clear that they did not have sex with men. This was impossible to verify, but I tried to detect whether they had ever been on the receiving end of anal sex by looking for traces of rectal infections like herpes. There just weren't any.

I wasn't completely naïve about this. I had a friend, Willy, who was gay, and who had worked in Abidjan, Côte d'Ivoire, in the early 1980s for a management consulting firm in West Africa. He had sex with plenty of local men. Practically every time he was back in Antwerp he came to me with some florid new genital infection that he'd picked up. I asked him if he was paying for all this sex, and he said no—he claimed that his sex partners were African men, and they were having sex with another man out of choice rather than financial gain. So I did know that there was this kind of underground gay scene in some African cities, at least in West Africa. But my patients truly seemed completely unrelated to it. It was a mystery.

Meanwhile Nathan Clumeck, a young ambitious physician from St. Pierre Hospital in Brussels, who spent some time in San Francisco, was also seeing patients from Central Africa with the same mystery syndrome. We had several dozen cases between us. In May, a French team of researchers headed by Luc Montagnier reported that they had isolated a new retrovirus that was related to the syndrome. By this time about 600 cases were reported in the United States— in homosexual men, Haitians, intravenous drug users, recipients of blood transfusions, and people with hemophilia. Because of the latter three categories, a probable mode of transmission via syringes or exchange of blood became evident. The homosexual connection posited a possible sexual transmission; the Haitian link was much more enigmatic. After a few unfortunate and inaccurate names such as GRID (Gay-Related Acquired Immune Disorder) and 4H disease (for homosexuals, heroin users, hemophiliacs, and Haitians), it was agreed at a meeting in July 1982 to use Acquired Immunodeficiency Syndrome, in brief, AIDS, which from an acronym became a word.

None of our patients in Antwerp were intravenous drug users or Haitians. We also had no patients with hemophilia: Belgium's supply of the blood product Factor 8, which hemophiliacs required to keep from bleeding to death, was still secure from the infection, as only domestic blood products were used and in a more conservative way than was then the practice elsewhere. But we did have what looked like AIDS patients. Together with Nathan Clumeck and a few other people, Henri and I founded an informal group where physicians who were seeing these patients could come together and share advice.

Then Jan Desmyter, a professor of virology at the Catholic University of Leuven created a National AIDS Commission. Actually, in typical Belgian style, three groups were formed: a Flemish one; a francophone one; and a federal, "Belgian" one. (I attended meetings of the Flemish and Belgian groups.) The rationale was that funding for certain topics—such as patient care—came from the federal government, while prevention campaigns were paid by the regions.

With most of our patients coming to us from Central Africa, I felt it was urgent to go there and take a look at the situation on the ground. If we were seeing 100 people from Central Africa coming to Belgium with this new illness, there might be thousands who couldn't afford the flight or obtain a visa. Nobody had done that—nobody had checked out what was happening in Zaire. Of course there were doctors in Central Africa, but except for a few surgeons reporting an increase in aggressive Kaposi's sarcoma in Zambia and Uganda, there were no reports from Zaire, Rwanda, or Burundi, the countries of residence of most of our patients in Belgium.

The problem was money. Nobody in Belgium was interested in funding research on this disease. The European Commission's grant for the Nairobi project was earmarked; I couldn't just use it to investigate AIDS in Zaire instead.

In August 1983, I went back to Seattle, to attend a conference of the International Society for STD Research. I spoke with Dr. James

Curran, the head of the CDC's AIDS Task Force. I said we urgently needed to take a look at what was going on in Africa and I asked him for money. He's a great scientist and a good man, whom I admire greatly, but he was simply too busy dealing with the epidemic in the United States, and even more so it seemed with fire-fighting the non-stop political crises that it was causing in the Reagan years. So, Jim simply had no time to follow up on our conversation. (Later he became the strongest possible supporter of our work on AIDS in Africa.)

Then in September I went to the International Conference for Infectious Disease in Vienna. By this time we had firmly identified 40 patients with the new syndrome in Belgium, 37 of them from Central Africa. I spoke with Tom Quinn whom I had met in Seattle where we both worked with King Holmes, now an infectious disease special-ist at the National Institutes of Health (NIH) in Washington and at Johns Hopkins University. We had also been in touch since then about chlamydial infections. He had recently completed a short visit to Haiti to take a look at the AIDS situation there. Tom took me over to see Jack Whitescarver and Richard Krause, who was then the director of the National Institute of Allergy and Infectious Disease, which was the leading US agency for basic AIDS research.

Right there in Krause's hotel room, I made my case. And right there, he said, "OK, I'll give you a hundred thousand dollars. You can go to Kinshasa, we'll make it happen. But there'll be just one trip. And we will be doing it together."

Tom Quinn and I set a date in October to go to Zaire. We agreed to meet in Antwerp first, to lay out our plans. He was going to bring at least one colleague from NIH, and I asked Henri Taelman to come along, so we needed to get everyone on the same page. Also, in the back of my mind I was thinking, This time, I'm going to be the team leader—because right or wrong, I felt that with Ebola our lab had been the first one to come up with the problem and isolate the virus, but the CDC had taken over the whole operation as they had the money and the experience. Tom was fine with that; he had a lot of extremely useful experience with parasites and STDs in gay men, but he had never been to Africa.

But Tom worked at the NIH. And within the American health

bureaucracy, there was something of a turf war on AIDS between the NIH, in Washington, and the CDC, in Atlanta. When the CDC got wind of our planned Kinshasa trip, they decided to send their *own* investigator to Zaire. Luckily it was Joe McCormick, the man who had investigated Ebola in Sudan, and he phoned me to talk it over. I saw that I had fallen into an institutional rivalry that could become very toxic, and I suggested we should all go together. Luckily the US Secretary for Health and Human Services had also recently ordered the CDC and NIH to collaborate more: this definitely helped.

We all met in Antwerp a few days before our planned departure for Zaire. Despite the almost palpable presence of clashing agendas, this meeting went fairly smoothly except for the heavy-handed intervention of the director of the Institute of Tropical Medicine, who declared solemnly that "we Belgians" knew the Congo—we knew "these people." Therefore I, Peter, should be team leader. I was hugely embarrassed by this, but although my US colleagues looked at my director with disapproval they indeed proposed that I should be the team leader. The NIH might not have accepted someone from the CDC and vice versa. I was an outsider; they could use me to bridge a difficult mix.

In the Sabena DC-10 on our way to Kinshasa on October 18, we sat together, and agreed on an action plan, even on what we would do with the specimens we collected, and who would figure on the publications coming out of the studies. I had just bought a small Brother typewriter with a small memory and printer, and we all signed a detailed agreement without any dispute.

WHEN WE LANDED at Ndjili airport, I could not help but think of my first visit, exactly six years earlier to investigate the Ebola outbreak. This time I was much better prepared, had much more confidence in myself, and also felt I was coming back into familiar territory. But the excitement of discovery in the air was equally there. There was the usual mob scene at Kinshasa airport. I shepherded everyone to the Fométro, where I had stayed in 1976; Jean-François Ruppol arranged our stay, as always helping as much as he could by also providing precious transport for the duration. We didn't actually have any kind of official government permission to do research on AIDS in Zaire, and without it we could be thrown out of the country; I was hoping that he would help us with that, too. The first evening, we had dinner in an Italian restaurant, Chez Nicolas, across the street from the Fométro office, to discuss the situation and to draft the questionnaire we would use to ask people about possible risk factors and their sexual practices.

Ruppol, Taelman, and McCormick were all old hands in Africa, but none of them was really at ease with publicly discussing sexual issues; they went red with embarrassment, especially when the conversation devolved into a discussion about the rumor that a famous American actor had been hospitalized for putting a hamster in his anus. Tom Quinn has a very loud voice, and at one point I looked up and realized that the entire restaurant had fallen silent. Everyone was glued to every detail of our conversation. So within about 48 hours the entire expatriate community in Kinshasa knew that a research team had come to Zaire to look at a weird sex disease.

Actually, it was thanks to Joe that we finally received the government permissions we needed to start working; his friend Dr. Kalisa Ruti was the chief of staff at the Ministry of Health. We went first to Mama Yemo Hospital, the largest hospital in Zaire. Dr. Bila Kapita, a skinny cardiologist who was head of Internal Medicine, gave us a tour of the vast and filthy compound.

When I was at Mama Yemo in 1976, when we were checking for Ebola patients, it seemed squalid enough. But by 1983 the conditions had grown far worse. Some of the buildings had literally collapsed, there was garbage rotting all over the courtyard—this was a *hospital!*—and when we walked into the wards, there were patients absolutely everywhere, two to every metal bed, with more on thin, soiled mattresses lined up along the floor.

Kapita was a small and austere man with a heart of gold, always a discreet smile, raised by Swedish missionaries in Bas-Congo province, clearly highly competent and dedicated to the people in his care, and investing in the development of the village he came from. A rock of integrity. Later I spent some time with him in his remote village, where his home was the only house of bricks and where he was investing most of his earnings, besides ensuring a solid education for his children. He had gone to the trouble of putting together a pile of files for us, representing patients he had seen and who he now thought might have had AIDS. This was October 1983, and he said he had been seeing such patients for a few years. But nobody had ever put it together and done something about it.

It was a really tall pile of paper. We agreed to take a look at it later, and then Joe, Tom, Henri, and I began to examine some of the patients. They were mostly twenty-five- to thirty-five-year-olds, with enormous weight loss, intractable diarrhea, and that ghastly, glassy-eyed look. Many of them had dramatic itching, with skin symptoms that had not been described in the literature. They had a lot of sores in their mouths—yeast infections and very ugly herpes sores—and eye infections. A few had Kaposi's sarcoma markings, especially on their legs, and many were breathing very superficially; perhaps the respiratory distress stemmed from tuberculosis. There was also quite a bit of cryptococcal meningitis, which we knew was a marker of AIDS. Kapita told us that their symptoms were remarkably aggressive: they progressed with startling speed and seemed not to respond to treatment.

We all were silent and staring at each other. Then Kapita opened the door into the women's pavilion and we took a look at another huge ward that was overflowing, quite clearly, with exactly the same thing. That morning we saw 50 or more cases of what we thought to be AIDS, though we still needed laboratory confirmation to be sure of our clinical impressions. And in 1983 that was a lot, because fewer than 2000 cases had been reported worldwide, and a lot of those people were already dead.

When we got out of there, I took a deep breath, as I was nearly breathless. I remember it well—a physical sensation that was so strong, I wrote it down. It wasn't the happy, tingling energy of scientific discovery. There was curiosity, of course, and an urge to find some kind of solution, but also the overwhelming feeling that we were facing a truly momentous catastrophe. And I suddenly realized that this epidemic would take over my life. It was my aha moment.

I recalled the nightmare that had haunted us in 1976: that Ebola would hit Kinshasa. Now I was back, and this new epidemic *had* hit Kinshasa. And given everything I knew, or thought I knew, this was going to be a lot more fatal than Ebola. AIDS was largely invisible, and I knew that meant it might be uncontrollable. Ebola was just the overture. This time, I knew, we were looking at the worst epidemic I could imagine, the greatest assailant I would ever face, something that would absorb all the energy that I could throw at it, and far more.

In my mother tongue, Dutch I wrote in my notebook: "Incredible. A catastrophe for Africa. This is what I want to work on. It will change everything."

CHAPTER 11

Projet SIDA

S O THAT WAS it: a second trip to Zaire that changed my life. The Ebola epidemic had transformed me when I was in my twenties; and now, seven years later, with this trip to Mama Yemo Hospital in Kinshasa, I was transformed again.

I sat on the bed in the room we were sharing at the Fométro that night and wrote down the thoughts that came to me as I faced the prospect of devoting a huge portion of my professional life to pursuing another lethal epidemic in Central Africa:

PROS:
INTERESTING AND NEW

- *Huge problem*
- *Making a difference for people*
- *Prestigious*
- *Exciting research*
- *Lot of publications and possibility of developing a long-standing program in Zaire*

CONS:

- *Several trips a year to Zaire, in addition to Nairobi*
- *A lot of administrative fights in Zaire, Belgium, with the Americans*
- *Mediating permanent conflicts*
- *Constant reports to the NIH*

I tried to dissect things down to bullet points, to very simple questions. But these are often not that useful in decision making, as was the case here. I didn't need the list; I already knew the answer in my gut. It was one of those very rare moments in life when you can almost physically feel the trajectory of your life shift. I had met something unknown, enormously powerful, that I, with my experience in Africa, and as a microbiologist, was in many ways equipped to hunt down. I knew I was going to pursue this thing as far as I could.

Still, the list that I came up with was clear. This was going to be a passionately exciting adventure—an opportunity to influence the course of history—but it would also mess up my professional and personal life with way too much travel and create enormous political and bureaucratic tangles.

Indeed, the next page in my notebook contains observations about a meeting we had the next day at the University of Kinshasa with Professor Jean-Jacques Muyembe, now the dean of the medical school. He was a good man and a very able scientist, but the university was in dire straits professionally and financially, dependent on rapacious officials in the Ministries of Health and of Higher Education. I knew him from Ebola days, as he had led the first team that went to Yambuku before the internationals arrived. He asked us for subsidies, scholarships, a budget to help set up a group on AIDS work, reagents, and also a commitment to produce *two* publications, so that the staff from the University of Kinshasa would also get scientific recognition. So the complications of working in a country struggling with poverty and failed governance came up right away. This meeting also exacerbated my own feelings of impotence: I knew that Muyembe's requests for help were all legitimate and yet I was unable to do much to assist him.

We needed to start collecting and examining blood samples. We set up a small lab at the Cliniques Universitaires with Sheila Mitchell from the CDC doing cell counts by hand. There was still no accepted laboratory test for the cause of AIDS. A team headed by Professor Luc Montagnier of the Pasteur Institute in Paris had identified the virus causing AIDS—he called it lymphadenopathy associated virus (LAV)—from a gay man who had traveled in the United States. But there was still no serological test for "LAV" available, and there was dispute about whether it was the cause of AIDS: Robert Gallo from the US National Institutes of Health claimed to have independently discovered the virus causing AIDS, calling it HTLV3. (Later it became clear that his virus was the same as Montagnier's.) Still other people theorized that the cause of AIDS was not a virus but some combination of various toxins.

Thus, initially the best marker for the virus was the ratio of T lymphocyte "suppressor" cells and "killer" cells, and all of them had to be counted manually. A little later an energetic young French researcher, David Klatzmann, showed that the human immunodeficiency virus, as the cause of AIDS would be called, selectively killed T lymphocytes with CD4 receptors, which are like the traffic cops of the immune system. Following Klatzmann's discovery, we no longer had to measure T helpers, just CD4s. And later still, we had the antibody test. But in 1983 it was still all far more complex and indirect.

We stayed in Kinshasa for five weeks, taking samples and working out a clinical case definition, because we knew that people would tell us, "This thing you've found in Africa—it's not AIDS, it's immune deficiency, maybe it's something to do with malnutrition or parasitic infections." We were working in an area of obvious diagnostic uncertainty, and we wanted our data to be unchallengeable, rock solid so that what we called a case of AIDS was, beyond dispute, a case of AIDS.

By November 2 we had about a hundred cases from Mama Yemo Hospital and the University Hospital that we felt were probably AIDS, but we were certain about 38 of them: 20 males and 18 females. Ten of them died during the study period, and 8 more died before the end of 1983, giving a 47 percent fatality rate within three months. They had striking clinical features: profound weight loss, with punishing, intractable diarrhea of unknown origin that seemed completely resistant to treatment: you don't often see that kind of diarrhea in adults. They were also plagued by persistent fever; headache; cough; difficulty in swallowing; oral thrush; swollen lymph nodes; dramatic itching with goosebump-type skin lesions; cryptococcal meningitis; herpes; oral candidiasis; and bilateral pneumonia. Sixteen percent had disseminated Kaposi's sarcoma. Twenty-five percent showed past or present syphilis. Men reported a lifetime average of seven sex partners, while the women (who were younger than the men, and almost all divorced) averaged three. The chronology suggested female-to-male transmission as well as male to female, and though this wasn't hard evidence, it was the first suggestion of female-to-male transmission. We could find no suggestion of homosexuality of drug use.

We also did a rapid overview of the hospital records, using cryptococcal meningitis as a marker, as the ubiquitous and normally innocuous fungus *Cryptococcus neoformans* only causes severe infections such as meningitis in people with severe immunodeficiency. And we found a few cases dating back to 1975, though it was impossible to confirm that they were AIDS. There was about one case per year until 1979 in each of the hospitals—University Hospital, about 40 minutes' drive from downtown, the Clinique Ngaliema, the Clinique Kinoise, and Kitambo Hospital, as well as the massive Mama Yemo, which was the only one that offered free medical care. But since 1980 each hospital showed more than 30 cases per year, which suggested the real boom in AIDS infections in Kinshasa might be roughly simultaneous with the one that appeared to be underway in the United States.

One day I did a very stupid thing: something I had warned I don't know how many hundreds of students never to do. I *recapped* the syringe that I had used to draw blood. I tried to put the plastic cap back on the needle before throwing it away. Such a pointless gesture. (It must be something to do with the Flemish obsession for neatness.) And I missed. I stuck the needle into my finger. I watched the blood pool up from the tiny puncture wound and hastily pressed it as hard as I could, hoping to squeeze out every drop of blood. There was nothing else I could do except disinfect it and move on. There was every reason to suppose the man whose blood I had just drawn had

AIDS: he was in a terrible state. But there was no way then to know whether he was infected or I had been infected.

On my way home I flew to Johannesburg to speak at an Infectious Disease conference at the University of Witwatersrand. I could talk of nothing but AIDS and the epidemic we had just seen in Kinshasa. There was just one AIDS case in South Africa back then: a gay white man who had probably become infected while traveling in the United States. These were well-trained physicians I was talking to, eager to learn about AIDS, fascinated by what I was telling them about the outbreak in Zaire. But no, they kept telling me, no: they were certain, there was absolutely no unusual immune deficiency in South Africa at all. (Today we know that they were correct. Although later South Africa was swamped by the world's biggest AIDS epidemic, in 1983 the virus had not yet hit the country.)

When I got back to Belgium I spoke to Tom Quinn, who had left Kinshasa earlier, to attend a World Health Organization meeting in Copenhagen. He said the whole conference was about AIDS in Europe and North America. Africa didn't figure at all in the picture, and there was no discussion of AIDS among heterosexuals who didn't use drugs.

Early 1984 I sent the blood sera we had gathered to Montagnier and Françoise Brun-Vézinet in Paris, so that they could take a look at the antibodies, checking them against the so-called LAV virus that they had identified. Even though Tom and Joe were American, there was no dispute about sending our samples to Paris when I suggested it following a brief encounter with Montagnier at an EC meeting on my return to Europe.

One of the blood samples we sent to Montagnier's team was from the man whose blood briefly mixed with mine when I made the stupid error with the needle-stick. And I also sent them my blood. I was really scared.

I sent the sera under code, and I was the only one who had the code. Montagnier's lab had no way of knowing which samples were from suspected AIDS patients and which ones were healthy controls, so in some sense this was just as much a test of the validity of his research as it was of ours. When he phoned me with the results, in February 1984, he seemed as nervous as I was. He went down the list—*sample number 2, positive; sample number 3, negative*—and I checked them against the code. Oh my God! That was it! He had a test! Montagnier's positives included just about all the people with clearly manifested clinical signs of AIDS: 97 percent. And although some of the people who had no symptoms were also positive, that result was not necessarily false: they might be asymptomatic carriers of the virus.

It was a very important and thrilling moment. And to me, equally thrilling was that my blood came out negative. The man whose blood briefly mingled with mine was antibody positive but I was clear. The relief was almost too much to take. It was a real life lesson for me and, ever since, I make sure that every HIV test performed by any team of mine involves the least possible waiting time before the result is given to the patient. This is not a routine procedure where you can tell people, "Come back in two weeks." The anxiety is simply unbearable.

Coincidentally, it was about this time that I read *Shadow on the Land*, a great book by Thomas Parran, a US surgeon general in the 1930s. He brought syphilis out of the closet; back then you couldn't even say the word "syphilis" in polite conversation, not to mention discuss its transmission. He estimated that well over 1 percent of the US population was infected, and it was Parran's drive for public awareness about syphilis, just as much as the discovery that penicillin could cure it, that drove the shadow from the land. (By the end of World War II, the US Public Health Service estimated that 1 in 10 Americans would acquire syphilis in their life time.) The book was an eye-opener for me. I had no clue that the Western world had so recently had such a huge syphilis problem, and I had never really thought deeply about the nature of bigotry about the disease, and the lethal effects such denial could have. (In 1998 I was awarded the Thomas Parran Award by the American Sexually Transmitted Diseases Association; this moved me greatly.)

Some people in Europe often clearly looked on AIDS as God's way of saying you shouldn't be a homosexual. The discrimination against AIDS patients was horrible. To me it recalled my childhood afternoons at the Father Damien museum, mulling over the hideous and medically unjustifiable stigma against leprosy.

I went on a live TV show with a colleague general practitioner from Antwerp, Dirk Avonts. We had painted a piece of broomstick in pink—it was pretty big, like a foot and a half tall, so it would show clearly on camera—and without giving any advance warning to the TV crew, Dirk showed how to put a condom on. That created quite a scandal and a flurry of letters to newspapers: how could we be permitted to broadcast such obscenity? My point was we needed to take this kind of shame out of the equation.

It wasn't until July 1984 that our paper with the Kinshasa results appeared in *The Lancet*. Initially it was rejected as being "of local interest only." (For another, later paper I submitted to the *New England Journal of Medicine*, an early referee wrote as sole comment: "it is a well-known fact that AIDS cannot be transmitted from women to men.") People had already developed the mindset that this was "just" a *gay* disease. I never understood why a virus would care about the sexual preference of its human host, because I applied what Stanley Falkow had told me when I was working in his labs: put yourself inside the pathogen. From the perspective of a virus, what is sex between human beings but contact between mucosal surfaces? It may not sound very romantic, but that's the contact that makes the virus jump from one cell to another to perpetuate its own life. I don't think the virus cares whether the sex is good, or about the color or gender of the person who inhabits that mucosal surface. Granted, some types of intercourse may be more efficient than others but none was exclusive. So I was always puzzled by this dogmatic insistence on AIDS as a homosexual disease.

Meanwhile, I wrote up a $600,000 grant proposal for the NIH that was about 70 pages long, laying out a whole research plan for a three-year project to study what was happening in Zaire. We were all very excited about it. Six hundred thousand dollars—total—for a three-year program seems like so little today, but I was just an associate professor in those days, and I made $1000 a month at the exchange rate of the time. The major point was that our brief experience in Kinshasa already made clear that AIDS was, at least in certain conditions, a heterosexual problem. That meant that there was really an enormous potential for harm across the population as a whole.

We needed to clarify that, and look at risk factors in a very systematic, in-depth way. Also, we could already see there was probably at least some mother-to-child transmission, and this was completely new to us. A third point, perhaps more controversial, was the span of the problem we'd seen, which suggested that the disease could have been around in Central Africa for longer than in the West, even though it didn't look that way at first. Fourth, we needed to understand the course of the disease in Africa. Was it the same as in the West? For example, it already seemed from our experience with AIDS in Belgium that Africans had less *Pneumocystis carinii* pneumonia and Kaposi's sarcoma, and more cryptococcal meningitis, than their European counterparts, but our sample was relatively small, and we did not know whether these findings were representative of what was going on in Africa.

We planned to establish a lab at Mama Yemo Hospital, with facilities for hematology, microbiology, and immunology tests including analysis of lymphocytes. We would do a full immunologic profile of patients who looked like they had AIDS and compare them with healthy controls, surgical patients, and people with TB, and various parasitic illnesses, so we could develop a solid case definition of AIDS in Africa. We would study potential risk factors—sexual activity, blood transfusions, needle exposure—basically, an epidemiological study just like we'd done with Ebola. And we would do a prospective study with family contacts and sexual contacts of the patients, to look at their clinical and immunologic status over time, and whether HIV could spread through casual contact in households in an environment where people live very close to each other in overcrowded houses and are constantly exposed to bites of all kinds of insects. Finally, we planned a major study of AIDS in children.

The proposal sailed through various committees and everything looked fine until suddenly, toward the end of January 1984, there was silence from the side of the NIH. The CDC had decided to start their own program in Kinshasa and had recruited the state epidemiologist of New Mexico—a doctor named Jonathan Mann—to do the job.

The first I heard about this was a phone call one afternoon in early March from Jonathan Mann. He said he was on his way to Kinshasa to set up a CDC project on AIDS. I wanted to say, "WHAT?" but didn't. But he asked if he could stop by my office in Antwerp on his way there, and of course I agreed. So I picked him up at airport in Brussels, and although I was very tense initially, he turned out to be a very charming man, rather diffident, physically something between Albert Einstein and Groucho Marx, with an intense, interested manner, almost like a psychoanalyst. He told me right away that he'd never been to Africa and he was clearly nervous about it. His French was very good; he was then married to a Frenchwoman. So we hit it off reasonably well, and we agreed that we would have no problem working together.

I joined him in Kinshasa at the end of March. I introduced him to various people, and I gave him a copy of the proposal that I had written up with the help of Tom Quinn and Joe McCormick. Going around the hospitals, it was clear there were new cases of AIDS: Bila Kapita, at Mama Yemo told us he suspected about another 100 since we had left less than four months before, with two new patients with cryptococcal meningitis turning up every week.

In April I received news from the NIH that my grant was not accepted. Later I found out that Jonathan blocked it for reasons that I can understand now since he was going to head up what would rapidly become the largest biomedical research project in Africa. Happily it took several years before I learned this, and by then I had developed enormous respect for him. He was a very complex personality—as an individual, rather insular and a control freak—but he had an incredible mind in terms of linking things that had not been linked before, like human rights and health. He had studied at the famous Sciences Po school in Paris, and combined political analysis with the public health aspects of AIDS; he strove extremely hard to move the field toward justice for the downtrodden in a way that was completely unique. He became an extremely skilled diplomat with a long-term vision, and on the other hand he had no tolerance for all the bureaucratic nonsense and inaction that is so characteristic of international agencies.

But at the time, the salient information was that the NIH had decided to drop me completely. They would partner directly with the CDC, and they selected Skip Francis, an African American immunologist who worked for Tom Quinn, to go to Zaire and work with Jonathan. So now I had no money for the work that I so badly wanted to do. However, Jonathan agreed that the Institute of Tropical Medicine could become a partner in Projet SIDA (SIDA is the French acronym for AIDS). We would be in charge of clinical studies, an area that he wasn't much interested in. The proviso was that I had to come up with the money to fund our work.

I began contacting pharmaceutical companies for funding the necessary infrastructure for clinical work—$10,000 here, $5000 there. And I found a young energetic doctor, Bob Colebunders, a really good clinician from Antwerp who was willing to go there for us full time, for not much money. I applied for a grant from the European Union, and from the Belgian Medical Corporation, and my old friend Jean-François Ruppol, in Kinshasa, introduced me to the head physician of the Banque Belgo Zairoise. For each of several years I went to see the elderly CEO of this bank, who was known as Le Chevalier (Knight) Bauchau, at the bank's headquarters in Brussels, where everything was freshly polished ebony and you could actually *smell* the colonial era. It was part of the *Société Générale*, where my father's father worked, long ago; it was also, still, the main bank in Zaire and I became one of their charities. Every year Le Chevalier Bauchau handed me a personal check for 100,000 or 150,000 Belgian francs—a personal check in my name—and he solemnly pledged the bank to support us logistically in Kinshasa.

So this became my capital, and the Institute of Tropical Medicine officially became a partner in Projet SIDA, a phenomenal research project and one of the things I'm most proud of in my life. It laid out all the ABCs of AIDS in Africa, fast and solid, and when, a few years later, the *New Scientist* did an analysis of the scientific literature on AIDS, papers coming from Zaire were the most often cited scientific publications on AIDS in the world.

It wasn't until October 1984 that Projet SIDA really began. We had a triumvirate overseeing it: from the NIH, Tony Fauci, the head of NIAID; from the CDC, Jim Curran, the director of the AIDS Division; and from the Institute of Tropical Medicine, me. Jonathan Mann and the whole project became accountable to us. So in a way

I was bumped upstairs, although in practice we Belgians could not hope to provide the financial heft that the Americans did. We divided up the labor: the CDC was roughly responsible for the epidemiology; the NIH for the laboratory; the Belgians for the clinical aspects. So Bob Colebunders and I were specifically responsible for describing in detail the clinical spectrum of HIV infection in Central Africa, as it was not known then how exactly AIDS manifests itself in a completely different environment than in the West in terms of nutrition, the interaction with other frequent infections, and genetic makeup. All this should lead to better clinical diagnosis and ultimately treatment. We also often found ourselves caught in the middle of the complex relationship between the two American agencies, whose modus vivendi was not always harmonious. (This was also true of the Armed Forces Institute of Pathology, which joined us later.)

In practice our work overlapped greatly and at the end of the day we all worked very smoothly together. We agreed that we would publish everything together, and that all studies would be designed and executed jointly. And I argued that we couldn't just use the endoscope, the bronchoscope, and all the other equipment we were bringing in, to do studies. We needed to provide a service to people in the hospital, and we also needed to invest in training Zaireans. Actually this was contrary to NIH and CDC regulations in those days (no longer today) because they could only fund research—clinical medicine was considered development assistance. But I insisted that Bob Colebunders—who was moving to Zaire with his wife, a nurse, even though he knew I only had enough money initially to pay him for six months—be there also as a service provider in the internal medicine ward of Mama Yemo, working with Dr. Kapita. We just didn't tell anyone else about it for a while.

It was on that trip that I got formal approval from the Zairean authorities to set up all this work and nailed down funding from the Belgian Development Agency. We set up the lab, which Frieda Behets ended up running. She was the Flemish woman living in Kinshasa whom I knew from my Ebola days; incredibly hardworking and determined, you felt she could parachute anywhere and survive in almost any circumstances. She became a superb manager of the project. Then there were Bosenge

Ngali and Eugene Nzilambi Nzila, two very young Zairean doctors who could cut through government bureaucracy very nimbly and knew how to connect with people. They were invaluable. Ngali later became the first director of the Zairean National Aids Programme, the first on the continent. Nzila in particular was a lot of fun, in addition to being a clever guy. His last name in Kikongo meant "the wrong path," which became a running joke, and he was a *sapeur*, a Zairean dandy, who wore impeccably tailored suits. He and I spent many an evening on the terraces of Matonge, where there was always good music—a genre evocatively named *sekous*, from the French *secousse*, "shake."

Kinshasa was again thrilling but it had an edge to it. I was staying at the Fométro—I always did, I never had any spare cash for hotels—and at night, often in the daytime too, I was constantly stopped at road barriers by police or military trying to shake me down for a bribe. I never gave them any money, but it could become unpleasant, particularly at night if they were drunk. One day I was arrested at Ndjili Airport and put in a room with some secret policemen, who accused me of smuggling diamonds, while my plane for Brussels was boarding. They finally let me go before the plane took off, but after that I put my principles aside. At a next visit to Kinshasa I went to the *Grande Chancellerie des Ordres Nationaux*, the institution that directed the Order of the Leopard to which I had been named in 1977 by the grace of President Mobutu. Unlike every other institution in Kinshasa, this ran on greased and soundless wheels; everything was in perfect order and spotless, and they immediately found my file. They issued me the card immediately, in the bright green color of the ruling party and signed by Mobutu himself. After that, any time I was stopped or harassed I showed the card, and from then on, I didn't even have to open my suitcase at the airport; they just saluted and stood aside. But at times I wondered whether I too had been corrupted by the corrupters.

WE BEGAN AN important household contact study. Can you get HIV infection from close, nonsexual contact? What about insect transmission—lice, mosquitoes? We didn't *think* it was mosquitoes, especially because we were then seeing hardly any HIV infection in children, who were severely affected by malaria, which is transmitted by mosquitoes. But with AIDS, almost none of the questions yet had answers: everything needed to be checked out. We found no evidence whatsoever of nonsexual household transmission, which was reassuring.

Projet SIDA also pioneered mother-to-child HIV-transmission studies. There were early indications from the United States that a then unknown proportion of infants born to women with AIDS would also develop AIDS, and nearly uniformly die with opportunistic infections. There were so many infected women in Kinshasa, and they had very high fertility rates, so this seemed like an immediate priority. We did the study in the pediatric ward at Mama Yemo Hospital, Pavilion 7, on every hospitalized child and a healthy sibling. Many children had symptoms associated with AIDS, but in the absence of quite advanced laboratory tests, diagnosis of HIV infection in infants and children can be difficult, even today. Then we began just collecting specimens, banking them, in anticipation of the day HIV tests became available; we knew several companies were working on them. (This work grew in importance under the aegis of Jon's successor, Robin Ryder.)

Clinically, the biggest problem was diarrhea: intractable, debilitating, inhuman, and humiliating. People stank, they were too weak to stand up, lying in this evil waste, and it went on for months: I had seen cholera but that is far more acute and of short duration. AIDS patients died alone. People—friends, family—were afraid of them. People knew very quickly there was an epidemic going on, and there was stigma, rejection. This affected me, as I think it affects every doctor who works with AIDS patients. It wasn't just about the enormous scientific curiosity and excitement, it was about people, our patients and others.

Jonathan began organizing surveillance for AIDS in Kinshasa to see whether the epidemic was expanding. We began working with blood banks, struggling to secure the blood supply. As a first step we looked at who the blood donors were, keeping their sera, because there was no test yet. There was a small blood bank at Mama Yemo

Hospital, with 30 to 40 donations a day, but they were either professional donors, paid for the service, or family members. The blood bank at many African hospitals is just a poor man at the door.

Then mid-1985 we got a first batch of the prototype enzyme-linked immunosorbent assay (ELISA) test. I can't remember how many it was, but no more than a few hundred tests. With the kind of prevalence we were seeing, just by painstakingly counting T-cells and CD4 cells, where could we start? A test didn't give us any hope of curing anybody. The most useful, direct application seemed to be to screen blood transfusions: there you knew you would be certain of preventing at least one new case of infection. So we began with that.

We also began to follow up on people we had considered to be "healthy" controls back in 1983, but who in the initial evaluation by the French research team were found to be positive for the virus. In some cases it took a long time before they fell sick, but they all did, and they all died. So, the results of their HIV antibody tests were not false positive, but an indication of dormant HIV infection.

MAMA YEMO HOSPITAL had become the referral center for all the AIDS patients in Kinshasa. I was spending a lot of time there, three or four trips a year. Jonathan Mann and I worked smoothly together, but we were very different men. His world in Kinshasa consisted of the base he set up at Mama Yemo Hospital, the US embassy, the American Club, his kids' school, and the Ministry of Health and home. We had our arguments now and then. For example, in the early days he prohibited us from telling people that we were taking their blood to test it for AIDS; we were supposed to say it was for a study on malaria. I argued that we should tell them. Actually that's a requirement of any ethical board: you should tell people what you're doing with their body fluids. But it was Jonathan who negotiated with the Zairean Ministries, and he argued that they wouldn't permit it.

It may have been true. Jonathan was an astute diplomat, and he made this groundbreaking enterprise acceptable to the Zairean authorities, who were then in denial about AIDS, as was about every other government in Africa, and very ready to accuse foreigners of racism. And he held it together, too, with the warring factions of the NIH and CDC.

There was one other argument between us. I knew there would be trouble because he took off his glasses, and began fiddling with them with the little toolset that he had; this was something that he always did when he was tense. Then he hemmed and hawed and said, "I'm very concerned about you going out so much." Jonathan could be judgmental, and it seemed like he was insinuating that just having a beer, or going out dancing, was not sound conduct. I said, "I highly recommend that you do too, and see real people: they're having fun, and most of the time just talking and dancing, but it's important that you see that." Moreover, I thought it was good professional conduct to socialize with our Zairean colleagues. I felt it meant that socially, politically, and in terms of the epidemic's vectors and trajectory, I could understand a little better what was going on in Kinshasa.

CHAPTER 12

Yambuku One More Time

I N JUNE 1985 the first International AIDS Conference was staged in Atlanta, Georgia. By this time 17,000 cases of AIDS had been reported, but more than 80 percent of them were in the United States. I attended, along with Bila Kapita, Wobin Odio (a Zairean professor of internal medicine), and Dr. Pangu, who had become the principal adviser to the Zairean minister of health. They were the only Africans present; in fact, practically the only black people. I was their interpreter, and because there was already the feeling that AIDS had originated in Africa, there was kind of a buzz around them. But they clearly felt insulted and shocked by the allusions to our work, and to the insinuations that were being made—that African patients were actually closet homosexuals, that they were having sex with monkeys. Dr. Kapita, in particular, was a man of such respect, such rectitude and dignity, that he was really very offended and angry.

There was major resistance at this conference to accepting the fact that HIV can be transmitted from women to men. People—and many were *scientists*—conceded that maybe it can be transmitted from men to women, but in that case it must be anal intercourse. I remember a discussion in front of our poster with some people from the New

The five missionaries who died from Ebola hemorrhagic fever in Yambuku, 1976 *(Sisters of the Sacred Heart of Mary, 's-Gravenwezel, Belgium).*

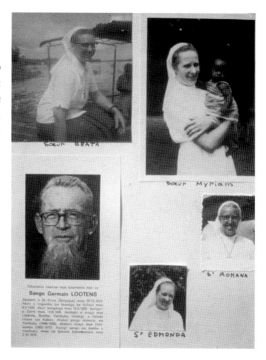

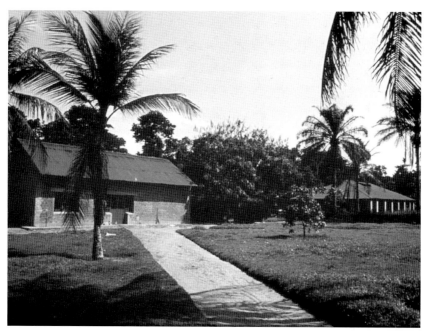

Yambuku mission hospital, 1976 *(P. Piot).*

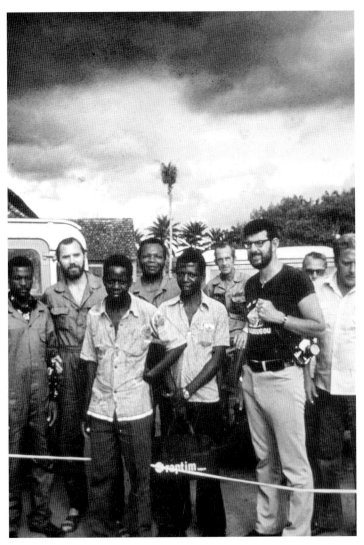

Arrival in Yambuku on October 20, 1976: with Joe Breman,
Pierre Sureau, Jean-François Ruppol, Jean-Pierre Kott,
Masamba, Nurse, Sukato (Ebola survivor) *(J. Breman).*

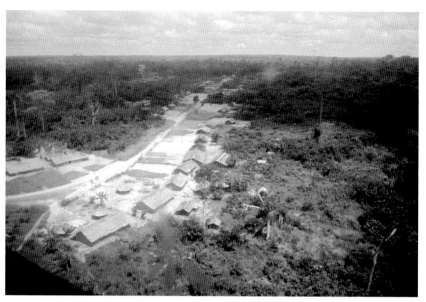

Village near Yambuku showing close contact with forest *(P. Piot)*.

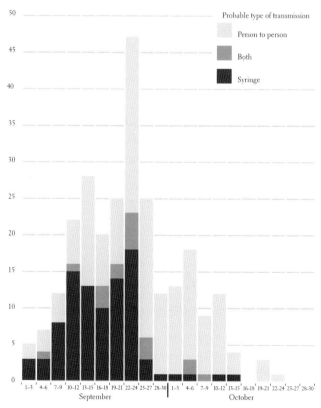

Cases of African hemorrhagic fever by date of onset, Equator region,
Zaire, Africa, Sept. 1–Oct. 30, 1976 *(P. Piot)*.

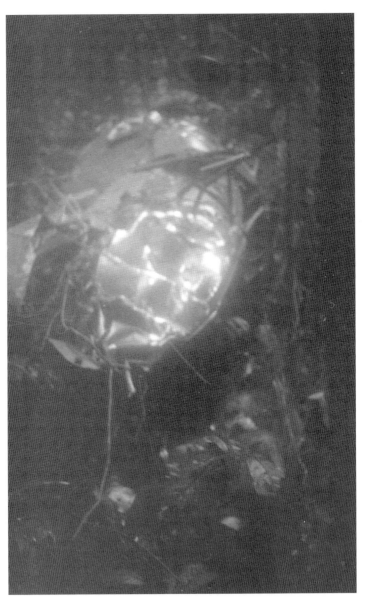

Crashed Allouette helicopter with dead pilot, 1976 *(P. Piot).*

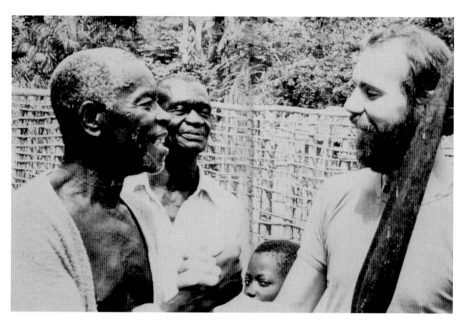

A farewell present from Yamotile Moke, 1976 *(P. Piot).*

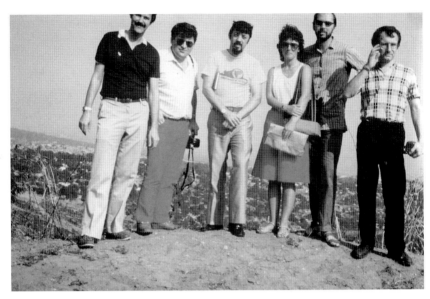

Kinshasa, October 1983: with Tom Quinn, Chris Bets,
Joe McCormick, Sheila Mitchell, Henri Taelman *(P. Piot).*

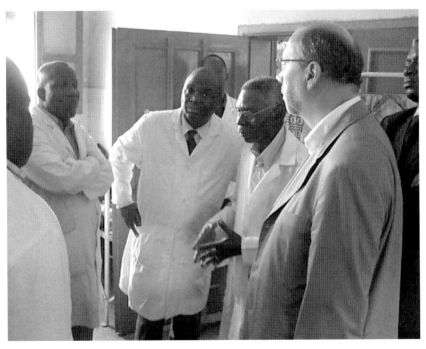

Dr. Joseph Bila Kapita and colleagues at
Kinshasa General (ex Mama Yemo) Hospital, 2008 *(H. Larson).*

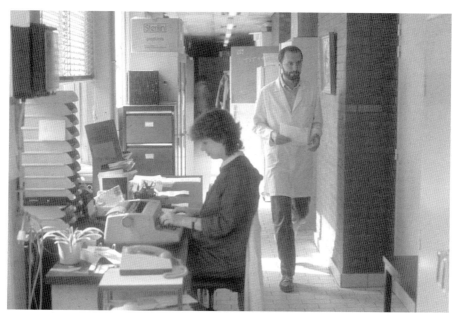

The corridor of my lab at the Institute of Tropical Medicine, Antwerp, with my assistant, Yvette Baeten, 1983 *(Antwerp Institute of Tropical Medicine).*

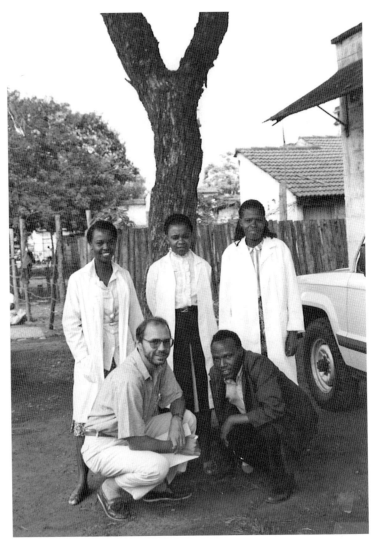

Taking a break from a sex worker clinic visit, Kenya, 1986 *(P. Piot)*.

York Health Department who insisted that heterosexual transmission was absolutely not possible.

There was also a big debate about testing. I remember the stickers proclaiming "NO TEST IS BEST," and noisy demonstrations. The logic was that a positive test only meant discrimination; there was no upside, because there was no treatment. And since everyone was supposed to use condoms all the time, there wasn't the benefit of protecting another person's health. I was puzzled. I saw their point, but also how useful it would be to know who is infected with HIV to protect themselves and others. That was the first time I encountered AIDS activism. It didn't yet exist in Europe, much less in Africa.

On a more positive note, I met Jean William "Bill" Pape, the Haitian infectious disease specialist who had begun looking at an epidemic of people dying of diarrhea in 1981, before AIDS was even identified. His group, GHESKIO, in the Cité Soleil, in Haiti's capital Port au Prince, was doing really pioneering work, and although they had funding from Cornell University, it was always a Haitian-driven project. His team is still at the forefront of both clinical care and research on AIDS in Haiti. We Zaireans bonded with him because we were from the developing world too; I wasn't really a Zairean, or from a poor country, but in this context I felt that I was, because it seemed as though we were alone in realizing that AIDS could be an even greater threat to developing countries than it was for the West.

IN OCTOBER 1985 I participated in a first meeting on AIDS in Africa itself, in Bangui, the capital of the Central African Republic. It was a small gathering of Africans, Americans from the CDC, French scientists, and myself. We all crammed into a meeting room of the Pasteur Institute of Bangui. This was at a time when the Africa office of WHO desperately did not want to get involved in anything to do with AIDS. Because, faced with a clear unfolding catastrophe for public health, WHO still had been inactive, except for its offices in Europe and the Americas, since originally it saw AIDS as a problem of wealthy countries only. And WHO Director Halfdan Mahler had recently told reporters in Zambia that "AIDS is not spreading like a bush fire in Africa . . . it is malaria, and other tropical diseases, that are killing millions of children every day." (To be fair to Mahler, he later became a strong supporter of AIDS work, and even told the United Nations General Assembly in 1987 that AIDS was a major threat to the health of the world.)

It was only with great difficulty that Dr. Fakhry Assad, the director of WHO's Division of Infectious Disease, managed to organize the meeting at the Institut Pasteur in Bangui, together with Jonathan Mann. The main outcome was a practical case-definition of AIDS, so that everyone in Africa could make a diagnosis: this would help us get a better idea about the distribution of it. And also, quite simply, it was the first time Africans were talking to Africans about AIDS. *"I'm from Dar es Salaam, you're from Kinshasa, our countries are neighbors, are you seeing the same thing I'm seeing?"*

Our discussions were an extraordinary mix of comparing notes, discovering similarities and differences, and formulating hypotheses about where this all started—only interrupted now and then by a staccato of heavy rain and mangoes hitting the metal roof. Oddly enough, because of the English/French schism that runs through Africa, once again I often acted as interpreter. It was truly a historic meeting, not only because it was the first of its kind in Africa, but also because in quite a few countries it triggered AIDS control activities by participants at the meeting. A new community was born: the community of African AIDS researchers. I was a proud member of it.

BY THIS TIME, 85 countries had reported cases of AIDS to WHO—even China had a case, which meant the epidemic was present in every region of the world. WHO was under pressure to take much more vigorous action. Halfdan Mahler approached Jonathan Mann, and he and Jonathan agreed to set up a new program at the WHO Headquarters in Switzerland. Jonathan left Kinshasa for Geneva in the spring of 1986.

His departure was a blow to Projet SIDA, because Jonathan was someone you didn't replace easily. In just 18 months he had constructed an incredible organization in Kinshasa, a project that was already publishing groundbreaking work and was poised to do studies of crucial importance for the future worldwide fight against HIV. But I could see his logic. He was a visionary, someone who liked to create things, and he was keen to play a global role.

There was certainly a need for it. AIDS was becoming an angry issue; there were laws for mandatory testing of immigrants, a lot of discrimination in the workplace. The president of the German Federal Court of Justice had just said it might be necessary to tattoo or quarantine HIV-positive individuals, and in some countries—the Soviet Union, Cuba—anyone found positive was confined to what was essentially jail and often punished for being a homosexual.

Jonathan Mann was capable of working to turn that around, in terms of public awareness and raising the intelligence level of governments.

In April, Mann and Halfdan Mahler scheduled a meeting of donor countries in Geneva, to raise enough money to get the new Control Program on AIDS off the ground. I was present: despite my total lack of experience regarding international diplomacy, I was representing Belgium, at the request of the Belgian Development Ministry, as nobody there knew anything about AIDS. Jonathan was very nervous about how things would go, so he and I had cooked up a plan: I would try to be the country representative who would speak first, to kick things off and set the tone of the meeting.

Of course it was Mahler, who was the host, who made the opening remarks, and what he said was basically, "Even though we're here to raise money for AIDS, and thanks for coming, don't forget there are so many more important health problems in the world." Talk about a fund-raising strategy; you could see Jonathan's face going green. So then I stood up and stoutly pledged Belgium to do something extremely vigorous but suitably vague. Basically: "We welcome this program, which is badly needed, and we will fully support it." And then the United States jumped in: "We fully agree with the representative of Belgium."

It was fine: the donor country governments carried it through, and they raised over $50 million. But among some people at WHO— who in the past decade had abandoned "vertical" health programs aimed at single diseases, plugging away instead at primary health care across the board—all this probably reinforced the feeling that AIDS was a competitor for their limited funds.

Part of the problem with WHO was and still is systemic: it was an inborn error of structure. The regional directors of WHO (there are six) are elected by the Ministries of Health of their regions. Thus they have political legitimacy that in a sense is as large as that of the director-general of WHO in Geneva, who is elected by the same member states. Although the director-general is nominally their boss, the regional directors lead their regions in a very sovereign way. Many were fundamentally hostile to new ideas. These men refused to give up control over their regions to a new centralized AIDS program in headquarters in Geneva. They would be Mann's nemesis.

DR. ROBIN RYDER, a curly haired, infectious disease specialist who worked for the CDC, replaced Jonathan as the director of Projet SIDA. Robin thrived in Kinshasa, laughing all the time, joking with everyone: he was a convivial man, as well as being very good at his job. He expanded the project enormously, until there were over 300 people working there, and he organized huge cohorts to study various aspects of HIV infection. He was also meticulous. Running such a large office in Kinshasa must not have been an easy thing, and he was lucky to have Frieda Behets to do the job. Logistics alone were a major headache, in a city where the phone almost never functioned. It was Robin who really fueled the whole project to create a proper blood bank. By this time, our estimate of HIV prevalence in Kinshasa was 3 to 4 cases per 100 adults. And we were still seeing plenty of transfusion-related HIV infection at Mama Yemo Hospital: about 1000 cases a year; more, in that one hospital, than in the whole of the United States at the time. This was not a research issue but it was an ethical one, and it was Robin who got the German international aid agency, GTZ, to set up a real blood bank and staff it.

Typically, an hour after someone gave blood it was being used in surgery. So the blood bank needed to use rapid tests rather than the then-more-accurate but slower ELISA. However, the rapid tests were now coming onto the market in a situation of pure anarchy: not all were reliable, and developing countries had no ability to certify or approve them. My lab in Antwerp began doing quality control tests on the rapid tests, funded by the AIDS program at WHO. We put together a serum bank, with sera from people well-documented as infected with HIV, and others with "problem" sera—patients who had autoimmune diseases such as lupus, which may give false positive to HIV tests, or from countries with endemic malaria, another key infection that we knew sometimes led to false results with the early HIV antibody tests.

However, some people in Kinshasa continued to be infected with HIV via blood donations, because technicians weren't available to do the testing at night and on weekends. We could see that almost all of them rapidly became infected with HIV. A blood transfusion was clearly much more likely than sex to transmit HIV, and the resulting immune loss also seemed to be much more rapid and devastating.

However, the majority of people with HIV in Kinshasa were infected through sexual contact, and it was important to design interventions to prevent heterosexual transmission. Based on the principle to start where the problem is greatest and where you can easily reach people at risk, we decided to try to prevent HIV infection among sex workers and their clients. The Matonge district in Kinshasa was the obvious place to work. So Marie Laga and Nzila set up a clinic for prostitutes in Matonge, based on our experience in Kenya. Matonge wasn't exactly a red-light district—there was a lot else going on there too—but there were plenty of bars and *dancings*, and all day long you could hear music in the streets, the hypnotic whine of the Congolese guitar. Nobody could sit still; the nurses would all be swaying to the music, there was laughing and chatter: it was a great atmosphere for a medical center.

We educated sex workers about AIDS—especially condom use and how to negotiate it with their clients and partners. We offered medical care, not only for sexually transmitted diseases, but also in general for the women and their children. We tried to comfort the women with HIV infection—at the beginning of the project a staggering

26 percent were positive—and in those days there was no treatment for HIV infection. We lost many women, who left behind too many orphans to be taken care of by their extended families. Many of these children ended up on the street. It was heartbreaking, but we were powerless in the absence of any treatment. Our center soon became a popular place with the whole neighborhood. After a few years, there was a significant decline in new infections.

Ryder was a pediatrician, and he was also instrumental in pioneering studies of mother-to-child transmission of HIV, at a time in the 1980s when it was not clear how HIV was transmitted to neonates and infants, and what the risk factors were. In Kinshasa, HIV-infected pregnant women were transmitting HIV to their babies with a frequency of 40 percent, compared to 5 to 10 percent in the United States. We also did a significant amount of work on cofactors for sexual transmission of AIDS. It was becoming clear from our work in Nairobi that genital ulcers from chancroid and chlamydia can favor the transmission of HIV. The high prevalence of poorly treated sexually transmitted infection in many urban populations of Central Africa was creating a highway for heterosexual transmission, multiplying its efficiency. This was of crucial importance for future programs to prevent the transmission of HIV, because it meant that by treating other sexually transmitted infections, we could hope to reduce the incidence of HIV.

Bob Colebunders's team and his successor Jos Perriens were among the first to unravel the connection between tuberculosis and HIV infection. They found that over 20 percent of patients with tuberculosis in Kinshasa also had HIV, much higher than in the general population. The connection was immune deficiency, which makes people vulnerable to tuberculosis disease, just as to other infections. Because infection with *Mycobacterium tuberculosis* is so prevalent already in developing countries, the AIDS epidemic generated in its shadow an epidemic of tuberculosis that became the leading cause of death in AIDS patients in Africa. Among other things we also showed that the then used treatment for tuberculosis in Zaire did not work for patients with dual TB and HIV infection, and developed a more effective treatment. Colebunders also discovered that a particular type of urticaria-like skin rash was diagnostic for HIV in Central Africa, as is shingles in adults. Projet SIDA was an apparently unending source of new discoveries: we did more groundbreaking work in a year than most research projects in Europe could hope to uncover in five years. Every year Jim Curran from the CDC and I met in Kinshasa with Tom Quinn, representing the NIH, to review the scientific highlights, a moment of pure joy for the brain. We got along extremely well: there were great celebrations with all staff in Matonge, with live music, and Jim Curran cracking memorable jokes. It felt like one large family. But there was also some institutional positioning, and as the poor cousin, I had to use pretexts of "human capital" to attempt to demonstrate that we Belgians were contributing equally to the Projet SIDA budget, whereas the US government was actually paying the lion's share.

MEANWHILE, WE KNEW that there was also AIDS in Nairobi. We had seen cases among the prostitutes we treated at our clinic. But until the HIV antibody test was commercially available, we couldn't do proper testing on a wide scale; we were receiving batches of prototypes, but we were sending all those tests to the Kenyan blood banks. So we banked sera. Working with Joel Breman and Karl Johnson on Ebola had taught me not just to properly preserve all the blood samples we gathered but also to be very careful to have meticulous administration, so we would know who was behind the sera: gender, age, circumstances. That is the type of bureaucracy that I favor. I now had an incredibly valuable library dating back to the early 1980s.

When the ELISA test for HIV antibodies appeared on the market in 1985, we were astonished that 9 percent of all the patients coming to us in Nairobi with sexually transmitted infections had HIV virus in their blood. (This being a rather specific sample of people, it didn't necessarily have great bearing on the prevalence in the whole population.) Among prostitutes who came in, the figure was over 60 percent: a stunning figure, at the time unparalleled anywhere in the world. Most of these women came from the Kagera region in Tanzania: this was some of the first evidence that the epidemic radiated out from the Lake Victoria region. What had been a smart survival strategy for these women had become a death strategy when the HIV epidemic emerged.

Using the banked sera, we could actually trace when the epidemic in Nairobi started. In 1980, none of the men we saw with sexually transmitted diseases had the HIV antibody. In 1981 it was already 3 percent of men, and 6 percent of women—a little higher among prostitutes, specifically, but not much: 7.1 percent. You could see it was spreading like bush fire. AIDS was a new thing in Nairobi, and it had hit the ground running. Compelled by these results, we decided to add AIDS research to our project in Nairobi, with a major focus on HIV infection in prostitutes. We set up a clinic in the Pumwani district, which was basically a slum that concentrated a large number of sex workers. We used a couple of rooms in the municipal health office; there were goats and sheep and a permanent market of all kinds of second-hand clothes and shoes just outside. You could buy only a left shoe, or only a right one.

Elizabeth Ngugi, the former head nurse, became a key figure, something between a community leader and a mother for these women who were despised, rejected, and badly treated by everyone, men and women. It was thanks to her that the project later achieved its life-changing work with some of these women, and it was in Pumwani that I perceived the incredibly powerful way that they could organize themselves, despite their lowly status. Even before AIDS, groups of women had banded together to contribute to health care or other emergency needs for their peers, and now Elizabeth helped them to set up more consistent groups for support and care.

I USED TO drive around Kinshasa myself; negotiating the chaos of the streets was actually kind of fun, and in any case I had no spare funds to pay a driver. But once, driving to the prostitute clinic in Matonge, I was followed by three men from Mobutu's fearsome secret police, the AND. Then they overtook my car, blocking me; they pulled me out of the car and searched it. When they found the slide projector that I had intended to use for a training session for the nurses, they mistook it for a video camera and accused me of being a Pakistani journalist.

A *Pakistani* journalist? I might have laughed, but with my hands against the car I was too preoccupied with other emotions. I told them I was a scientist, a member of Mobutu's Order of the Leopard, but they just laughed at me and said they were taking me to AND headquarters—which would mean serious trouble, possibly for days. I pleaded with them to take out my wallet—they could have the cash I was carrying—and check for my Leopard ID. When they found it, they muttered about the photograph, but then the atmosphere switched in the second: they slapped me on the back, and laughed, and wanted to know all about my work in Matonge.

"Why a *Pakistani* journalist?" I asked them, and they said it was my beard, and my tan: I didn't look *completely* white. The whole episode was surreal, just another weird pothole in a normal day's work in Zaire.

I HAD BEEN helping Jonathan Mann set up his program at WHO in Geneva: I helped him identify people who could work in his new Control Program on AIDS, and set up advisory committees with the few scientists working on AIDS in those days. His right hand was Dr. Daniel Tarantola, a French veteran of many public health programs, including smallpox eradication, and unsurpassed for his organizational capacity (and humor). We had met in Nairobi and hit it off immediately. Daniel's brainchild was the short-term national AIDS plan that Jonathan wanted every country to adopt. The main idea was that by establishing a plan, AIDS would be discussed in the Ministries of Health, a budget would be allocated, money raised from donors, and as many countries as possible would finally start HIV prevention programs (treatment was not yet an option in the 1980s). They would take a clear look at the epidemiological situation and develop a program for "social marketing" of condoms, which meant that rather than go for boring public health–type messages, they would use the techniques of consumer marketing to promote a social good. Additionally, it involved developing distribution networks that meant you didn't have to go into a pharmacy to buy a condom, but could buy one in small kiosks and at ambulant vendors together with soap and matches and lightbulbs.

With few exceptions, such as Uganda, the majority of African governments still either denied the reality of the epidemic or showed a cynical skepticism, accepting international aid without making much of an effort to fight the virus. In rich countries AIDS was associated with homosexual behavior, prostitution, or intravenous drug use and it was difficult for them to acknowledge these realities in their own countries. When confronted with studies showing very high levels of infection they denounced them as biased samples or said that their country was struggling with far more important health issues, which for most African countries at the time was absolutely true. However they did not see the epidemic that was spreading silently: in most countries outside Central Africa, people had been infected with HIV too recently to be ill or die; it takes on the average eight years after infection before one develops AIDS.

Zaire was, I believe, the first country to adopt a national AIDS plan; Ngali left Projet SIDA to become director of the plan. He began distributing condoms to the women who sold drinks and cigarettes and cola nuts at stands set up outside bars and nightclubs, or those just walking around with trays on their head. They were called the *marchés ambulantes*, "the walking markets." They made a little profit on their condom sales and it was a much more effective way to reach people. Mobutu's party had developed a very effective way of reaching people through traditional groups—theater, dance, and other entertainment—and Ngali worked the AIDS message into that process. With Population Services International (PSI) we developed a cool brand of condoms, "Prudence," "pour l'homme sur de lui-meme" (for the self-assured man), with the slogan "Confiance d'accord, mais prudence d'abord" (Trust is fine, but prudence comes first). It worked. Prudence condoms became very popular in Kinshasa. HIV prevalence in the city in 2010 is hardly higher than 25 years before, and it may be that these early prevention programs had a real impact and saved many lives.

Music was key. Franco Luambo, from the TP-OK—Tout Puissant

Orchestre Kinshasa—Jazz Band, was one of the most popular singers in Kinshasa. He wrote a song, "Attention Na Sida," and people danced to it in every nightclub. "*Use radio, TV, newspapers / To tell the people about AIDS / We have to tell them how to protect themselves / We must all fight AIDS . . .* " Then he died of AIDS, in 1989, and a copper plaque with his name on it was fixed to the tall stone pyramid, "Le Monument aux Artistes," on the Place de la Victoire. By the early 1990s almost every name on that pyramid belonged to a young and talented musician, and almost every one of them had died of AIDS. All the plaques have been stolen now, but the bare, stubby pyramid remains: a slightly surreal reminder of yet another terrible loss suffered by Central Africa.

Ngali confided in us the kind of pressure he was under to kick back part of his budget to officials from the Ministry of Health and other cronies of the regime. He was a principled man, and he worried a great deal. It is a high-risk project, to be an honest man in Zaire; a few years later, he died in a mysterious car accident.

When Mann laid out his scheme for every country to issue a short-term plan for fighting AIDS, his idea was to short-circuit the resistance he was encountering from the WHO regional directors by sending consultants to each country who were directly responsible to WHO headquarters. Each consultant would take a look at the current AIDS situation and how it was being dealt with, and specifically epidemiology, clinical management, lab services, blood banks, and condom availability and promotion.

Jonathan asked me a couple of times to join his team at WHO Headquarters, but I was not ready yet to make the leap from fieldwork, research, and seeing patients, to the more distant policy level— as much as I had become convinced that policy was key to stopping this unfolding epidemic. I did, however, go to Ghana for WHO as a consultant, to help set up the Ghanaian AIDS Plan, in a team led by Lev Kodhakievich, a Russian who had worked in smallpox eradication. The Ghanaian government initially was suspicious and we had to wait for a week to receive permission to work, which we received thanks to the intervention of Ghana-born Peter Lamptey, who established the AIDS program of Family Health International, to which

I became an adviser. In the meantime we visited some of the old castles along the coast, where dozens or hundreds of slaves were once crammed like produce into the basement, sometimes directly under the chapel or the airy dining room of the dwellings of their English, Dutch, or Danish masters.

Ghana didn't have a huge AIDS problem, except in one northeastern region. Just like the Tanzanian women in Nairobi, women there traditionally went to the capital or to a neighboring country, Côte d'Ivoire, for two or three years, where they would work in commercial sex and then come home with enough money to start a business.

We visited Kumasi, the seat of the Ashanti King, who once ruled major parts of West Africa, and you could see how poor the people were in 1986 in Ghana: in the market people were buying *half* an onion, because they couldn't afford a whole one, and no hotel rooms were complete—they either had no windows, no running water, or their restaurant menus were virtual, with most items not available. We ended up combining the whole trip with a training program for lab technicians on how to do HIV antibody tests, because although fewer than 3 percent of prostitutes who had never been out of the country were seropositive, 51 percent of prostitutes who had recently been working in Abidjan, the capital of Côte d'Ivoire, had the virus.

IN JUNE 1986, the International AIDS Conference took place in Paris, and the whole event was dominated by the standoff between Gallo and Montagnier. America versus France; which man had isolated and identified the HIV virus.

There was no real doubt in my mind that the French were the first to discover the cause of AIDS, even if Gallo had greatly contributed to the development of the HIV antibody test. But this very chauvinistic conflict discredited the whole field for several years: people thought AIDS research was not really about science, but loaded with ego and personal ambition. It was not until 1987 that the two teams came to a compromise, and even then it had to be negotiated by officials close to presidents Reagan and Mitterrand: political figures who belonged nowhere in a dispute about science. In 2008 Françoise Barré-Sinoussi and Luc Montagnier received the Nobel Prize in Physiology or Medicine for the discovery of HIV—Bob Gallo should have shared the honor.

Nzila and Ngali flew with Mann to Paris, but what they really wanted to see was Zaire's old colonial overlord, tiny Belgium. So I invited them to stay at my place in Antwerp. It was magical to see Belgium through their eyes; and we staged a truly memorable evening at a wonderful café—The Sweet Name of Jesus—run by a Zairean near the cathedral.

I WAS INCREASINGLY becoming a manager, and I enjoyed it. It was not only about budgets and administration, writing up reports so we could get funding, but also to bring on ideas, lead people, translate science into policy, and negotiate collaborative efforts. In Nairobi I helped someone structure a hypothesis, laid out a research project, and then I met them again three or six months later to check how it was going. That may have been the most efficient way to work, but it was less and less hands-on. In Antwerp the lab had grown from 20 to well over 100 people, and I became part of the senior management team at the institute. I was putting together a group on AIDS and STD so there would be much more interaction among clinicians, epidemiologists, and the key people in the microbiology lab. I was also still running the STD clinic, which had morphed from a part-time office beside the rodent housing in the Institute of Tropical Medicine to a much bigger, full-time affair, with three physicians and a nurse. We also moved to a higher floor, with access through the front entrance rather than a back door, and signage that announced where we were and what we did—sexually transmitted diseases—in letters big enough so you could read them.

I helped start the Flemish Center for AIDS prevention and various self-help and support groups for people with HIV. I was involved in numerous consultancies involving clinical, epidemiological and lab work, not just on AIDS but also on tuberculosis, reproductive tract infections in women, and low birth weight. I was doing studies with new antibiotics as well as studies of the new vaccines for hepatitis

A and hepatitis B; of sexual behavior; of programs to *change* sexual behavior. I also had master's and PhD students: the institute already had a master's program in Public Health that focused on the organization of health services, but in the mid-1980s I devised a second master's program called Disease Control that taught techniques of outbreak investigation, epidemiology, and program management.

I was traveling to Nairobi, to Kinshasa, and to the United States. And then there was my family.

I also invested much time in training people—increasingly in Africa itself. Thus, with Ibrahim Ndoye, Souleymane Mboup, and Awa Coll-Seck—all stars of AIDS, public health, and medical research—I organized an annual course on STD and AIDS control in Dakar, Senegal. Many alumni of that course became top AIDS leaders, such as the elegant Ethiopian dermatologist Meskerem Grunitzky-Bekele, and the Senegalese activist As Sy, who became regional directors for Africa in UNAIDS.

I was basically running around like crazy. Like my grandmother once said, citing a mordant Flemish proverb, "Peter, your ass can't sit still." I was almost addicted to this frantic lifestyle, and felt with such devastating health problems there was no time to lose. And there was something else I badly wanted—needed—to do.

I often urged Jonathan Mann to authorize a trip back to Yambuku, to the Catholic mission where the Ebola epidemic had broken out 10 years before. He always refused: he felt, I think, that if we found high levels of HIV in Equateur province, where President Mobutu was born, it would be politically explosive, and he was also frankly frightened of security conditions outside the capital. But now Mann was gone, and Henri "Skip" Francis, Tom Quinn, Joe McCormick, and I decided to pull out the sera that had been carefully banked from the Ebola epidemic: they were still correctly coded and neatly preserved in freezers at the NIH, the CDC, and in Antwerp.

Out of 659 sera, we found 5 villagers who in that remote and isolated region had been HIV positive in 1976, 10 years before: a prevalence of 0.8 percent. We had their names and location. If we could find those people—at least discover whether they were alive or dead—then maybe, we thought, we could learn a lot about how this disease worked over time within the individual. And by conducting another population-based survey, we would have a unique picture of the speed with which HIV diffused within a rural population.

So in August 1986, at the age of thirty-seven, I went back to Yambuku. Skip Francis came along too, as well as Marie Laga, laboratory technician "Kash" Kashamuka, and Eugene Nzilambi Nzila. (Later Dr. Kevin De Cock, a Belgian epidemiologist from the CDC, whom I had met five years earlier in Nairobi, performed additional studies in the region.) It was very moving to return to a place that had been so formative, and to do it in such good company. Skip was great, observant, and humorous, eager to see more of Zaire than just Kinshasa; Nzila, the dandy from the nation's capital, and Kash, from the eastern Kivu, were off-balance and full of self-deprecating humor in a region they had never been to. Both looked to me for guidance: they might be Zaireans, but I was the one who knew my way around the place.

The fact was, everything in Yambuku was exactly the same. If anything, the road was worse, and the river port of Bumba had disintegrated a little more. Father Carlos had created a small health center and school, but Nogeira was closed, I remember—entropy settling in. At the health center and hospital, they had seen only a sporadic patient with AIDS, and I didn't think they would have missed an epidemic of AIDS like the one going on in Kinshasa. Some people recognized me, and I noticed that when they spoke about the recent past they would say "before Ebola," "after Ebola," so that the epidemic was present in many things: "My son was born before the epidemic." In a way I suppose we shared that, because that was how I thought about my life, too. And it was how my parents and grandparents talked: something happened before or after the war of 1940–1945.

At the same time, I found myself better appreciating the beauty of the place: it could so easily have been a paradise. But there had been fighting, marauding bands of soldiers, and life was not good, you could see that.

At the mission hospital in Yambuku, there were now boxes of disposable syringes and a full-time doctor: the medical operation was clearly in much better shape. The atmosphere was strained, however.

There were two Fathers living there; one, about sixty, went about in black leather *lederhosen*—it was quite incredible, in that heat—with a sleeveless T-shirt, and plastic boots in case of snakes. He had a long white beard, so above the neck he looked like a missionary and below like an eccentric character. I once heard him thundering at some of the villagers: a domineering tone that the sisters appeared to dislike almost as much as I did. It was a very curious setup: four Flemish women and two Flemish men living a few feet from each other, alone in Africa, for decades, and often bristling with dislike. But women were not allowed to preside; and they must confess to these men.

We identified all five of the villagers who had tested positive for HIV 10 years before. Three had died of what could have been AIDS, but two were surviving without any medical care at all and no discernible symptoms: a fifty-nine-year-old woman and a fifty-seven-year-old man. The man had a low CD4 count, so we thought it was likely that his immune system was beginning to fail. We isolated the virus from them and clearly it was the same as the virus in Kinshasa. Until then we had not known you could live so long without showing symptoms of AIDS: the disease had been discovered only five years before, so there was no way of knowing it. But because we had banked and coded our Ebola sera so carefully, we were able to do this, what amounted to a kind of medical archeology.

We found six current hospital patients who had AIDS, in the Yambuku mission and in the small Lisala and Bumba hospitals. They had nonspecific symptoms and were dying. But among the general, healthy population, we found the exact same prevalence of HIV infection in the blood samples that we took as we had back in 1976: 0.8 percent. In other words, the population of Yambuku was less affected than the Swiss canton of Geneva, which was showing 1 percent prevalence at the time among pregnant women. This told us that something like HIV can remain endemic at a very low level in a population, if conditions are not there for intense transmission.

Another interesting finding was that just about everybody who was HIV positive had traveled outside the region, or had a spouse or sexual contact who had. So typically, somebody was infected by going to a city, and maybe they then infected one or two people in a lifetime. But that was it, because in this very traditional region the number of sexual partners was, as far as we could gather, much lower than in Kinshasa or, as a matter of fact, than in Europe or the States. There was also less sexually transmitted disease of all kinds. The large number of injections for medical reasons or to vaccinate also did not seem to have led to the spread of HIV. In terms of the origin of AIDS, this meant it might have been around for decades or perhaps even a century, because if there is no amplification of risk there can be a very slow rate of transmission, like a barely flickering candle. Applying the Anderson and May formula from chapter 5, the basic reproductive rate $R°$ was around 1 for at least a decade.

We published our work in the *New England Journal of Medicine* in 1988; Nzila, I'm proud to say, was the first author. Today we know HIV hasn't been around for centuries; based on genetic diversity analysis, we know it could have originated in the 1930s or perhaps even 1900s, probably in west Central Africa north of Congo, but it can't be much older. But since that time I have felt it is wrong to speak about AIDS in Africa unless I also make it clear that there are many Africas, with different AIDS epidemics, with very different social factors at work.

It was also quite poignant to leave Yambuku, to sip a last glass of vermouth with Sisters Marcella and Geno and wake up one last time to the sound of the sisters' sweet morning hymns drowning out the frogs and birdsong. I told myself I would go back again one day, and vowed to keep in touch with Father Carlos. I'm glad to report that he has satellite-connected e-mail now, and a website, and that the Belgian King Baudouin Foundation (of which I was chair of the board) recently awarded his parish 400,000 euros for water supply and high school education. He has set up a small hydroelectric power station, to provide the town with a little electricity, and I still nourish a plan to return for a visit, just to see how things are going, how I can help, and to share a beer.

CHAPTER 13

The Unfolding of an Epidemic

A FTER I RETURNED to Antwerp, I moved my family of three to Kenya for six months. I wanted to invest more in the project there and start a few studies: I wanted to do something myself, rather than fly in and out and have other people doing it. Also, I felt I would have better ideas, a better feeling for the sociology of the epidemic, if I really lived the personal, day-to-day experience of life in Africa, not via whistle-stops and secondhand knowledge from books or data. But I didn't want to spend even less time with the children, and Greta and I both felt the experience of living abroad would enrich the kids' lives. It seemed like if we ever wanted to do it, we should do it soon, because any later and it would be too disruptive to their education.

We moved in December 1986. In addition to working on the research project, I taught at the University of Nairobi. We put the children in the Dutch primary school: their schoolbooks were exactly the same as the ones they had had in Antwerp, which was comforting. The Kibera slum was just down the hill from our house, and my son Bram would disappear there for hours with a bunch of other kids: he was constantly playing in the sewer system, and he would come home in unspeakable filth with some new animal in his pocket—a chameleon or a snake or some insect.

While we were in Kenya, an article was published in the *Guardian*, a British newspaper; it said there was plenty of AIDS in Nairobi, and that prostitutes, in particular, were heavily infected. Frank Plummer, our Canadian project director, and I had asked the reporter not to mention our names, because we were worried about the government's reaction: Kenya relies heavily on the tourist trade, and was concerned that publicity around AIDS would keep tourists away. But the Ministry of Health didn't need to read our names in the article to put two and two together. We were summoned to the offices of the permanent secretary of the Ministry of Health, where members of the Home Ministry were also present, and after a short meeting we were accused of spreading false rumors about Kenya, and told that we may be expelled. Frank and I had certainly not expected such a violent reaction, and in our naïvete did not see how facts can be subversive. When comparing notes after the meeting we became convinced our phones had been tapped, though we never had proof of that. After a full day of nerve-wracking waiting in an anteroom at the Ministry, and drinking plenty of good Kenyan tea we were told the verdict: we could stay and continue our research, but should refrain from any interaction with the media. We were relieved, and made some half promise. But we had learned our lesson and also realized we needed to communicate much better with the authorities, who were not that well informed about the results of research going on in their own country, as unfortunately can be the case in Africa. This episode also taught me once again that AIDS is imminently political—as Jonathan Mann had told me numerous times, but I had then often thought he exaggerated.

We agreed with the Ministry that we would share our results, and show what we were doing. So I invited Dr. Wilfrid Koinange, the director of Medical Services, to visit our clinic for sex workers in Pumwani, as he had said there was "no prostitution in Kenya." A few weeks later Dr. Koinange did visit us, and although he made no comment, I think he saw the value of the work that we were doing (and also that there is indeed prostitution in Kenya). In any case, we had less trouble with the authorities after that, and Kenya now has a well-functioning national AIDS control program.

We returned to Europe in the late spring of 1987, smuggling in one perfect Jackson chameleon that Bram could not bear to part with. (I carried it through customs under my hat.) On my return I had to spend too much time with turf issues around the allocation of AIDS funding to various universities in Belgium, and hated it. Worst of all, my friend Willy was very ill. He had developed AIDS before I went to Nairobi, and I had hospitalized him in Henri Taelman's ward before I left. But now his situation was far worse, and his brain was affected. Willy was in his early thirties. He was a fairly cynical person, but he didn't want to die. As he grew sicker we talked about death, about the meaning of life, and of this illness. The hopelessness of AIDS in those days is difficult to express. There were no real treatments, nothing major I could do for him. But I felt then that I was a real physician, not only a clinician who treats an infection: it reminded me strongly that medicine is as much about caring as about treating.

As a psychologist or a counselor I had no more qualifications than someone you'd meet at the barber. Yet I accompanied many AIDS patients. I say "accompanied" instead of "treated" because that's what it felt like: I accompanied them down their road. I stopped seeing patients in 1993 after I moved to Geneva, but of those I saw until then, every single one is dead. Almost all were people my age or a little older; some of them were friends of people I knew; and it really consumed me. I had studied medicine because I wanted to fix people's problems, and this felt like the complete opposite.

I was frustrated by my inability to have a meaningful effect and not always sure how to cope with the intimate information that patients were sharing with me. The things people tell a doctor when they are rejected and dying bite very deep. In some cases, this may have been the most intimate relationship that these people ever had with somebody. And nobody knew. These were not things I shared with others, even my closest friends.

I saw partners, I saw wives, I saw women who learned that their husbands were gay and—oh, by the way—also had HIV. Sometimes

I had to tell people that they, themselves, were also HIV positive. After struggling to find the right words, I realized it was best to tell them straight out: "I've got bad news." You can't break that statement down or make it incremental. It's already a shock. Then I delivered the information: "Your test is positive." I could practically hear a big bang go off in their head and knew they couldn't hear me anymore. In the beginning, I tried to say far more, but then I realized that there was no point. I scheduled another appointment, so that we could talk it through later. Preparing for such a conversation would nearly always keep me awake the night before, as I could only think of the death sentence I had to communicate, and the devastation I was about to announce. Some were angry at me, some cried, a few were relieved, most were speechless. This was far more difficult and emotional than writing a grant proposal, having a manuscript rejected, or dealing with interagency politics.

Because of our good collaboration with Nathan Clumeck's group in Brussels, we also started to connect patients seen in the two centers, which at this point saw the majority of people with HIV in Belgium. This is how we put together a cluster of women with HIV, who were mostly connected with each other through sex with the same man, who had kept a diary of his very active sex life. We interviewed and tested most of his partners, and as much as possible their partners. This was not only a very delicate undertaking, but sometimes also a drama. We found that 11, or 56 percent, of his 19 female partners had become infected with HIV, and that one in eight regular male partners of these women had subsequently become infected with HIV. Two women had slept only once with this HIV-positive engineer from Burundi, who died before we had unravelled this deadly cluster of sexual encounters. None of the women considered themselves at risk for HIV. It took a few years to contact all the individuals and put the puzzle in order. In the late eighties there were still skeptics about heterosexual transmission of HIV, particularly from women to men and outside sub-Saharan Africa. In 1989 we published what is still the largest documented cluster of heterosexuals with HIV in the *New England Journal of Medicine* with Nathan as the first author.

In nearly all ways the situation for AIDS patients was even more hopeless in Africa than in Belgium, because even palliative care, never mind pain management and intensive care, were rarely available to AIDS patients.

Then came a glimmer of hope. At the end of 1986 a clinical study showed that azido-thymidine (AZT)—developed in the 1960s as an anticancer medication but never licensed—slowed the progress of AIDS. Six months into the clinical trial 19 patients receiving a placebo had died, but only 1 person in the group receiving AZT had done so. In March 1987 AZT received approval from the US Food and Drug Administration, becoming the first-ever medication to provide proven treatment for AIDS.

An electroshock went through the still-small world of AIDS doctors. While ramping up production, Burroughs Wellcome began to distribute small quantities of the drug. I had worked with the Burroughs Wellcome team in Belgium doing tests of acyclovir, for herpes, so I knew exactly whom to contact. Thus simple networking ensured that our Belgian patients began receiving treatment at the same time as patients in New York and San Francisco, before the drug even came on the market.

The cost of treatment was $7000 to $10,000 per patient per year. In Belgium this never became the heated political issue that it did in the United States, because patients didn't actually have to pay such sums: they were picked up by the social insurance system. But I was very aware of it, and of the implication that our patients in Africa would simply never be able to afford to be treated.

Still, in the beginning we celebrated. We were relieved and optimistic. And our patients improved; they put on weight, got up and walked, and some even ran and went back to work. But after a while it became clear that this improvement was only temporary. AZT had serious hematological side effects, and worse, the virus mutated so fast that viral strains became resistant to the drug. We were back to square one for saving lives.

IN GENEVA, MEANWHILE, Mann was fighting bureaucracies maybe more even than AIDS. He put AIDS on the public health agenda, and he put the public health agenda on the stage. He had fantastic political skills and a real gift for explaining. He mobilized money and made sure that basically every developing country had a national AIDS program, had some funding, and had started awareness-raising about AIDS and how to avoid it. There was enormous resistance from governments on all continents due to a combination of denial of risky sexual activities in their societies, the perception that this was a Western disease, and the concern that too much attention for AIDS would undermine their struggle with a plethora of other serious health problems. And then there are those whose priority is not their people's well-being, but accumulating personal power and wealth.

I became the chair of the Steering Committee on Epidemiology and Surveillance of WHO's Global Programme on AIDS, where I was glad to rejoin several epidemiologists for whom I had great affection as well as respect, such as Jean-Baptiste Brunet from France, John Kaldor from Australia, and Roy Anderson from Great Britain, besides the other capable members of the group. We met regularly in Geneva, and advised on the epidemiological work of the AIDS program. We were uncertain of WHO's methodology to estimate numbers of people with HIV and with AIDS in the world—a difficult task under any circumstance, but even more so in the early days of the epidemic when few individual countries had reliable data. They were initially using what is called a Delphi survey—when you have no data but ask experts to give their best guess, basically, and then you take an average—and later mathematical models that predicted peaks of the epidemic that some populations already had surpassed.

Later it turned out that the numbers from WHO were, in fact, grossly underestimated for Africa and Eastern Europe, and overestimated for Western Europe and Asia. But my point was not so much that they were inaccurate—few of us could have claimed to do better with the data at hand—but that we should not have claimed to be able to provide solid estimates at all. (This changed enormously in the following decade, and by the way, UNAIDS' data are, in my humble opinion, the best and most solid data on any health problem in the world.)

I persuaded the Belgian Development Ministry to start another project in Burundi: a small version of Projet SIDA that did some baseline research, epidemiological surveys and training, and started prevention and care programs. And Kevin De Cock, my Belgian friend in CDC, began a research program in Côte d'Ivoire: Projet RetroCI. We agreed to work together, and Peter Ghys from my group in Antwerp worked there with Kevin full time.

The Ivoirian capital Abidjan was particularly interesting in that it showed evidence of HIV-1 (the same type of the virus that was in the United States, Kinshasa, and Nairobi), but also of HIV-2, a second type that had been discovered in Senegal by Max Essex, from Harvard, and Souleymane Mboup, a Senegalese professor of microbiology and one of Africa's leading scientists. It became clear that HIV-2 could cause the same AIDS symptoms that HIV-1 did, but it appeared to be less virulent and was spreading less rapidly. Nonetheless, by 1990 AIDS became the leading cause of death in Abidjan, and HIV-1 the predominant HIV type. (Projet RetroCI later played a major role in the introduction of antiretroviral therapy in Africa, besides delivering excellent science, training, and HIV prevention.) By this time, you could actually watch the epidemic spreading: countries falling ill, hospitals overcrowded with AIDS patients, companies losing highly trained staff. In some parts of Uganda and Tanzania, there were already so many AIDS orphans that their grandmothers simply couldn't cope.

THE THIRD INTERNATIONAL AIDS Conference was held in Washington in 1987, and I was asked to speak at the opening. This was a very big deal for me, and I was planning to announce to the world unequivocally that there is heterosexual transmission of HIV, indeed a lot of it. Robert Gallo was speaking, and Vice-President George H. W. Bush was going to speak next. I was waiting my turn, sitting in the front row of the conference room at the Washington Hilton when—just like in one of those nightmares—I realized that I had left my speech in my hotel room upstairs. I raced out. When I got back Bush's security people didn't want to let me in. Finally I made it, just in time to watch as people hissed at Bush and turned their backs on him, in protest against President Reagan's plans for more extensive HIV testing programs. I never thought of myself as someone with undue respect for authority but I believe we should always let people speak, even if we disagree. We can protest before or after. I did agree to a large extent with the protesters' points, though: the US government could do much better on AIDS, from funding research and prevention programs, to countering AIDS-related discrimination. This was the year that ActUp was founded in New York by gay AIDS activists. Together with other activist groups they would become a very vocal and effective force to accelerate research and access to AIDS treatment, and were soon an integral part of the growing AIDS "movement." Washington was the first of a long series of protests at AIDS conferences, and I myself sometimes became the object of them. AIDS activism in the eighties and nineties could be loud and out of control. Nowadays we've sanitized these protests: conferences arrange a short window so the activists can go ahead and make their points. In Washington in 1987, police with long yellow rubber gloves arrested AIDS activists outside the Hilton on Connecticut Avenue. We have come a long way.

By this time, the European Union had set up a Task Force on AIDS, and was beginning to send money to fund AIDS-related projects, as a form of emergency development aid. Lieve Fransen, the Flemish doctor who had worked in our research project in Kenya and then moved to Antwerp to earn her PhD, was running this task force. One day she called me and asked whether I was interested in developing an AIDS control program in Lubumbashi, the capital of Shaba province in southeastern Zaire.

This project wasn't about doing research. It was about doing what needed to be done: provide a safe blood supply, try to improve the public health service in general by training people, and rehabilitate the medical lab so they could properly diagnose. It was the work of a nongovernmental organization, and I was an academic. Nonetheless, when I thought it over I found that I wanted to do it. I wanted to do something practical about AIDS, with direct impact on public health. Instead of studying reality, I wanted to actually change it.

The first thing we did once the project actually got started, in 1988, was to refurbish the public health laboratory, which meant new equipment and an architect—even the roof had to be rebuilt. I became like a manager of a big operation, though Drs. Kambali Magazani from Zaire and Geert Laleman from Antwerp ran the project on-site. All kinds of things went wrong, from using rapid tests for blood that were sensitive to fluctuations in temperature and had a short shelf-life to incorrect readings. Things broke and shifted and rotted. I quickly learned that funding was not the only hurdle to an organized project, and not just in Africa but everywhere.

I remember a midwife at the hospital. She had AIDS: fungal and herpetic infections in the mouth, intractable diarrhea. There was a Tanzanian pathologist and he told me that in 15 years he had never seen anything like the swollen lymph nodes he was now seeing daily. There clearly was AIDS in Lubumbashi, and I felt I was watching the epidemic move in, but it was doing so in slow motion. HIV prevalence was low—something like 3 percent, compared to the 6 percent we estimated in Kinshasa—and the incidence, the measure of *new* infections, didn't seem to be explosive. The big question was, Would it stay this way?

We were 1000 miles away from Kinshasa, deep in southern Africa. The Shaba province (and Lubumbashi) is a kind of panhandle that sticks way down south into Zambia in an awkward, artificial-looking shape. And yet, in the Zambian copper belt, just across the border, the prevalence of HIV was far higher—over 15 percent—and it was spreading much more quickly.

Since colonial times the miners were permitted to live in Lubumbashi alongside their families. The Belgian mining companies built family housing and schools, they hired the sons of miners. It was a different setup from the system that mining companies created in Zambia, with tens of thousands of single men away from their families, living in hostels, doing a terrifying dangerous job, with recourse to prostitution often their sole sexual expression. Was this the explanation for the difference in HIV levels? We still do not know. Again I realized that there was not going to be one AIDS epidemic in the world but many different ones, depending on behavior and culture, and that any kind of solutions that could be put together were going to have to be tailor-made.

IN 1988 MANN organized a major ministerial conference in London that was attended by 115 ministers of health, more than had ever gathered on a specific disease. Before that meeting, Minister Ruhakana Rogunda from Uganda was the lone voice who in a dramatic speech at the World Health Assembly in 1987 had called his peers to face the reality of AIDS on their continent. Even though many attending the London meeting were still in denial about the scale of the problem in their own countries—and several came from governments that had pledged to shut out foreigners with HIV—all of the ministers signed off on a declaration backing the human rights and dignity of people living with HIV. This had not been a foregone conclusion by any means. Since Mann's arrival in 1986, WHO had been giving governments a range of services, from technical help with drawing up three- to five-year AIDS plans, to funds for new laboratories and training programs for medical professionals; it was even fund-raising from Western governments to support AIDS programs in poor countries.

The budget for the Global Programme on AIDS had grown bigger than any other single program at WHO, but it was raised directly from donor countries: it didn't come from WHO's general budget. The name itself, Global Programme on AIDS (GPA), emphasized that this was not a temporary or short-term emergency. Jonathan Mann also established a Global Commission on AIDS with highly respected political and scientific figures, to protect him, I think, from the political pressures.

Halfdan Mahler's term of office as director-general of WHO came to an end. He had received multiple complaints about Jonathan from irate ministers of health who felt pressured to address AIDS but the two of them had developed a good working relationship, with a lot of mutual respect. Hiroshi Nakajima, formerly the WHO regional director for Asia, was appointed as the new director-general. This was a whole different story.

Mann had done something very unusual for WHO since the

eradication of smallpox. He directed his short-term plans straight out of headquarters: he completely bypassed the regional offices and sent his staff and temporary consultants to each country. This really was the only solution, otherwise in many countries there would have been virtually no movement to ward off the epidemic. But in doing this he created powerful resistance against him from the regional directors who control around three-quarters of the WHO budget.

Jonathan had the guts and political acumen to convene a meeting of the Global Commission on AIDS in Brazzaville—the city that hosted WHO's regional office for Africa—in essence forcing the regional director to confront the reality of AIDS in Africa under the impatient eyes of eminent persons from across the world. This is when I met one of Asia's marketing geniuses, Senator Khun Meechai Viraidya from Thailand, who was a member of the commission. We got to know each other when I was looking for someone of my height to ask to lend me fresh clothes, as my suitcase had not arrived (and neither had Jim Curran's). Meechai immediately gave me a suitcase full of all I needed, and we became friends for life. Meechai was a businessman, politician, and community leader—an entrepreneur in many respects, and above all a superb communicator. He became the architect of Thailand's successful AIDS program, imposing 100 percent condom use in commercial sex, which was flourishing in Thailand. This ultimately led to a decline of HIV in the country—one of the very early achievements in HIV prevention in the world.

In the meantime HIV continued its spread over the world, discriminating nowhere. The Soviet Union reported its first case in 1987, and in November 1988 I went to Moscow with a team of Belgian AIDS experts to share our experience with our Russian colleagues, who were very concerned about further spread of HIV in their vast country. Until then all AIDS patients from the USSR had been hospitalized, often for months, in the Institute for Infectious Diseases in Moscow. While Dr. Vadim Pokrovsky, the top soviet AIDS epidemiologist, was showing us around in his institute I suddenly saw three Africans at the end of the corridor. I tried my luck and shouted, "Bonjour!" The three men rushed to me, happy to be able to tell their sad story in a language they mastered far better than Russian. They were students at Lumumba University from Burkina Fasso and Burundi, had tested positive for HIV on arrival in Russia, and had spent several months in what was basically quarantine, even if they were in good health. I promised I would bring up their case with the authorities to see if they could help these students. Just like small Belgium, the Soviet Union was confronted with multiple entry points for HIV. Little did we know at the time that Russia and the former Soviet republics would experience a still-growing HIV epidemic driven by injection drug use.

It was my first visit to Moscow, and I don't pretend I fully understood what was going on, particularly in the quite secretive days of the Soviet Union. But there was clearly change in the air among health colleagues, who were eager to connect with us. It was already bitter cold, but the people were warm once we socialized.

IN ANTWERP, OUR lab started using simple techniques to look at pieces of the genome of all kinds of isolates of HIV-1. At some point these strains had been grouped into A, B, C, D, and so on, based on the sequences of the envelope gene, and there was a great deal of discussion of their relative pathogenicity and how you could develop a vaccine to protect against them all—a still-unresolved challenge. When in 1989 members of my team, Bob De Leys and Martine Peeters, isolated two very unusual HIV-1 strains from a couple from Cameroon, the genetic variation of HIV appeared to be even wider than we thought. The woman was nineteen and both she and her husband had persistent generalized lymphadenopathy, but their serum gave only faint bands in the confirmatory Western blot test. The virus that we found in it was very aberrant. (We called it ANT70, though it is now known as Group O: Group "Oh" not Group "Zero.") It had major differences with all the known strains of both HIV-2 and HIV-1, and was particularly divergent in the envelope glycoprotein. Sampling indicated that 5 to 8 percent of HIV-1 infected individuals in Cameroon harbored the Group O variant, but five additional strains of HIV-1 subtypes (A, B, E, F, and H) were also found. It seemed that in Cameroon and surrounding countries such as Gabon, the greatest diversity of HIV strains were circulating, suggesting that the virus had had more time to diversify there than elsewhere.

This was not good news. Already we were dealing with HIV-1 and HIV-2: two viruses that created the same pathology but that were genetically quite distinct. We already knew that people could be infected with both different families of HIV viruses at the same time. If, in addition, strains within each of these families diverged to this degree, we were in trouble; it would tremendously complicate the development of a vaccine against HIV infection.

Per molecular clock calculations, Group O seemed to be the oldest virus strain yet identified. It may be even older than SIVcpz, a virus closely related to HIV-1 that Belgian microbiologist Martine Peeters had also found in a pet chimpanzee named Amandine in Gabon. (SIV denotes a *simian*, or monkey, virus and cpz is for chimpanzee.) That discovery came more or less by chance, when Martine and her French husband, Eric Delaporte, were screening monkeys and apes for HTLV human T-lymphotropic virus (a virus that can cause T-cell leukemia and myelopathy/tropical spastic paraparesis in humans). They were working in Franceville at a medical research center funded by the French petroleum company ELF-Aquitaine, and we maintained close contact with them from Antwerp (they sent us samples of gonococcal stains). All of us were stunned when an apparently healthy chimpanzee was found to have a virus almost identical to human HIV. In fact the chimpanzee virus so closely resembled HIV-1 that initially Martine's publication was refused: there was disbelief that this was possible; the viruses were so similar that reviewers assumed it must be due to a lab contaminant. When Martine was back in Antwerp working in our team, she found a second SIVcpz in a chimpamzee named Noah, living in the zoo in Antwerp. He was healthy as was Amandine and is now living in a chimpanzee hotel in the Netherlands.

Many viruses have species-jumped at some point, and these are the viruses that overwhelm their new target group with epidemics, because no immunity has yet developed against them. So this research contributed to exploring the complexity and diversity of HIV, and to showing that its greatest diversity is in west Central Africa, specifically Cameroon and Gabon. I don't like the term "Ground Zero," which suggests a single, explosive event: the transition from ape virus to human virus was more like a kind of seepage. But this place is probably where it first happened.

In addition we found an extremely rapid rate of gene mutation, faster even than the flu virus. We did a lot of work on characterizing virus isolates, and following particular strains as they grew in various populations. For example, in Thailand there seemed to be several, fairly separate HIV epidemics under way, in gay men, heterosexual prostitutes, and injection drug users.

Could we find any kind of antibodies that would neutralize every possible strain of HIV? Some antigen, some piece of envelope protein, that could be a clue to help develop a vaccine? We began working on it in the late 1980s. It was painstaking work—monks' work. And it came up with no practical results. (It was not until 2010 that researchers found any such antibodies.) The reality is that a lot of scientific research goes nowhere. Medical researchers have a saying: if you want quick results, become a surgeon.

In other areas at least, we were getting results. Studies in Rwanda by Philippe Vandeperre, and in Nairobi by Pratibha Datta, Joan Kreiss, and Joanne Embree, told us that children who were breast fed by HIV-positive mothers had a higher rate of infection than children who were not, particularly for women who were newly infected during their pregnancy. This confirmed our suspicion that recent infection led to a high viremia and far higher probability of transmission, but it also indicated that HIV was transmitted through breast milk more often than we had previously thought.

Frank Plummer in Nairobi made another fascinating observation. Some of the prostitutes who had been attending our clinic in Nairobi for years—women who were well known to us, who had literally had thousands of sex partners, and indeed several bouts of sexually transmitted disease—did *not* become infected with HIV. It was almost a Sherlock Holmes–type of observation—the dog that *didn't* bark—but once he started thinking about it, it popped up again and again.

We came up with about two dozen women who appeared to be immune to HIV. Despite counseling, they didn't always use condoms. But either their immune system was better equipped to recognize HIV-infected cells and remove them, or they had fewer target cells for HIV to infect in the first place. The good news was, the women's constant exposure to the HIV virus reinforced their ability to fight the infection. The bad news was, if their exposure was stopped, even for a matter of weeks—if they took a break from sex work and returned to their villages—they lost their immunity. Frank and his team are still working on this immunological exception, and one day it may bring a clue to the development of a vaccine.

Other sex workers, the so-called elite controllers in research jargon, were infected with HIV, but they were somehow generating the ability to hold the viral load in check. Only with such a huge cohort of people, following them closely through time, could these observations have been made. Research still hasn't figured out how to reproduce this ability, but disentangling this other immunological puzzle could open the door for how to develop a real cure, meaning that HIV can be eliminated from the body, or kept under control without permanent antiretroviral treatment.

The Nairobi team was also the first to make a seminal observation that would revolutionize HIV prevention over 15 years later: we found that HIV-positive men were far more often not circumcised as compared to HIV-negative men (in Kenya some men, such as the Kikuyu, traditionally are circumcised, whereas others, such as the Luo ethnic group, are not). Because male circumcision is intimately connected with religion, culture, and ethnic origin, the subsequent multiple observational studies could not exclude that the association was a confounding one. Also, the majority of European and Asian men are not circumcised, and yet there was not this major HIV epidemic as in Africa. We had to wait for three controlled trials in South Africa, Kenya, and Uganda to prove beyond doubt that male circumcision protects men from acquisition of HIV.

These were the years of relentless scientific progress in AIDS, but I felt time standing still and running out at the same time—in particular in southern Africa, where we needed every possible prevention intervention to reduce the continuing horrific spread of HIV.

CHAPTER 14

Changing of the Guard

I N MARCH 1990, Jonathan Mann sent a brief fax to a few dozen of his key allies in the fight against AIDS. He was quitting WHO. The news shook the AIDS community like a blast of icy air. Jonathan was our moral leader; for some he had acquired the status almost of a savior. But he couldn't take Dr. Nakajima's interference any longer. The new director-general of WHO, and therefore Mann's boss, was now controlling Jonathan's travel, public statements, high-level contacts, and budget. In a way some of this could be perceived as normal practice: the Global Programme on AIDS (GPA) had become like a state within a state at WHO. Moreover, Mann was the the public spokesman of AIDS, in fact, to some degree the public spokesman for world health in general. But Mann's AIDS program had to be independent, because that was the only way to jump start HIV prevention programs in as many countries as possible, especially when many of them did not perceive the urgency. A number of donor governments withdrew backing from Mann and started to set up their own bilateral programs, after becoming critical of internal management in GPA and Jonathan's human rights rhetoric. I guess that Jonathan felt backed up against a wall so he choose to leave rather than to try to change the system from within.

A few weeks later Michael Merson was appointed as director of the Global Programme on AIDS. Merson had been at WHO for over a decade, running the program on diarrheal diseases and respiratory tract infections—two of the major killers in the world. He was highly respected in public health circles and was a solid manager, but he had little knowledge of AIDS at that time or of any of the constituencies and activists who were such important actors in the AIDS community. The first thing he set out to do was "normalize" the GPA in WHO's structure, and introduce proper accountability. Since GPA was set up in a minimum of time as a new type of global emergency response, it had all the strengths and weaknesses of a start-up, with the culture of a small nongovernmental organization. This was obviously not sustainable and corresponded less to the needs of the AIDS response after a few years. He faced a working environment that was incredibly hostile: GPA staff rallied against him because they thought he was Nakajima's man, and I admit that initially I felt the same way.

Soon after Merson was appointed I went to Geneva, as chairman of the Steering Committee on Epidemiology, to ask what his plans were and whether we should continue. And I found that unlike some people in the AIDS world, I immediately liked him. He was from Brooklyn, and he had a very different outlook on life from Mann, the Boston intellectual. Merson definitely did not have Mann's charisma, but he was dogged. I found him very connected to reality. Jonathan gave thoughtful and important speeches on human rights, but he hadn't been very engaged with program delivery, and Mike was all about finding the most effective way to impact people on the ground. He was more like an engineer than a philosopher, and to me it was obvious that we needed both.

IN MAY 1990 riots broke out at the university in Lubumbashi. I wasn't there; I hadn't been back for months. But I grasped the situation: President Mobutu used the copper mines of Shaba as his personal treasury, and he was not popular in Lubumbashi. Mobutu's Civil Guard had shot dead several dozen students during demonstrations. According to the Belgian daily *Le Soir*, more than 50 people were killed. Belgium reacted by suspending all funding for Zaire except humanitarian aid, and demanded that an international commission of inquiry be set up. Tit for tat, Zaire expelled several hundred Belgians and cut off diplomatic relations. The EU cut off funds. We had to pull out of Lubumbashi.

We left money for salaries so the local staff could keep working, but we never managed to get the project back off the ground. It had lasted barely two years. We had clearly saved some lives, because now they were screening blood, and there was a functional lab, although that was plundered during the riots. Still, I knew we hadn't worked there anything like long enough for the system to become self-sustaining.

International development programs are highly dependent on a safe, peaceful environment, as well as on the whims of the donor. And although in this case I agreed, politically, with the opinion of the EU to withdraw funds from Mobutu's regime, I also saw that the result was that six months later, blood was no longer being screened for HIV in Lubumbashi. I had tried to send as many tests as possible, being creative with my research budget in Antwerp, but there was a limit to what I could do about the salaries.

A FEW MONTHS after his appointment, Merson asked me to help him develop some strategy ideas for the GPA. At the time we were working a lot in Nairobi on sexually transmitted infections and their role as a portal for transmission of HIV. We had lengthy discussions about the fact that WHO had two completely separate departments for sexually transmitted diseases and for AIDS; they did not collaborate. The sexually transmitted disease department was headed by André Meheus, my old friend from Antwerp with whom I had gone to Swaziland. I tried to get him and Mike together, but although André had a staff of three and GPA had hundreds, André felt that as the nominal head of the world's efforts to fight sexually transmitted disease, *he* should have been in charge of AIDS too. Just as he had when Mann was in charge, he constantly challenged Mike Merson's authority with donors and with WHO's executive board At the same time, AIDS professionals ignored the wealth of experience in preventing classic sexually transmitted diseases, rather arrogantly claiming that AIDS is totally unique and that everything had to be reinvented. I proposed that WHO merge the programs, and I brokered an agreement that GPA's board approved. André's department was made a division of GPA and this made him answerable to Merson. Ultimately the two men came to a decent working relationship. I did not realize it at the time, but I was becoming a kind of health diplomat.

I was named to committees at the European Union, the US National Institutes of Health, to councils at WHO and in Belgium and France, and in Florence in 1991 I was elected president of the International AIDS Society, the association of AIDS professionals. I was laying out agendas for research, evaluating other people's work. I was becoming part of the global AIDS establishment. I think I was quite hard on people working with me—*what is the question we are trying to answer?*—pushing our discussions until the question was staring stark at us. In science, asking the right question is key to finding a relevant answer, just as in life it is the path to wisdom. Sometimes research is like creating a flint: you have to tap it the right way until you find the sharp cutting tool inside the rock.

I reviewed the work of my juniors every six months. Had we maintained quality work? In the very messy world of field studies, had we done the job the way we'd intended? When the time came to break the code and correlate results, or analyze the data and find any kind of statistical associations or their absence, you had to maintain a sure hand. Some people underdo it; they do important work then fail to draw the interesting conclusions. Others go for drama, and that is even worse.

Money came in; work went out. But my administrative skills were definitely at their limit. I had over 100 people working for me in Antwerp alone, and budgets for all kinds of different programs to manage, often with several donors, each with their own rules and conditions. At one point I received a monetary award for my research, and instead of putting it into Nairobi or Kinshasa as I would usually have done, I invested in a much-needed three-week executive course in management at Harvard (everybody else was from private corporations). Like many academics, I was very disciplined with research but a terrible manager of people; my style was very ad hoc and impulsive, pushing problems away until the last possible minute, creating (though I had never seen it that way) stress and chaos. At Harvard I learned to be much more systematic, seeing my staff and collaborators regularly, asking for their feedback, giving positive reinforcement. It was an excellent course, which has helped me a great deal to this day.

IN THE LATE eighties a group of African scientists organized a Society for AIDS in Africa. They asked me to be part of the founding group, which I took as an honor. There had already been three conferences on AIDS in Africa in Europe—the first one organized by Nathan Clumeck in Brussels in 1985, and only one in Africa, in Arusha. The African society was now keen, and I fully supported them to organize these conferences on the African continent to allow scientists from the region to exchange experiences and foster collaboration, as they had far less opportunity to do so at international conferences. Dr. Bila Kapita badly wanted it to happen in Kinshasa. I felt we owed him an enormous, unrepayable debt. Although Kinshasa's conference facilities were not great, to say the least—and despite the mounting political trouble in Zaire—I agreed to organize an international conference on AIDS and sexually transmitted disease in Africa in October 1990, which would be the second to actually take place *in Africa*.

We raised enough money to rent the *Palais du Peuple*, a convention hall graciously donated to Zaire by China and where Mobutu's party held its meetings. But we didn't have much money left over, and particularly needed some to host African participants. So for the first time I had dealings with the market in foreign exchange. I went to the diamond district in Antwerp—tiny shops that are the center of the world diamond trade—where Zaireans had more or less obscure dealings with diamond traders. I had over a hundred and fifty thousand Belgian francs (then about $50,000) with me in cash; it came from the nonprofit foundation of the department.

I had been given the name of a man. I gave him the money. He told me to come back the next day and he would give me the sum back in zaires (the Zairean currency). I was flummoxed and asked for a receipt. Of course he laughed at me: there are no receipts in this kind of market. Still, the next day he handed me the zaires: a small bag full of bank notes. This procedure multiplied by about three the budget I would have had if I had converted it at the official exchange rate.

So I flew to Kinshasa with money packed inside my underwear and socks. Normally every article was meticulously picked through by customs people looking for bribes, but I used my special Order of the Leopard card, and got through customs without a problem.

When I got to Kapita's place he told me the budget that *he* had been promised from the government hadn't arrived yet. The whole thing was looking like a disaster. But a couple of days later a man from the National Bank arrived, with no warning, at Kapita's house with a suitcase full of freshly printed zaires. So this was our budget for our international conference: a bag and a suitcase of cash. Ultimately we had a surplus as far more participants showed up than we had planned, meaning higher income. We used all the benefits to refurbish some of the hospital wards at Mama Yemo Hospital in Kinshasa, construct a clinic in Kapita's home village in Bas-Congo, and to support further education of young Zairean doctors.

I asked the prostitutes from Matonge to prepare food for the conference; I figured it would be a nice income-generating project, and an alternative to sex work. We budgeted enough food for 1000 people; this was how many we were expecting to attend. (In fact, 1500 showed up.) And we decided to have a big party with one of the hundreds of local live bands. But logistics were a nightmare. We had block-booked the Hotel Intercontinental, but it turned out the manager was new, fresh in from Florida, and had no idea of how to operate in Kinshasa. The day before the conference opened people who had reserved rooms were being made to double-up and some were turned away, because the desk clerks were accepting bribes from people who had no reservations. So I made a deal with the manager: I gave him a bottle of whisky and a carton of cigarettes and he gave me the codes of the computer reservation system. I sent the desk clerks home with pay and put Jan Vielfont, my creative and unflappable assistant in charge.

Still, many people had to share rooms. Then the morning that the conference was due to open the WHO regional director showed up. To say the least, he had not excelled in promoting AIDS awareness among his ministers of health and was not supportive of GPA. But I guess our conference was looking like a big deal—it was attracting plenty of reporters—because now he wanted to speak at the opening. I just smiled and said, "Certainly, your Excellency," as I saw this as an opportunity to bring him on board. We needed a broad coalition against AIDS, not just people like me. I gave him the bedroom of the suite I was using as an office. He slept on the bed and I slept on the sofa in the sitting room.

Everything that could have gone wrong went wrong those few days: there wasn't enough food and even the conference bags were stolen. But it was a strong and good experience, because Africans were talking to each other about the problem of HIV, completely frankly. Africans were making the presentations. Amidst a buzz of intellectual activity good science was coming out of Africa. Both Projet SIDA and the Nairobi group made some of the better presentations, and I was proud to give a prestigious platform to our younger colleagues. For the first time some serious global media coverage focused on AIDS in Africa—until then it had all been on AIDS in the West.

AIDS CONFERENCES WERE not only a challenge to organize but one actually threatened my life. In the spring of 1992, I was on my way to the first conference on AIDS in the Maghreb in Marrakech, Morocco—a breakthrough in a region that had never confronted AIDS, nor sexuality in its many forms. After less than an hour the Royal Air Maroc pilot announced in French and Arabic that he had to land the plane for "security reasons." I was traveling with my good friend Michel Caraël, a journalist and social scientist from Brussels with whom I published several papers and books, who immediately said, "Peter, a terrorist attack!"

I said, "No, Michel, he means *technical* reasons," and continued to work on my presentation for the conference, sorting out my slides (no PowerPoint yet!), as this is what I used flights for: to work and read.

But suddenly a voice resonated in Arabic through the plane's loud-speakers, visibly causing panic among the Moroccan passengers, who all looked to the back of the plane. I turned around and saw a man standing there, shouting. He had a cigarette in one hand and some-thing else in the other. A passenger told me that he was a Palestinian who wanted us to go to Baghdad and had requested the liberation of Palestinian prisoners in Israel.

Now I was scared. What to do? The crew told us to stay in our seats, and were magnificent in their handling of passengers who were praying aloud to Allah or God, passing their small children toward the front of the plane. (The passengers were mostly Moroccan immi-grants in France and Switzerland, and many were on holiday with their children.) The crew also sneakily raised the temperature in the plane, to sweat out the terrorist. Then the pilot said that we would fly to Tripoli, Libya, and we circled in the dark above the Mediterranean for what seemed like an eternity. Michel said, "I'm going for the guy! I'm over sixty, I'm Jewish, and he'll kill me first—I've got nothing to lose!" I blocked him from standing up and then returned to my pre-sentation, trying to concentrate—a kind of denial technique, I guess. My other neighbor, a twenty-year-old Swiss woman started getting out of control, not with fear as the rest of the plane, but she became sexually aroused, repeating all the time "Quel beau mec" (What a cool guy!). I told her to shut up, but as Freud taught us, the human psyche has many circumvolutions.

Then we started our descent, and the rumors intensified. Some people recognized Malaga (in South Spain), others were 100 percent sure that we were approaching Tripoli, others saw the Mediterra-nean coast of Morocco. We landed in complete darkness. My heart was beating at superhigh speed, my mouth was dry, and my bladder was exploding. Someone announced that all Arabs could leave the plane, and the others must stay. Oh no, now what? Then someone took my hand and said, "Viens, mon frère" (Come, my brother). It was Guy-Michel Gershey-Dammet, the head of the National AIDS Program in Côte d'Ivoire. While I pulled Michel, the Jew, with me, I mumbled "Waha, waha" (all right, all right) and "Al hamdelila" (God be pleased)—my adolescent trips to Morocco now a lifesaver.

Trying hard to look Moroccan, we ran out of the plane. We were pushed into large armored cars, still in the dark, still not knowing where we were. I was holding hands with both Michels, wondering what would happen.

We were in Casablanca military airport. Troops stormed the plane and killed the hijacker; nobody else was badly hurt. We were driven away and immediately put on a plane to Marrakesh, where we landed after midnight—and there, no support, no apologies, no nothing from the airline or authorities, just a routine wait for our luggage and a struggle for a taxi. Remarkable. In the hotel, I heard what had happened from my old friend Jean-Baptiste Brunet, the head of AIDS at the French Ministry of Health, who had been seated in the back of the plane. A smoker, he had passed cigarettes to the hijacker, and said the man had boarded in Geneva with his arm in a plaster cast, which he had taken off in the toilet, returning with some kind of real or fake bomb device.

I couldn't sleep for two nights after that. I gave my talk at the conference like a zombie and went back to the airport, where I was told that my return flight was overbooked. No seat. This was really too much. I exploded. I yelled at the poor check-in person, "First I am hijacked, and now you are bumping me off the plane! What kind of company are you? I want to see the manager!"

Instead of the manager, two tall men with dark glasses lifted me up bodily and hustled me into a small room. I was shoved onto a chair, and they put a strong blinding lamp on my face and started pushing me—this was at least as bad as the shakedown at Njili airport in Kinshasa. They shouted, "What hijacking? What do you mean?" I told them what had happened, but they nearly accused me of being involved in the crime. Because of press censorship those days in Morocco, no media had mentioned the hijacking.

Finally they let me go, and I was put in first-class to Tanger and then to Brussels. So at least there was some compensation. The changes at WHO and the troubles of setting up conferences quickly faded.

• PART FOUR •

CHAPTER 15

An International Bureaucrat

T HE EPIDEMIC WAS getting worse and worse. My friend Joseph—Willy's partner, who had nursed him through his sickness and death—was also now desperately ill with AIDS, even though I had managed to get him AZT treatment. Everywhere I went there was nothing but AIDS, and nothing but bad news.

By 1991 HIV had infected over 20 million people around the world and killed over 5 million. In Africa AIDS was now the number one killer; every survey result was worse than the previous one. In 10 African countries more than 10 percent of the entire population was infected. Faced with the reality of dying infants, the blank horror of the term "AIDS orphans," hospitals full of dying men and women with AIDS, and much needed professionals passing away because of AIDS, I felt completely impotent. How long could I continue just studying this unfolding disaster? Asking intellectual questions and jetting about to research their possible answers no longer felt like the most useful thing I could do.

I wanted to change the course of the epidemic, not just study it. I was throwing off a lot of my very Flemish underdog type vision of the world: the modesty that can be so fatal to ambition, the assumption that one individual can't really have an influence. Up to then I had felt as if I were still a student—asking questions, seeking, and learning. Now I wanted to act, to take what I could of that knowledge and use it for the world.

Mike Merson, just as his predecessor Jonathan Mann, had begun calling me, asking if I would join him at the Global Programme on AIDS at WHO in Geneva. I said no at first: I had never seen myself as an international bureaucrat. But Mike was persistent. He offered me a temporary arrangement, a broad mandate, a self-defining position as a special adviser. He suggested that I could take a one-year sabbatical from the Institute of Tropical Medicine. We were doing excellent work there, and in the projects in Nairobi and Burundi as well as in Kinshasa, but a year's sabbatical would give me the opportunity to take a step back and think things through.

Meanwhile the political troubles in Zaire, a country nearly as big as Europe, were growing ever more tumultuous as President Mobutu's kleptomaniac rule was under heavy threat from rebellions. In September 1991, exhausted soldiers who had been left unpaid for months mutinied at the army base near the international airport. The civilian population of Kinshasa joined the riot and generalized looting broke out. Homes, shops, and businesses were attacked and over 200 people were killed. France and Belgium sent paratroopers to evacuate thousands of foreign nationals to Brazzaville, the EU suspended aid again, and the United States withdrew all its programs.

Even at the best of times it was often impossible to phone Kinshasa, and of course in those days e-mail was not available outside CERN, the European nuclear research center near Geneva. But our American colleagues at Projet SIDA had a solid communication channel through the US Embassy, and so it was Tom Quinn, in Baltimore, who kept me informed through the weeks of violent plunder in Zaire. Our American and Belgian colleagues were safely evacuated, but Tom and I were concerned about the Zairean staff of Projet SIDA. We were really a big family; seven years of improbable adventures and shared frustration and jokes and joy had welded some intense bonds. Although both Tom and I were glad, in a sense, that there was an uprising against Mobutu, we knew that it could end in horrible bloodshed. There was also the risk that our labs would be looted and that all the work—the people under our care, the sera that we had banked, the data we had accumulated—would be damaged or lost.

It never occurred to me that Projet SIDA might close forever after our colleagues evacuated. I thought we would suspend our work for a month or so, but I couldn't imagine that this massive investment, by far the largest international research program in Africa, would simply end. However, Mobutu's death grip on power seemed unending. The troubles in Zaire continued. In November Tom told me that the US government had decided to pull the plug on the whole project. Our American colleagues would not be going back and all US funding was halted.

Frieda Behets and I tried to argue that we should maintain some kind of presence; in fact Frieda volunteered to *be* that presence. But she was paid by American money, and that meant American government insurance, American legal issues: the answer was no. Projet SIDA's major sources of income were the NIH and CDC, and there was nothing Tom could do about it; legally, his hands were tied. Projet SIDA, a program that had been producing remarkable work and was barely damaged by the looting, came to an end.

Both Belgium and the EU also withdrew all aid—meaning Jos Perriens, our Antwerp clinician, was no longer paid.

The Zairean staff of Projet SIDA tried to keep the program going to some extent, using leftover funds from the Belgian Cooperation Agency and from our department at the Institute of Tropical Medicine. Although our budget couldn't hope to match the shortfall from US funding, I was legally less hamstrung than Tom was and I kept some funds going for a while: Médecins Sans Frontières took over the prostitute clinic in Matonge, and we channeled some money to them. I also tried to organize fellowships overseas for the staff members who had university degrees: laboratory technicians and physicians. Several of them obtained PhDs, and are now in important positions in public health and development agencies and in pharmaceutical companies in the Democratic Republic of Congo, as the country is now known, and throughout the world. They were a remarkable

group of very smart and energetic young scientists, who would probably not have had an opportunity to grow scientifically and professionally without Projet SIDA. As for the thousands of blood samples,
when the situation in Kinshasa stabilized, Skip Francis picked them
up and brought them back to Bethesda.

But the program to screen blood collapsed. All our studies were
cut short. The cohorts we had carefully assembled for long-term
follow-up fell apart. As for clinical investigation—the bronchoscopes,
the diagnostic tools, the care we gave to patients—all we could do
was hope for the best and leave the equipment to Dr. Bila Kapita and
his colleagues at Mama Yemo Hospital. Kapita was stoic—he is not
the kind of man to express reproach—but I knew how bitter he felt
at this abandonment, and I admired his dignity. As of today he is still
in charge of Internal Medicine at the hospital; he is by any standard a
hero, and people with his integrity, commitment, and work ethic are
Africa's future.

The end of Projet SIDA broke my heart in so many ways. It was a
very sobering experience. I think it changed me as a person. I felt the
temporary nature of things.

The next time Mike Merson approached me was in December
1991, at a conference on AIDS in Africa in Dakar, Senegal. This was
by far the best organized conference on AIDS in Africa, thanks to
a dynamic team led by one of Africa's leading scientists, Professor
Souleymane Mboup, a brilliant and humble military microbiologist, a very sophisticated man who trained numerous West Africans.
Mboup was working with Max Essex at Harvard on HIV-2. He was
the primus inter pares of a remarkable group of Senegalese AIDS
experts, who were among the first on the continent to mount an open
and effective response against AIDS, with the full support of then
President Diouf. It was a first step toward "ownership" of the epidemic by Africa's scientific elite and proved highly successful. HIV
prevalence has been kept as low as 1 percent up to today.

The time was ripe, and Mike convinced me: I agreed to take a
sabbatical from my work in Antwerp. I moved the whole family to
Geneva for a year and began work at WHO's Global Programme on
AIDS in August 1992.

WHEREVER I GO, I integrate quite rapidly into the new environment, but at the same time I never feel that I am fully part of the system, one of many contradictions. It goes all the way back to how I felt growing up in my family, my village, my school. That semi outsider feeling keeps me sane, I think.

I didn't see the move to WHO as a radical change in paradigm for my work. I had been going to Geneva so often—every couple of months—that it no longer seemed like foreign territory. And I certainly did not feel that I had suddenly transformed into an international civil servant. I hadn't "sold out." I was an adviser, on a one-year contract.

In a senior position at WHO, I felt I could have more influence on the course of the AIDS epidemic than if I remained in Antwerp. In these days WHO seemed like a very rich organization, though its annual budget of $2 billion was less than that of many hospitals in Europe or the United States; but the AIDS program alone controlled $150 million, and it could reach almost anywhere in the world. In Antwerp I administered perhaps $1 million a year, and the number of lives I could hope to impact was infinitely smaller. I also wanted to learn how an international organization functions.

From the very first week in Geneva I was confronted with the dark side of WHO: because of a "preexisting condition," Greta was not eligible for full health insurance. That the World *Health* Organization would deny its employees something so crucial shocked me. Fortunately we could continue to benefit from Belgium's excellent health care system, but I was bitter about the failure of the employees' union to support my position. A few years later I would stage another battle with WHO's leadership, its health insurance, and the then head of the UN Joint Medical Service in Geneva to ensure that people living with HIV could be recruited as full employees with the same medical benefits as other staff; this took years of trench warfare.

In terms of my job, I had two immediate deliverables: I was to reorganize the research component of GPA and I was to oversee its newly created division for sexually transmitted disease—boost it, shift its management structure, and set its priorities. Suddenly the sexually transmitted disease section had far more money to work with than WHO had ever conceded to it before, and what I intended to do was set up some studies to look at how to integrate efforts to control sexually transmitted disease and HIV, because these were essentially the same populations and the synergistic relationships among the various infections were gradually becoming more clear.

I had heard of an interesting project that worked with prostitutes in a district called Sonagachi in Calcutta, one of the biggest red-light districts in Asia. At first blush, their approach seemed similar to the one used in Nairobi and Kinshasa, only on a much larger scale. So after I arrived at GPA, one of the first trips I made was to India. This was a shock and an inspiration. In those days there was hardly any HIV in India, but in discrete pockets of the population there was a high number of other sexually transmitted diseases, particularly among sex workers and their clients. (There was also an awful lot of denial: the then minister of health told me, "We don't do *those things* here.")

What struck me was the environment that they worked in. Prostitution was on a far larger scale, far more organized and also much more brutal, I think, than anything I had ever seen in Africa. Thousands of prostitutes were tightly packed in huge brothels, many under lock and key; some, in Mumbai, I later saw living in actual cages. Down dark alleys and up dark staircases were small rooms in which two women would receive clients simultaneously, with simple cloths hanging between their beds and children running around. They were often forced, initially, into prostitution by violence, and they were rejected by society as a whole. The misery was palpable. And the smell—I can smell it just writing about it—a stink of sewers and humidity and sweat and genital secretions.

This is the sexual misery of some of the world's poor. As in the Carletonville mines in South Africa, I felt bad both for the men and for the women, but mostly for the women. There was a lot of violence, because men drank before going to a prostitute and then they beat them up. The police raped them in exchange for letting the brothels operate. Their lives were appalling.

The project's organizer, Dr. Smarajit Jana, was an entrepreneurial

Bengali public health specialist who had just started working with these women, providing medical care for them and their children. He also helped them organize themselves into a union, driven and organized by the women themselves, to try to deal with sexual violence, set up groups for information and support, and impose both the use of condoms on clients and a degree of pressure on the brothel owners. The project also worked with the police to change their roles and end a culture of impunity for sexual abuse of prostitutes. It was impressive, and it worked in terms of disease prevention. At the time, this was a very innovative approach, particularly in a region where women had little power in society in general. This and later experiences elsewhere convinced me that we should not only offer good AIDS and STD care and condoms for sex workers and others at high risk but also general social support and protection from violence. AIDS is just one of their many problems, and often not seen as part of their struggle for daily survival, although it was literally about their survival.

Now I had money to provide that kind of support. I had transformed from someone constantly scrabbling for grants and donations to someone who had a budget to distribute. Actually it's not so easy to distribute funds for research: we needed to come up with a rigorous scientific protocol, one that would teach us something that could be applied to other projects in the world.

These days, a remarkable HIV prevention program called Avahan is taking this comprehensive approach a step further. It is run by Ashok Alexander and other former staffers from the McKinsey consultancy firm, with funding from the Bill & Melinda Gates Foundation. They added social marketing techniques to induce sexual behavior change and use of condoms, just as if they were selling soap—looking at their customers, their tastes, the package design, the promotion campaigns; they use feedback just as if they were salesmen, looking at where sales go up or down, taking regular surveys on peoples' beliefs and actions; they use microplanning and mathematical modeling techniques, mapping out in detail where the sex workers operate. Most public health programs lay down a five-year plan and don't deviate, but Avahan's approach has been extremely successful in bringing down new HIV infections across the most at-risk populations in India, working with India's successful national AIDS program. Sex in India, like most societies, doesn't have what's called a "normal distribution": most people have not much sex and a small group has a lot of sex, but every so often there's a link between them. So by focusing efforts on the peak populations—so-called core groups—there's basically a very cost-effective impact on the overall level of infection in the general public too.

This model is very much true in Asia and most other countries, although less, perhaps, in southern Africa, where because of the very high prevalence of HIV today, if you have sex for the first time at age eighteen there may be a 20 to 30 percent chance that your first partner is already HIV positive. In any case, in India overall prevalence has gone down through this work by the private sector working hand in hand with government action, reaching the prostitutes who are most difficult to engage with. It's a remarkable sight to see these ex-McKinsey men and women with MBAs squatting in the slums, talking to women who are among the lowest members of society. Most of the women don't even have a birth certificate, thus no identity. One of Avahan's first efforts is to make sure the women have a national tax card, a form of ID that allows them to open a bank account, and know how to use their mobile phones to transfer money into that account and send it to their family, where it's more difficult for their pimps or steady partners to lay their hands on it.

No well-written consultant's report or scientific article can capture the complex realities of both the lives of, say, sex workers in India and of the challenges of real-life AIDS programs, where the devil is in the details. Even now, whenever I visit a country or program, I make it a point to sit down with people on the front lines of HIV prevention and treatment, and with those we work with and for: be it sex workers, truckers, orphans, women in sweatshops, construction workers, various people living with HIV, drug users, homosexual men. In 2011 I spent half a day talking to sex workers in Mumbai—there wasn't much work for them that afternoon because India and Pakistan were playing a historic cricket match—and I asked, "What has this program done for you?" One woman responded very succinctly: "I am a person now." Not only could she manage her own money, but she was also in an organized group, so that if a client, or a group of policemen, beat her up she could call on other women for help. She could also be much more easily reached with HIV prevention messages.

Finally, because the vast majority of patients in India go to the private sector for medical care, and there is an enormous number of unlicensed practitioners of medicine, we decided to do a small study of what that meant in terms of current treatment for sexually transmitted disease, using dummy patients. We sent patients to doctors, claiming they had various manifestations of sexually transmitted disease, to see whether the physicians actually examined them and what they prescribed. Many physicians, it turned out, didn't even ask the men to drop their pants to look at their symptoms; and they often prescribed something completely useless. We added providing professional education to our list.

We needed a practical strategy. I recalled the work of Maurice Piot (no relation), whose work I had encountered in medical school. Working at WHO in the 1960s, Piot had analyzed the tuberculosis treatment protocol and uncovered its shortcomings. Although his results were published, his systematic process had been long ago forgotten. For our purposes, let's say 100 people have syphilis, and the first sign of that is a genital ulcer. Now assume 80 percent of people with a genital ulcer go to see a doctor. Maybe 80 percent of doctors, in such cases, prescribe a syphilis test. Then 80 percent of the patients do the test, pick up the result, go for a follow-up visit, and receive a prescription for treatment. Of those, 80 percent receive a prescription for the correct treatment, and 80 percent of those apply the treatment correctly, and are cured. We're already down to 32 people, and we've been working with some very conservative approximations. We needed to do better.

Classically, WHO would have concentrated on that final stage: writing treatment guidelines for selection of the correct antibiotic and the proper application of treatment. But there's a whole chain of events involved, including health-seeking behavior and adequate training for medical staff, which was being completely neglected. And the outcome of that neglect on the community is high transmis-

sion of disease, and, in the case of gonnorrhea or chlamydial infection the outcome for the individual may be sterility, lifelong pain, or
even death.

So when I got to Geneva I unearthed this old model and tried to
apply its lessons in Africa and in Brazil. We set up research projects
and developed and evaluated guidelines for detecting and treating
sexually transmitted disease in resource-poor environments, doing it
very systematically, just as I had in Swaziland, but now for all sexually
transmitted diseases. These became official WHO policy, and you
still see these posters of flow charts on the wall in primary health-
care clinics around the world. So in a way, just in doing that one
thing, we influenced the world and the way that millions of people are
cared for. The reality is that 90 percent of STDs can be treated by a
semiskilled nurse or midwife, and this frees up specialist physicians
for more complex cases while ensuring the care is properly delivered.
It is not particularly romantic or adventurous work, but setting up
policies and norms can have huge impact on people.

Next, I went to Zimbabwe to take a look at another high-risk setting for sexually transmitted disease, in so-called high-density urban
areas. In 1993 Zimbabwe had the highest HIV prevalence in the
world, with nearly 30 percent of pregnant women being HIV positive. In colonial times, every township was built around an administrative center, with a school, a health center, and a beer hall. The beer
hall was owned by the municipality and was a main source of income
for the town. Just by talking to people it became obvious that the beer
halls were the center for sex. They had two sections, serving Western or traditional beer. Traditional beer was served in plastic buck-
ets, with various sizes measured in gallons. Several people shared a
bucket, and when they got drunk enough they went off and had sex,
some of it paid for.

My idea was that it just wasn't good enough to wait for people to
appear at the health center with incredible abdominal pain, in the
case of women, or huge ulcers on their penis, if men. We should go to
the beer halls. Doctors don't usually do that. But I wanted to see condoms promoted in and around the beer halls—posters in the toilets,
baskets of free condoms, and various types of entertainment trying

to focus on prevention behaviors—just as we had done in the eighties in Antwerp and elsewhere to reach gay men in the bars. Today this seems like a very obvious idea, but traditionally in public health we expected people to come to health services instead of taking the services to the people.

Then I went to Thailand, where AIDS was beginning to ravage groups of sex workers, and their spouses and children as well as their clients. My purpose was to advise the government about whether to authorize a phase 1 HIV vaccine trial by Genentech, which was looking at a candidate vaccine. (For the cognoscenti, this was based on an antigen to the gp-120 component of the HIV envelope.) There was not much evidence available from animal models to inform the decision of whether to move into wide-scale human studies or which candidate vaccine to select. Thailand already had an active and high-quality biomedical research community, and the vaccine work was led by Professor Natth Bhamarapravati, a dengue specialist from Mahidol University, and young researchers from the Thai Red Cross, such as the infectious disease physician Prahpan Phanuphak and anthropologist Werasit Sittitrai. The need was certainly there, as Thailand then had Asia's most serious AIDS epidemic, with 4 percent of twenty-one-year-old army recruits being HIV positive in 1994. We agreed that there should be no substandard for research in Asia, that WHO would have to review all proposed study protocols before the Thai committee in charge would make a decision, and that the country should not engage in HIV vaccine trials without a strong involvement of the affected communities and a good communication plan. Following the visit, I brought a number of researchers together in Geneva to think about it, and the consensus, though not unanimous, was that we should move to early trials in humans—provided there were guidelines for safety and ethics. It turned out that this particular vaccine candidate did not protect against HIV infection, but when used in combination with another antigen, it may offer some protection, as found in another trial in Thailand in 2009. These results still require solid confirmation but, in any case, the immunization schedule is so complex, requiring multiple injections, that it is impractical for large-scale use. What matters at this stage is understanding whether protective immunity is feasible or not as a concept.

Vaccine trials are tricky: among other things, it is unethical to expose people to risk, so you have to set up a placebo group and a "vaccinated" group, and educate *both* about HIV prevention, knowing that someone, sadly, will take a risk sometime. What you're seeking to measure is the possible number of infections that could be avoided: an odd and difficult concept to quantify. Making global recommendations was the sort of work that only a multilateral agency could do, as it is in principle not bound by the interests of a particular nation or industry: convene the best people in the world; lock them up in a room with food, water, and an agenda; and have them come up with a consensus of recommendations, independent of personal interest. (This implies careful selection of the participants, obviously, and a clear understanding of possible conflicts of interest.)

At WHO I could set agendas, and one of my private obsessions in HIV research was vaginal microbicides. These are creams and ovules that women could put in the vagina (they already existed as very imperfect contraceptives). I felt strongly that to stop the heterosexual spread of HIV, we needed to find an effective prevention technique that women could control because they might not be able to insist that their partners use a condom. Microbicides had shown some indications that they could be effective to some degree in protecting against gonorrhea, and in 1988 I had received a grant from AmFar, the American Foundation for AIDS Research, founded by Elizabeth Taylor and Mathilde Krim, to begin looking at whether any spermicides could be effective against HIV. We had done a baseline study in Kinshasa and in Antwerp to evaluate spermicide use among prostitutes: Do they prefer ovules or vaginal tablets? Which product of spermicide do they prefer? Is frequent use associated with side effects? This was, I believe, the first study of microbicides for HIV prevention. It gave rise to a larger study of actual effectiveness by Joan Kreiss in Nairobi that found that use of a sponge containing nonoxynol-9, a spermicide, actually *increased* the risk of HIV acquisition in women, because it caused vaginal irritation and abrasions.

Still, I hadn't given up on microbicides, so when I got to GPA I convened a meeting of experts on the subject. We initiated a study with another product, which was another failure. This is how science advances—it isn't blind, but it falters and zigzags. It was not until 2010, after several studies had failed, that a vaginal microbicide gel containing tenofovir, an antiretroviral drug, was shown by the remarkable science couple Quarraisha and Salim Abdool Karim in South Africa to be about 40 percent effective if used once before and once after sexual intercourse. This proof of concept, indicating that the right microbicide could prevent HIV in women, at last opened the door for intense work to refine and intensify the gel to attain more complete protection.

Through my interest in a vaginal microbicide for the prevention of HIV, I met a genius of drug development, Paul Janssen, the founder of Janssen Pharmaceutics in Belgium. He had discovered more than 80 new medicines that made it to market—more than anybody else in the world. He was not only a master chemist and pharmacologist, but also a very erudite Renaissance man, who had thought about the big problems of history and society, and had a flair for opportunities. For example, his was the first Western pharmaceutical company to start a joint venture in China, in Xian, as early as 1985. Paul became an unfailing friend; we were each other's sounding board, and we had incredibly stimulating discussions about drug and microbicide development and how to bring medicines to the people in developing countries. His passion was to discover a simple and inexpensive treatment for HIV infection, if possible a cure, for use in poor countries. I could not always follow his drawings of chemical structures of potentially new molecules, and often had to look up what we had discussed in my pharmacology textbooks (this is before there was Google).

At my request, Paul invested in various pharmacological preparations of a vaginal microbicide. "Dr. Paul," as he was affectionately called by all his employees, died in 2003 in Rome when attending a meeting of the Pontifical Academy of Sciences to celebrate its 400th anniversary. A former student of mine, Dr. Paul Stoffels is now realizing Dr. Paul's dream by bringing new potent antiretroviral drugs—some of which we discussed at our meetings back in the 1990s—to market through Janssen of Johnson & Johnson. That is how long it can take to bring a new medicine on the market. Stoffels too is an exceptional entrepreneur. He founded the pharmaceutical start-up Tibotec, which my lab in Antwerp closely collaborated with early on. Tibotec developed not only new antiretrovirals, but also a much needed drug against tuberculosis. It was the first TB drug developed in over three decades, because the pharmaceutical industry basically had not invested in such research despite the increasing development of resistance.

In 1994 nearly every AIDS patient died. This was true all over the world, but in the worst affected populations in Africa, the suffering of patients was inhuman and people died much faster. They had no access even to painkillers or drugs to treat their opportunistic infections. As the Global Programme on Aids we could simply not continue to focus only on prevention: we had to provide solace to patients with AIDS and ensure that the treatment of opportunistic infections would become affordable. Janssen Pharmaceutics was the first pharmaceutical company willing to help. It offered millions of doses of ketoconazole for use in Africa.

Ketoconazole is an effective treatment for the painful fungal infections of the mouth and throat that make swallowing nearly impossible. This was a breakthrough: we had made a first, if very modest, step toward international support for care for people living with HIV. We still had to set up a distribution system to accredited hospitals in sub-Saharan Africa, which took much longer than I had anticipated. However, our biggest challenge to conclude the deal was not with Janssen, but with WHO's lawyers, who came up with one objection after another—the organization was not ready yet to deal with the private sector.

AFTER A WHILE I found that I was thriving at GPA, somewhat to my surprise, and that I was feeling useful. People took my advice seriously, and the officials I met (and hoped to influence) could have, at the very least, enormous nuisance power and, at best, could make important decisions. Brokering ethical guidelines for vaccine trials or recommending treatment guidelines for STDs meant that I could actually influence public health policy and shift health practice. Each step might be slow, but the ripples it created were extremely broad and their impact was real.

I started to become interested in decision-making at the highest level. I could see how political AIDS is, because it's not just a matter of making sure the labs function and the condoms are available and the drugs stay cold: you need the political heavy lifting to have an impact. Budgets must be voted, and political will and leadership are vital. I was still planning to go back to Antwerp, because I had no desire to become part of the WHO system. But I felt that, here and now, I could deliver something very specific: rigorously constructed research projects that bound together medical queries with social science to generate the best possible evidence for policy and decision making on AIDS. When Mike Merson asked me to stay on for another year, I agreed to do it.

Mike was by now embroiled in discussions with the UN Development Programme (UNDP), the World Bank, UNICEF, UNESCO, and UNFPA (the world population agency), along with a group of representatives from major donor countries and nongovernmental organizations, about how to transform the Global Programme on AIDS. This task force, set up in April 1992 by the GPA board, was frustrated by the lack of coordination of international work on AIDS. The positive news was the that the big agencies of the UN system had begun to set up AIDS programs when AIDS started to affect their areas of activity, but as is typical of the international development system, they were doing this separately, almost in competition.

There were some strong personalities in charge of this process: Jim Sherry at UNICEF, Elizabeth Reid at UNDP. They had their own views on what to do and frankly they worked at loggerheads, laying down different policy recommendations, sometimes accusing Mike Merson of not understanding the epidemic. And all the agencies were going to the same donors and saying give the money to *my* agency, not to *his*. The donor countries, meanwhile, could see that WHO's political and administrative modes of doing business were creating enormous inefficiencies, because routing everything through regional offices meant that a lot of money was stuck there. There was no question of corruption but often sloppy management and entrenchment: "If I'm not running this project, it won't happen." At the same time, major development agencies such as USAID and the UK's Department for International Development were setting up their own AIDS programs and were reluctant to channel their money through the multilateral system over which they had less control and which did not directly benefit their own international development organizations.

There was a lot of disenchantment with WHO, which was under attack for its weak management, although Nakajima was reelected as director in 1993 in controversial circumstances. This coincided with a move by many Nordic countries and others to reform the whole UN system, and re-creating a new world AIDS program became a big part of that. In addition, a number of developing countries, especially Uganda, felt that not enough money was coming into Africa to deal with AIDS: again, the bottom line was that AIDS needed a higher profile international organization. However, the other UN organizations wanted only a weak secretariat-type coordination: they wanted to continue to run their own shows. It was an unpleasant and conflicted process. But I was not involved in this gestation. I didn't feel emotionally or intellectually interested in it: I thought of it as Intra-UN equivocation. All I knew was Mike would disappear for a few days for some traumatic meeting with an interagency task force that was shaping the skeleton of a new UN program on AIDS, with a lot of drama and accusations of double-dealing and personal ego.

It was Hans Moerkerk who first approached me to become head of the UN's new, reformed AIDS entity. ("Entity" was the word employed, since even the word "agency" was the subject of bitter conflict.) Hans was the chair of GPA's board, since the Netherlands was the number one donor to AIDS. (The Dutch have a big development-aid budget, and they target it strategically: they don't just sprinkle it uniformly, they target a handful of issues and deliver a big packet.) Hans was a "nuchter"—as we say in Dutch—no-nonsense and stubborn Dutchman, who was in charge of AIDS at the Ministry of Foreign Affairs and had been at the forefront of the gay rights movement in his country. We had become friends over the years, when he negotiated more money for AIDS, sought resolutions against blocking people with HIV from entering countries such as the United States and China, and demanded stronger accountability for international assistance. He is a smart diplomat and activist all rolled into one. But I said no. This was not for me: I was not interested in becoming a UN bureaucrat.

Then Jean-Louis Lamboray, a Belgian public health doctor who had worked for the Belgian medical cooperation in Zaire, came to town. He and I had worked on setting up outposts of Projet SIDA in Kinshasa, where we could recruit people for our research projects, add a nurse or two, train them, beef up the lab, set up a functioning freezer. Jean-Louis had joined the Africa division of the World Bank, and he was probably the first World Bank person to be interested in the impact of AIDS on African economies. In fact in the late 1980s he organized a presentation for me at the bank in Washington. In my simplistic view of the world from Kinshasa, where I had seen the influence of the World Bank in Africa, and the failures of WHO, I felt that the bank was the international institution to get on board for the fight against AIDS. So I went to Washington to make the case. It was a complete failure. I was urging the bank to invest massively in AIDS control, but the audience was mostly economists and they blew me out of the water with arguments about cost effectiveness and return on investment. I had not come with a plan, with bullet points that said each specific action will save this many lives and thus produce this positive impact on the economy. I hadn't considered the hardnosed arguments you need to influence policy—a mistake I tried not to make again.

In any case, Jean-Louis represented the World Bank in this interagency task force preparing this new UN entity on AIDS. One day when we met for lunch he said, "We're going nowhere because there's no leadership and all the players are trying to undermine each other. We need a leader. What about you?" Again, I said, "You must be joking." Director of a UN agency? I thought this meant someone with great political clout, someone charismatic, who could move politicians to make decisions and mobilize donors. I didn't think these were my strengths.

But when I heard who the main candidates were, I thought, Why not? It was a mix of UN officials and politicians, such as Dr. Jesus Kumate Rodriguez, the then minister of health of Mexico, who was a friend of both Dr. Nakajima's and of James Grant's, the UNICEF director (who, incidentally, in 1990 objected to include a reference to AIDS in the Declaration of the Rights of the Child). Dr. Kumate was already seventy years old and quite conservative in his views on issues such as condom promotion. There was also Elizabeth Reid from UNDP, who was very committed to the AIDS cause, and other internal UN candidates.

I had real practical familiarity with AIDS on the ground. I knew quite a lot about a range of AIDS issues: epidemiology, microbiology, vaccines, policy, clinical, lab. I had a whole network of contacts and experts to fall back on, I was connected with activists, and I was fast acquiring experience at how to function within the UN. On the downside I lacked political experience and was not familiar with the ins and outs of the United Nations system—but that could also be perceived as a plus. So, I didn't one day wake up with the illumination that I wanted to direct a UN agency.

At the time in 1993/1994 I was going to Tokyo almost every month. I had made it a condition of my employment at WHO that I could continue to function—without pay—as president of the International AIDS Society, to prepare the first of the annual international AIDS conferences to take place outside Europe and North America. In those days these conferences influenced the AIDS agenda in a big way, and the work of structuring them meant you could spotlight specific aspects of the epidemic and key figures of the AIDS movement because that is what it had become: a movement. My agenda was to bring in more of a developing-country perspective to these conferences, as that had not been the case until now, and to bring in networks of people with HIV and community organizations because I felt strongly that this could not be just a conference of doctors and scientists: the people affected and the NGOs definitely had a major role to play in the AIDS response, and were often the driving force to obtain budgets and get things done. I also promoted caucuses, one on women because they were marginalized at these conferences, not only as presenters in plenary sessions but also in terms of women's issues. People were missing a whole dimension of the epidemic—not only heterosexual transmission, aspects of coerced sex, and risks in stable couples, but also how to ensure that HIV prevention programs would not perpetuate macho behavior.

Setting up the 1994 Yokohama conference was a huge headache, but it made me appreciate and like Japanese society, food, and culture. Japan bans prostitutes and drug users from the country, and nearly all Asian and East European countries even ban methadone—a form of substitution treatment for heroin addiction. We anticipated activists with big placards reading "I'm a junkie," possibly derailing all media attention from the substance of the conference to the protests. We needed to be sure everyone would be allowed entry into the country to participate in the conference and we needed to train police and staff in hotels and restaurants that you can't get HIV infection from serving someone at a table and so on. It was a huge opportunity to raise awareness about AIDS in Japan, where the AIDS agenda had been dominated by a scandal around contaminated blood substitutes for patients with hemophilia, and where traditionally the voice of marginalized communities has been very weak or even suppressed. I was the middleman between the official deciders and the international activist community, represented by the Canadians Richard Bruczynski and Don de Gagné, and a nascent Japanese NGO community, which included activist civil servant Naoko Yamamoto and my good friend Masayoshi Tarui, a professor of philosophy and expert on Immanuel Kant at Keio University. We convened every night at Daigo's, a bar—actually just a tiny counter for six customers—near Shinbashi train station. Since that time, whenever I am in Tokyo, I go to pay my respects to Master Daigo and drink a few glasses of his sake with the Japanese who used to work with me in UNAIDS, such as Hiro Endo, Tammy Umeda, Chieko Ikeda, and Aikichi Iwamoto.

Decision making was painfully slow. Then one day I was invited to a shadow committee. It turns out, decision making for the conference occurred in circles. You have a big circle, where nothing is ever really decided, but ideas and opinions are gathered. Within that is a smaller circle, the first shadow committee, where fewer people are seated but have more power. I got to a second shadow committee eventually, and I still don't know whether there was another, third, core group.

The conference was opened in great pomp by Crown Prince Naruhito and his wife Crown Princess Masako in August 1994, in Yokohama—after Nagasaki, the first port in Japan opened up to the world in the nineteenth century. It went very smoothly, although there were no scientific breakthroughs announced. These were the terrible years of HIV's continued, apparently unstoppable expansion—years of despair among scientists because of the lack of progress in research. During the conference I began talking to friends from all over the world (some of whom I hadn't seen for a while) to discuss whether it would be a good idea if I became a candidate to direct the new UNAIDS program—and if I were a candidate, whether I had any chance of winning. I found it was particularly my African colleagues who encouraged me, even pushed me. People like Ibrahim Ndoye, the head of Senegal's national AIDS program, Ugandans Noerine Kaleeba from the AIDS Support Organization TASO and Sam Okware from the Ministry of Health, and Winston Zulu, a Zambian activist living with HIV. They trusted that I would speak up for them.

I had a very strong bond with the NGO community and with "Positive People," as they were called, and they were also encouraging. Then I met with Franz Bindert, a German official whose main concern was that a European direct the new program. He said that if I were candidate, Germany would support me; moreover, because Germany held the rotating presidency of the European Union that semester, they would try to rally all EU member states behind me. I wasn't as familiar then as I am now with the backstage power calculations of international politics, but even so, I knew that this was big news. I also spoke with other possible candidates for the job, such as my old friend Helene Gayle, who was then head of AIDS at USAID, and is now president of Care International, one of the largest private aid agencies in the world. Helene had extensive public health and AIDS experience and was popular with AIDS community groups in

Africa. We agreed we would stay in touch, whatever happened, even if, as she predicted, "it would be dirty."

After the conference ended I took a week off in the Alps with my family and thought about the prospect seriously. I thought about how the new UN agency might work. I weighed the kind of impact it might have. Then I called Hans Moerkerk to tell him I would be a candidate to direct the new body. I added that I wanted to win.

CHAPTER 16

Sharks in the Water

G ENEVA IS A small town, and the UN is a big industry there. By mid-September the air was full of rumors about who would be nominated as director of the new AIDS program. Various AIDS constituencies and governments were becoming exasperated by the lack of progress by the cosponsoring agencies, and a consensus had emerged that the process wouldn't be able to move forward until a leader for this new entity had been identified. Most countries were looking for a political hot shot: a well-known figure, a bankable name.

The selection of this director started accelerating at various levels. The Netherlands and Germany formally announced that I was their candidate, soon followed by Denmark and then my own country. (In other words, I certainly was not promoted by my own country first, as is so often the case with candidates for top UN jobs.) As president of the European Union for the second half of 2004, Germany rallied the European Union behind me. Soon thereafter, and to many people's surprise my friend Ibrahim Ndoye from Senegal told me his government had officially decided to back me.

Ibrahim also told me that a marabout—a holy man—had slaughtered a bull for my success, just to be sure. And he sent me a special amulet by DHL, a wad of nonwoven cloth, tied up with thread. There's something inside it, though I have no idea what. As a scientist I'm kind of embarrassed to say this, but I have carried that thing beside a photo of my children in my wallet ever since; it has done a good job so far.

Slowly, but surely, support for my candidacy grew, including from nongovernmental organizations, which had become very vocal in the process. By now, every day brought new rumors about candidates. They destabilized me a little in the beginning, but I decided to keep my head cool and continue with my work at WHO, while quietly lobbying for the new position. I had nothing to lose: deep down I was still hoping that a more competent person than I could be found for what increasingly looked like it was going to be a brutal job. I also still had a job waiting for me back in Antwerp, as the new dean of the Institute of Tropical Medicine. On three occasions I was approached to renounce my candidacy and become the deputy of someone else— as, in the words of one official, they "would need someone to do the work." I thanked them politely and said that if they wanted me to do the work, I could just as well be the actual boss. At no stage did I feel it worth compromising, just to have a well-paid, prestigious job.

Quite a lot was at stake. It was by no means clear whether the new AIDS program would be a weak secretariat—basically a powerless coordinating administration—or a strong body that would, in effect, lead the whole UN system's effort against AIDS, with money and political clout. The task force of UN agencies was still paralyzed, still calling it an "entity," and there continued to be a high degree of animosity about the process. On October 6, a director from UNDP told me that if I were appointed, "UNDP and UNICEF would do everything they could to sabotage me." I suppose they saw me as a puppet of WHO, a technical guy from the medical establishment. Even if I hardly knew them, mid-level UNDP and UNICEF staff treated me with hostility. I'm still puzzled by their behavior, in which mediocrity was often matched by arrogance.

I began to actively campaign. In October I went to New York, to a meeting of the Economic and Social Committee, ECOSOC, a broad and often weak UN body that oversees economics and social affairs. I had never even heard of ECOSOC before, but it was the body with the mandate to formally establish the new agency. I also went to Washington, to visit the World Bank and see policy makers at the US departments of State and of Health and Human Services. In the eyes of the UN system Washington is kind of a lion's den because it is the powerhouse of the world and the largest contributor to UN programs, given the size of its economy. Even though some were implying that US support for the AIDS agency would depend on having an American as its director, I knew after my trip to Washington that I could work with the United States and vice versa.

Then, in a surprising turnaround, Dr. Nakajima and his regional directors at WHO said they would nominate me, together with Dr. Kumate from Mexico. Many Ministries of Health, which had been waiting for WHO's guidance, followed suit. I was then in a very delicate position: I didn't want in any way to be perceived as a pawn of Nakajima's; I had a very different vision on what this new program on AIDS should do. But I understood that without WHO's support no director would be successful.

The appointment was due to take place on December 12, 1994, at a meeting in New York of the executive heads of the Committee of Cosponsoring Organizations. A task force cochaired by Nils Arne Kastberg, a Swedish diplomat, Bernadette Olowo-Freers, a Ugandan diplomat, and El Hadj As Sy, a Senegalese NGO leader organized the process. They sent out what they called a "straw poll" to all governments and well over a hundred NGOs, asking them who they would like to see as director. (This was unprecedented, as far as I know, in UN history.) On December 2, I had lunch with Helene Gayle, and she said she was giving up her candidacy for personal reasons, and would support me. On December 5, the results of the poll came in and I was flabbergasted to see my name so prevalent among them. I did not know a soul in many countries nominating me. In the meantime, at an AIDS summit hosted by the French government, several countries said they supported my candidacy.

On the morning of December 12 I was drinking tea at the Belgian Permanent Mission across the street from the UN headquarters in New York when I got a call asking me to come immediately to the meeting of the Committee of Cosponsoring Organizations, which was deliberating on the new appointment. I had no idea this would be part of the process, but the principals of all six agencies—WHO, World Bank, UNDP, UNICEF, UNFPA, and UNESCO—wanted to interview me. I had never even set foot at the UN headquarters, and I didn't think to ask for the number of the meeting room. When I got to the building, the security guards wouldn't let me in, and I literally just ran past them. (This was before September 11!)

But then I had no idea where the meeting was. So I asked someone what floor the secretary-general's office was on; I thought a meeting that important, creating a new UN agency, must be on his floor, the 38th. Finally someone told me it was taking place in the basement—a bad level, I thought, to start a new career. I arrived half an hour late, a nervous wreck. I was asked a number of tricky questions, as each agency wanted to test me on their area of interest, sometimes in conflict with the viewpoint of another agency. The atmosphere was not pleasant. This antipathy had more to do with institutional territory than with my person as such. As individuals these were mostly decent and competent people, but the whole process of creating this new agency—whose mission was, let's not forget, to help people—was in fact driven by the urge for control and power.

I waited in a corridor for about 15 minutes and then someone came out and said I had been chosen. I went back in, everybody congratulated me, and then they promptly moved to the next item on the agenda. Although I was still digesting what had just happened to me, I realized that the discussions were basically aiming at undermining the position of the newly elected director—me. Dr. Jim Sherry, who represented UNICEF (the director, Jim Grant, was by now terminally ill), passed me a very small piece of paper with five words on it: "Peter. Congratulations, you poor bastard." Friendly and cynical at the same time—at least he was honest! I decided on the spot that I wanted to hire him.

Around noon Nakajima took me up to meet UN Secretary-General Boutros Boutros-Ghali, who formally appointed me. We shook hands for a photo; I never saw him again. We then went straight to a press conference where the first question was, "What is the position of this new UN program on masturbation?"

Another trick question. A few days before, President Bill Clinton had fired US Surgeon General Joycelyn Elders because, when asked whether it would be appropriate to promote masturbation as a means of preventing young people from engaging in unsafe sex, she replied, "I think that it is part of human sexuality, and perhaps it should be taught." Outrage ensued. Such a trivial episode; so surreal, that something like that could end a fine career. But I knew about it, and realized that the wrong answer could be the swift demise of my own, ultrashort career at the UN. So I responded to the reporter's question very blandly: "To a scientist it's very clear you need two to transmit the virus. Next question, please." I dodged the bullet—my political skills were already improving.

Then CNN asked me for a live interview for the world news, strung me up with some equipment, and the world was told about my existence and that of this new program that would stop the AIDS epidemic. So began the media whirlwind that would last for 14 years. There was no return possible, and I knew that. I went back to my hotel and wrote in my notebook: "I feel very lonely, with an impossible task."

THAT NIGHT I couldn't sleep: hundreds of thoughts tumbled through my head at once. Eighteen million adults and over a million children were estimated to be living with HIV already, and the curve was rising steeply. In the following 12 months, over 3 million more people became infected worldwide. China began reporting fragments of data in what was soon recognized as an epidemic of at least 30,000 to 50,000 people who had been infected when selling their blood in the central Henan province, through criminally careless medical practice. No country in the world could be called "safe" from AIDS, and it was absolutely unclear whether HIV would start spreading as fast through Asia as it was already doing in Africa—we simply did not have the information. There was no treatment. The lives of people with HIV could be prolonged, but they could not be saved. And there was not even the beginning of a real vaccine.

We needed a massive, very profound behavioral shift. People around the world had to learn to use condoms at every sexual encoun-

ter except confirmed monogamy—whether they be acts of prostitution, of homosexuality, or casual encounters of any kind. Injunctions
to "just say no" whether to curb epidemics of syphilis, smoking, gam-
bling, or heroin use—were ineffective.

Community-based programs like TASO (The AIDS Support
Organization) in Uganda, on the other hand, showed evidence of real
success. Noerine Kaleeba, a physiotherapist whose husband Christo-
pher had died from AIDS, founded TASO with the help of 12 others.
Noerine was a superlative communicator and organizer, with a vitality that her country badly needed; Uganda had just emerged from
years of civil war, only to be confronted with deaths from another
man-made disaster, AIDS. Like the White Ravens support group
whose board I had worked on in Antwerp, these programs helped
individuals in small and large ways, through acts of human solidarity
and compassion and they provided the street-level intelligence that I
knew was crucial to any kind of program for social change. They supported each other, helped each other to endure the sorrow of illness
and the mourning of loss.

Noerine's TASO organizers were also fun, joyful people, who
understood their society. For example, Noerine understood how difficult it was for people to even say that they were infected with HIV, and
developed the idea that you should select one safe person—perhaps
even a stranger within the TASO network—and share with that person until you were more at ease with the words necessary to informing
your partner. TASO also launched a very moving project of "Memory
Books," where parents with HIV would write down their lives in a
book, so that their children, once orphaned, would carry the fullest
possible memories of their parents. I will never forget witnessing a
conversation between a woman with HIV and her daughter, with the
mother recounting her life and discussing her unavoidable death with
striking calm and dignity. It was human strength at its best. I thought
then—not for the first time—that AIDS not only brings out the worst
in people, with rejection and discrimination, but also the best.

TASO grew and grew, and at last tally, had provided treatment and
support to 200,000 Ugandans with HIV and their families. Groups
like these are the unsung heroes of the AIDS epidemic, and I very

much wanted to sing them. In fact, I wanted to tie in community organizations like TASO to all the work we did, globally as well as within countries. People needed to realize that AIDS was different. In the worst-affected countries, AIDS transmission was a matter of national emergency, because it was clearly set to grow exponentially, and its long-term and ripple effects on society were exceptional. In contrast to most diseases that affect primarily children and the elderly, AIDS affects young adults, the productive and reproductive elements in society; their children are orphaned or infected, and grandparents then have to take care of them. Even if we could stop AIDS today—stop it cold—in terms of new transmissions, it would still have a massive impact on generations to come. The economic losses and social damage may go far beyond anything that we have seen with an epidemic in modern times, and nobody's going to resuscitate the parents of the 14 million orphans.

So we needed to get world leaders on board. All the UN agencies needed to pull together into a joint approach to AIDS programs, with much less duplication and far less back-biting. We needed to have more powerful responses to AIDS in every country. We needed to develop policy guidelines for HIV prevention and treatment: people were hungry for examples of policies with concrete results on the ground. I also wanted us to develop a more solid epidemiological data base. I didn't want us to actually *run* programs on the ground, as I felt strongly that this should be done by local governments, NGOs, and businesses, rather than by expensive international civil servants who may actually undermine local capacity by doing work that locals could do. But I felt we could have real value added in terms of coordination, evaluation, and policy guidance, because the supranational nature of the UN meant we could have a better view of what worked than anybody in only one country and that we should become the world's advocate for AIDS, mobilizing desperately needed resources. As I saw it, we might be small but we should be smart and powerful—a catalyst for support to developing countries.

All this and much more went through my head in that first sleepless night after I was appointed. The only real measure of our success would be in lives saved.

THE DAY FOLLOWING my nomination, I went to UNDP, UNFPA, and UNICEF (which are based in New York), as well as to some of the permanent missions to the UN. Immediately the discussions moved to battle stations. The heads of cosponsoring agencies had determined that the new AIDS program should be staffed by people on loan from existing agencies. In other words, I would get people whom they did not want to keep or people whose loyalties lay with the agency that was paying their salary. They also wanted the cosponsoring agencies to determine our budget envelope, which WHO would "administer." It was my belief that this was intended as a consolation prize for Nakajima, since in losing AIDS, WHO had lost its biggest program. Furthermore, the cosponsoring agencies wanted us to "coordinate" their work, but to have no programs on the ground. We would be a simple secretariat, as weak as possible. The impact we could have would be close to nil.

Now my mind was buzzing with questions of a wholly different kind. First, I wanted clear answers to two basic questions: who was my boss; and who had the right to hire and fire. The agency heads wanted me, as director of the AIDS program, to be accountable to them. But I argued—throwing around some big words here—that we were necessarily accountable to the people and, that, in UN terms, meant governments. My boss should be an executive board, on which should be represented not only governments but also people with HIV and NGOs. I wanted to feel answerable to the people who were on the front line. Such a thing had never been done in the UN, but for me it wasn't in any way ideological. I just felt I couldn't do a good job without them; anyone who was part of the problem needed to be part of the solution. I also felt that I could not at the same time coordinate the programs implemented by six UN agencies and be accountable to all six of them; it was a recipe for nonaction and nonaccountability.

Moreover, I wanted the new program to have a small but strong central core, and I wanted us to have offices in affected countries that would be in charge of all the UN's AIDS efforts, staffed by people whose one main commitment would be fighting the AIDS epidemic.

There were also a number of other key questions to thrash out: what size budget we would have at our disposal; how to channel it to countries and for which priorities; how to fully involve the various UN agencies; how to create incentives for them to act together in a harmonious way. It was going to be a long, long series of battles. I had only 12 months in which to define, structure, and staff a new UN organization: we were due to become fully operational in countries in January 1996. I suspect that WHO was convinced I could not pull all this off, and that after a year or so it would all just go back under WHO's control. So I kept a low profile and let them feel secure in that opinion, until such time as I would be strong enough to raise my head. As I had heard in Seattle, "The first whale to surface is the first to be harpooned!"

It was around this time that Kofi Annan sent me a note. He was head of UN Peacekeeping Operations back then, and I had met him to discuss the problem of peacekeepers infecting Cambodian women with HIV. (Later, of course, Kofi Annan became one of the most distinguished secretaries-general of the UN.) His note read: Congratulations, Peter, and now let me tell you a story. There's an old man who feels he is going to die. He tells his two sons to come with him into his fishing boat and row him out into the ocean. When they row so far that he can't see the coastline any longer, he tells them to stop and says, "Sons, let me tell you. The sea is full of sharks. So don't fall into the water. And if you fall into the water, don't bleed." Good luck, Kofi.

I've thought about that story many times as I've navigated the choppy waters of multilateral politics.

MY PRIORITY WAS to bring together a top-notch team to build the secretariat in Geneva and a few key countries. At first most of my core people came from the WHO Global Programme on AIDS, in particular the administrative staff, who initially were firm guardians of WHO orthodoxy. They knew how to move money and job descriptions through the system, but it took several years for them to develop a more can-do culture and shed their determination to follow WHO's habit-encrusted rules. I sought advice from trusted friends who had not been involved in the interagency negotiations, which I now had the dubious honor of chairing.

Dr. Seth Berkley, who was then working for the Rockefeller Foundation (now head of GAVI, the Global Alliance for Vaccines and Immunization), offered me the use of their center at Bellagio, in northern Italy, for a brainstorming seminar. So in February 1995 I invited a dozen people there for a weekend. It was a discreet little meeting, and we had agreed that there would be no record or report: this way people could speak their minds. I subsequently used this approach occasionally, particularly when I felt we were not progressing enough or when there was the need for a strategic reorientation. I wanted to hear from all kinds of people and take in what they thought we needed to do. Besides Berkley, attendees included Jim Curran, head of AIDS at the CDC; Jean-Baptiste Brunet, the young French epidemiologist with whom I had first visited Lubumbashi; Rob Moodie, an Australian public health specialist who had worked at Médecins Sans Frontières; Roland Msiska, the director of the Zambian AIDS Program; and Winston Nzulu, the Zambian activist who encouraged me to run for the job of director; Susan Holck, seconded from WHO, who introduced me to the labyrinth of the UN; Noerine Kaleeba, founder of TASO (which had just received the prestigious King Baudouin Prize for Development); and Werasit Sittitrai, a Thai AIDS activist with the Red Cross. Three representatives of development agencies instrumental in the creation of our new entity of UNAIDS also joined us: Jo Ritzen from Norway, Joe Decossas from Canada, and Hans Moerkerk from the Netherlands. Not a terribly representative group, but one I could rely on.

Basically we designed the core functions and structure of the new program. The first task was going to be to develop solid data on HIV and AIDS, worldwide, from Albania to Venezuela. This wasn't just for policy purposes. Sure, sound epidemiological data and mathematical modeling are essential to any kind of program, scientific or sociological: they predict, they illustrate, they are the baseline for evaluating the impact of what we do. They also give power: if you're trying to coordinate the work of many actors, it's key to be at the hub of knowledge. To make AIDS a higher priority in terms of policy and budgets, we needed an unimpeachable reputation for solid facts; they make the news, and they give credibility.

But although hard evidence would be the basis for our policy and advocacy, we decided that, with the exception of epidemiological estimates, we would not engage in research as GPA had done. It seemed to us that we would have no comparative advantage against major AIDS research funders with huge budgets, such as the US National Institutes of Health or the European Commission, and that it could divert from our core business. So our first core functions besides political and resource mobilization were knowledge translation, policy development, the evaluation of policies and action on AIDS, and dissemination of real-world good practice regarding AIDS.

Clearly our program had been set up to coordinate the UN system's response, but I strongly felt that coordination for coordination's sake is not only a brain killer but also would probably lead the new program to focus exclusively on administrative and political processes, with hardly any impact on people's lives. It was neither my strong point nor my interest. I felt our most important test would be how well we could support the response against AIDS in countries, on the ground: this was how I wanted to be judged. All of us agreed that if we were just a Geneva-based headquarters, we would be irrelevant, both for governments and for the people, and we would fail. So who should we work with: The Ministry of Health? of Finance? The office of the president? The nonprofit private sector? Business? Community groups? Religious entities? Where would our office be based? How would it relate to the rest of the UN system, and other administrative/political bodies?

Thus we planned a series of regional consultations on every continent, to be organized by Dr. Purnima Mane, a tiny, energetic woman from Mumbai with an infectious laugh, originally a social scientist specializing in gender issues and a real powerhouse. I saw these meetings as a kind of customer research: we wanted to bring together a wide range of actors, from governments and academics to people with HIV, and ask them, "What do *you* think will work?" They would also serve to try to wake up local leaders and provide an opportunity to market the new program and to recruit staff.

Finally, we picked out a name for the new program during the Bellagio meeting: UNAIDS. The working title had been "Joint and Co-sponsored United Nations Program on HIV-AIDS": you couldn't even figure out the acronym. "UNAIDS": that says what it is. My then fifteen-year-old daughter Sara designed the logo: a red ribbon over the UN logo, as straightforward as a teenager can be. But when I went to the first formal meeting of the cosponsoring agencies in Vienna and proposed the new name and logo, there was an instant bracing of spears. I ultimately won the case, but it was a struggle, and this pattern became a very familiar one. Sometimes the issues involved were trivial, but I often felt like Gulliver: hobbled and hamstrung, when what I needed was help. At the end of the Bellagio meeting I asked Rob Moodie and Werasit Sittitrai and Noerine Kaleeba to join our staff. It was a real act of faith for them, and I am still grateful that they took the professional and personal risk to come in and help build something that really only existed in a few UN documents. Rob organized our country work, Werasit our prevention activities, and Noerine marshaled community-based action.

Dr. Susan Holck, Mike Merson's former right hand, was key at helping me maneuver through the UN and the endless coordination meetings of the first six months. Then Sally Cowal, a former US ambassador with a long history of postings in various countries, joined as director of External Relations. Sally was dynamite: one of the first female US diplomats who could stay on after she got married (until 1972, married women were banned from the US Foreign Service), she brought us some much needed diplomatic savvy, even though patience was not her greatest feature. She was good friends with some heavy hitters in the US government.

My senior team was complete when Dr. Awa Coll-Seck, an infectious disease professor from Senegal, joined us as head of policy, strategy, and research. Awa was one of those strong West African women, brave and pragmatic. She had pioneered AIDS care in her country and was a cofounder of the Society for Women and AIDS in Africa. (She became minister of health and then head of Roll Back Malaria.) I also asked Jim Sherry, whom UNICEF had tried to use as a kind of killer dog against our program, to change sides and become my special adviser, as I felt that my lack of experience of the UN system and of multilateral politics might prove to be a major handicap. He was a real political operator, with the capacity to see through apparently innocent proposals at a glance, and was of tremendous help in building a broad coalition against AIDS.

So by April I could count on a dynamic and totally committed team. We felt we could move mountains. Each of them then recruited the best possible people in their respective fields. We recruited people from a wide range of backgrounds—academia, economics, journalism, activism.

Quite early on, I also ordered media training for all the senior staff, including myself. I wanted UNAIDS to speak clear, loud, and with professional skill. We needed to catch the media's attention and use it as a foghorn—a massive, permanent amplifier. I thought about how astutely Jonathan Mann had done this, translating the problem to journalists, ordinary people, and politicians: getting them to see what they had to do. In contrast I was, initially, frankly useless at interviews, particularly on live TV. I found them terrifying; and I was still a typical academic, accustomed to stating the problem, discussing what methods you use to examine it, and what the conclusions might be. By the time I reached my main message most people had switched to another channel.

The media training was an eye-opener, an awful experience: the trainers videotaped us in fake interviews, and played them back so we could see every excruciating hesitation and mistake. Then they told me to forget everything I might have learned ever since medical school about the scientific method. Throw it away. Cut to the chase—when you start talking, begin with your conclusion. If there is still time left, know exactly what other message you plan to deliver. Carve the message out so it's clear. And always mention the "brand": UNAIDS. I found this first experience of professional communication illuminating; it was as if I had always been waiting for it. And I think I became quite good at the job of coming up with messages and campaigns and themes: Making the Money Work; AIDS—A Problem with a Solution, The Three Ones, and so on.

Retrospectively I made a mistake when I agreed that our program could be housed within the WHO campus. I also should have broken more radically with their bureaucracy. The old WHO Global Programme on AIDS was still operational, and it was very uncomfortable to cohabitate between the past and the future: It also didn't help that many of their staffers knew they would be losing their jobs. I will be forever grateful to Stefano Bertozzi, an American physician and economist, who was a master at neutralizing the tactics that were deployed by Nakajima and some of his regional directors to undermine us. After Mike Merson left WHO to become dean of Public Health at Yale University, Stefano Bertozzi had the unenviable task of closing down GPA and that included firing several hundred people. Stef was a man for all seasons and all tasks—a brilliant, if sometimes absent-minded, man and the finest multitasker over the age of thirty whom I have ever met. I sought his advice on major professional issues since we met in Kinshasa in the early nineties (He is now director of AIDS and TB at the Bill & Melinda Gates Foundation in Seattle.) But together, we wasted too much time fighting with the Nakajima administration, which would flex its power over almost every issue, from recruitment to procurement and travel.

There was also constant, never-ending friction with the cosponsoring agencies. It started the second week of January, when I called a meeting of colleagues in charge of AIDS in the six partner agencies to discuss how we would work together. This was a sobering experience. When, at the start of the meeting the facilitator asked participants the classic warming-up question about their expectations for this meeting to define the new program, the UNDP representatives bluntly said, "No expectations whatsoever." The tone was set.

To everything I proposed, the task force of UN agency representatives at first responded no. I had to recoup, get political and diplomatic support, and go to their principals, who were far more open and reasonable than their staff but initially made little effort to stop their tiresomely bad behavior. In fairness, it was not all ill will; much of this opposition had to do with different institutional cultures—people were not used to thinking outside their own organizational box. But the constant bickering was extremely draining. I remember one meeting where WHO, UNICEF, World Bank, and UNDP could not even agree on what the words "program" and "programming" meant.

WHO wanted to keep all the technical work under its control. The World Bank emphasized in a memo that the "Bank would assume no liability" for UNAIDS and wished to have "as little involvement as possible." So throughout my tenure the best-case scenario was essentially a juggle between conflicting oppositions, avoiding the disaster that would ensue if there were ever a united front of all UN organizations against us. Asking for consensus in our favor would have been utopian.

Today I know that we were far ahead of our times in terms of working across the very diverse United Nations system, with its nearly 50 agencies and organizations covering about every aspect of society and governance. We were trailblazers for what is now a much more unified UN system than in the midnineties. But at times I truly felt I was meeting the worst aspects of human nature. For people working in the UN to be so wrapped up in issues of turf and ego and bureaucratic politics, in the face of a human problem so terrifying, well, it was deeply demoralizing and profoundly unethical. It made me angry and more determined at the same time. My skin grew a little bit thicker every day, and I reminded my team that we should not be deterred by bureaucratic guerrilla warfare, but build out the organization, solidify support outside the system, and never forget that we were privileged to be working on one of the most important challenges of our time. That kept us going.

I missed contact with people on the ground and with people living with HIV, and decided that my first public appearance as executive director of UNAIDS would be among them. So in March, I attended the seventh annual conference for the Global Network of People Living with HIV/AIDS in Cape Town—the meeting taking place for the first time ever in Africa. By then, 850,000 people were believed to be HIV positive in South Africa alone: approximately 2 percent of the population. I spoke at the opening, together with Thabo Mbeki, then Nelson Mandela's deputy president. He gave a remarkable speech, and although he was a little stiff, I thought we had a good rapport. I

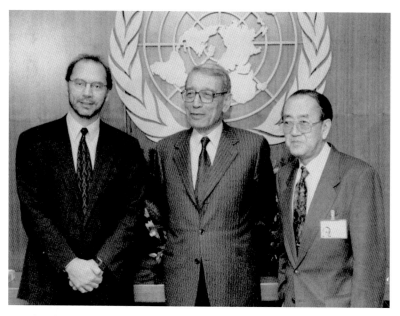

The day of my appointment as executive director of UNAIDS with Boutros Boutros Gali and Hiroshi Nakajima, December 1994 *(UNAIDS)*.

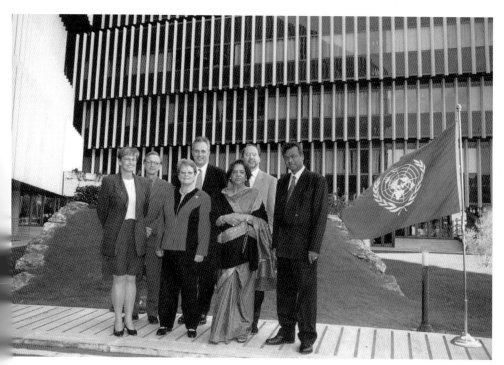

The UNAIDS Committee of Cosponsoring Organizations, Rome, 1999 (Carol Bellamy, Gro Harlem Brundtland, Mark Malloch Brown, Nafis Sadik, Mat Carlson) *(UNAIDS)*.

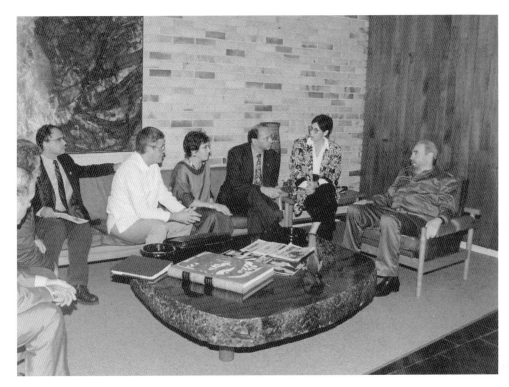

In Fidel Castro's private office, Havana, 1999 *(UNAIDS)*.

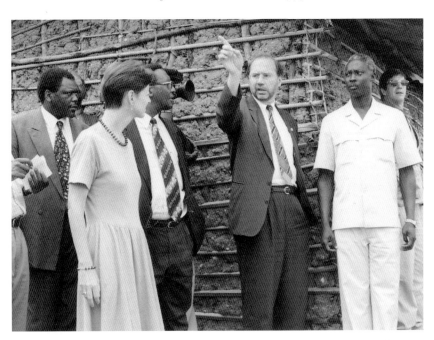

Visiting a refugee camp in Burundi with Kathleen Cravero, UN resident coordinator, and later deputy executive director, UNAIDS, 1999 *(UNAIDS)*.

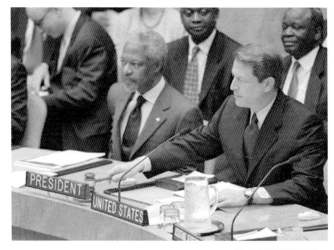

First ever debate on AIDS at first session of millennium of UN Security Council with Vice President Al Gore and Kofi Annan, January 2000 (*UNAIDS*).

Exploring the truck cabin during a visit of an HIV prevention program with truck drivers in New Delhi, 2000 (*UNAIDS*).

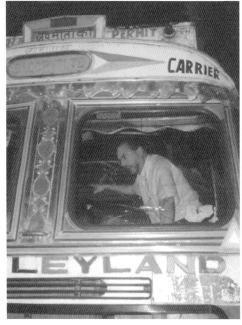

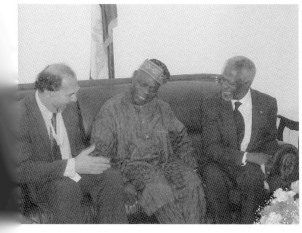

A relaxing moment while preparing for the OAU Special Summit on AIDS in Abuju with President O. Obasanjo and Kofi Annan, 2001 (*UNAIDS*).

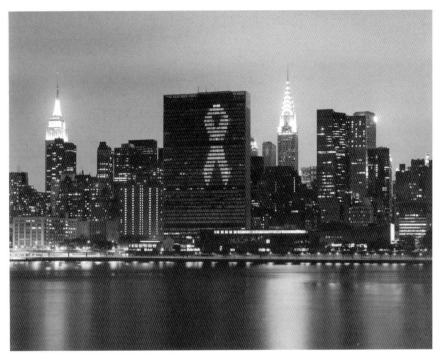

The red ribbon on UN Headquarters for the UN General Assembly Special Session on HIV/AIDS, June 2001 *(UNAIDS)*.

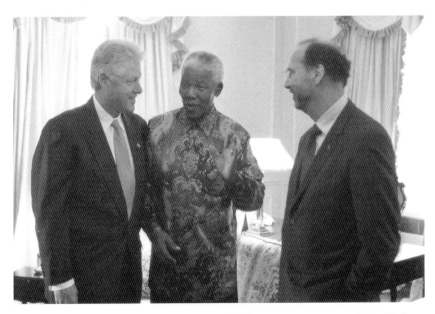

Discussing AIDS strategy during the Children's UN Summit in New York, 2002, with former Presidents Bill Clinton and Nelson Mandela *(UNAIDS)*.

Meeting with sex workers association (WATCH) in Kathmandu, Nepal, February 2003, just after losing the election in WHO (UNAIDS).

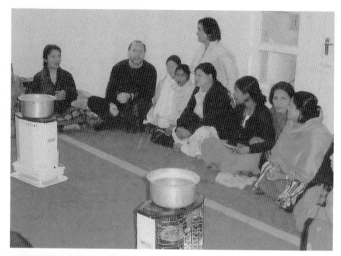

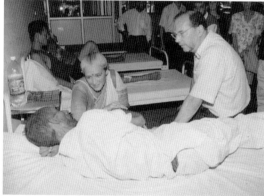

Visiting with a patient with AIDS, together with Nafisa Ali. Ashraya Holistic Care Center in Rajokari, India, 2003 (UNAIDS).

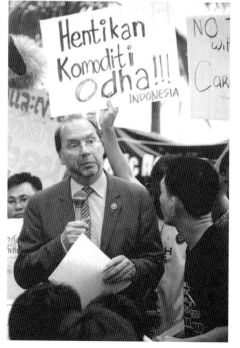

Heckled by AIDS activists at the International Conference on AIDS in Bangkok, 2004 (UNAIDS).

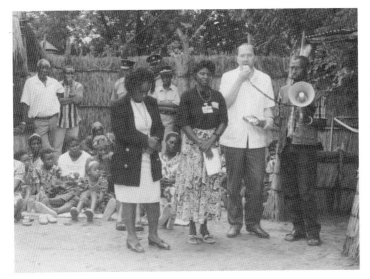

Livingstone, Zambia, 2003: addressing a community gathering on AIDS *(UNAIDS)*.

Returning from rehabilitation-through-labor camp for women in Guongdong Province, 2004 *(UNAIDS)*.

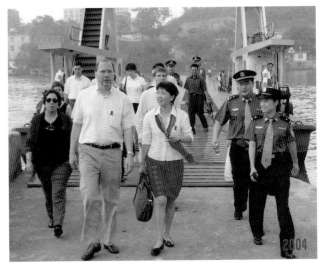

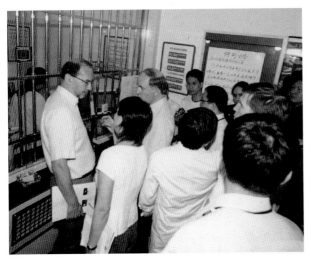

Visiting a methadone maintenance clinic in Yunan Province, with Ambassador Randal Tobias, 2005 *(UNAIDS)*.

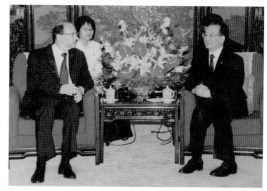

Meeting with Premier Wen
Jiao Bao, June 2005 *(UNAIDS)*.

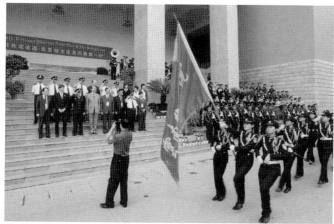

An unanticipated review
of the troops at the Yunan
Police Academy in Kun-
ming, 2005 *(UNAIDS)*.

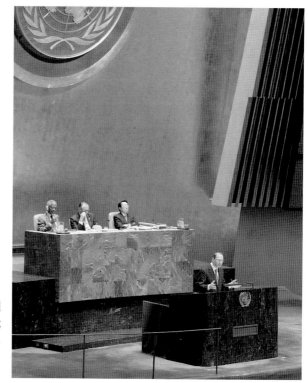

Addressing the UN General
Assembly in New York, 2005
(UNAIDS).

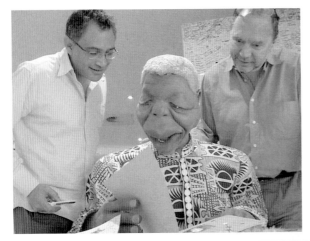

Together with Zacki Achmat, founder of TAC (Treatment Action Campaign) at the Nelson Mandela Foundation, Johannesburg, 2008 (*H. Larson*).

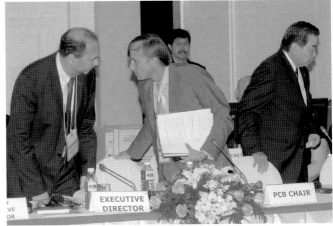

My last UNAIDS Board meeting with Ambassador Mark Dybul as chair, December 2008 (*UNAIDS*).

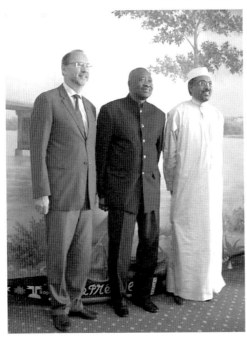

Formal photo with President Amadou Toumani Toure and my successor Michel Sidibé, Bamako, Mali, December 2008 (*H. Larson*).

was impressed by his sharp mind and thought he would be a strong, perhaps key ally for us. (Sadly the future proved me very wrong.)

Those were historic days in South Africa. The ANC had taken power barely a year before, following the end of the apartheid regime that had ignored the looming HIV epidemic. There was immense hope of a better future for all. During this visit, I had intense discussions with AIDS activists and people with HIV from the country and all over the world. I met some remarkable people, each of whom made history in their own right—from Quarraisha Abdool Karim, who was struggling to set up a national AIDS program at a South African Ministry of Health still dominated by the old guard, to Edwin Cameron, an Afrikaner gay man living with HIV who is now a justice at the Constitutional Court. The AIDS activists' expectations of UNAIDS were enormous—completely out of line with our resources—but I returned to Geneva re-energized and more convinced than ever that a successful response to AIDS would not be possible without restoring the health and dignity of people with HIV. I was determined to make that our core goal.

I headed back into the trenches of political rivalry. As it turned out the UN member states did not agree on the mission and structure of our new program. So despite my total lack of experience in this field, I had to try to broker political agreement among governments with hugely diverse interests. UN civil servants are not supposed to interfere with political processes, but if I hadn't gotten directly involved, the agenda would have ground to a halt. It was a superfast learning curve, but fortunately I could count on a number of friendly diplomats in the New York missions of countries such as Belgium, the Netherlands, India, Brazil, Uganda, Canada, Sweden, and the United States. One of my main allies turned out to be Ambassador Richard Butler, the Australian president of ECOSOC. He was a bulldozer, very committed to UN reform in the sense of agencies becoming more transparent and more accountable to member states, and he felt the UN agency heads were trying to pull a fast one. He pushed through an ECOSOC resolution that made it clear that I was principally accountable to the member states—not the cosponsoring agencies—and set up a "Programme Coordination Board" to oversee our work.

People were running around with calculators, working out which countries should be represented on the board; it ended with 22 countries, 5 each from Africa and Asia, 2 from Eastern Europe, 3 from Latin America and the Caribbean, and 7 from Western Europe and North America. Once again, I was adamant that the board include representatives from community groups and people with HIV. Not surprisingly, China and Cuba objected strongly to membership by nonstate actors. But unexpectedly the Netherlands also had objections, because they felt that only states legally represent people and can be held accountable. With a promise that this would not be a precedent for other UN governing bodies, five nongovernmental organizations were invited to take part, one each from Africa, Asia, Latin America, North America, and Europe. This was the first of a still unfinished series of exceptions made in the name of the urgency and exceptional nature of the AIDS epidemic. UNAIDS is still the only UN body with nongovernmental organization representatives on its governing board, albeit with no voting rights. (The NGOs, led by As Sy from Senegal, actually rejected voting rights, as they did not want to be held accountable for every decision made by UNAIDS.)

Thus on July 3, 1995, the Economic and Social Council of the United Nations unanimously voted to establish the Joint and Cosponsored United Nations Programme on HIV/AIDS. This resolution was our founding charter, and it laid down language that I could work with. For example, WHO would not "administer" the UNAIDS budget but would give "administrative support" to us. Trying to explain this kind of hair-splitting nuance to friends, I could see they thought I had gone insane—how could I waste my time on something so petty? But by now I knew that in international relations, every tiny word could make a huge difference.

We had hired staff, listened to people, strategized, and set down a legal foundation that I could work with. Now I had to raise money. But at the first meeting of our Programme Coordination Board, in July, there were major disagreements over our budget. I think some countries saw UNAIDS as a way to cut their contribution to the UN and expand their own, bilateral programs on AIDS. I was asking for $140 million for two years. (This was, incidentally, far less than what

Mike Merson's budget at GPA had been.) I felt strongly that we should have a small number of UNAIDS staff in countries as advisers and coordinators, but that we shouldn't directly pay for national staff and cars: governments needed to take responsibility for AIDS programs as part of their own agendas. So I reduced expatriate staff and cut the four-wheel drive cars and per diems. I wanted to see a Kenyan person coordinating AIDS work in Kenya, paid by the Kenyan government. (Of course donors wanted this too, as this was a time of declining aid budgets after the end of the Cold War.)

Still donor countries were divided about what UNAIDS should do. The United States felt we should implement AIDS activities on the ground, and the United Kingdom argued that we should be limited to a small group of coordinators and knowledge disseminators in Geneva. Developing countries and NGOs wanted a large budget, the majority going to their activities: When I became aware of the intense lobbying by the United Kingdom and other donors in the board room, I feared that the board would decide on a budget that would make it impossible to do our job. I asked for time out. This was one of those moments in life where I could not give in. I walked right up to the lion's den.

As the delegates milled around the atrium I went over to Dr. David Nabarro, who represented the United Kingdom; he was a capable and influential man, but he was also the main opponent of our budget. A circle with half of the delegates formed around us, and you could have heard a pin drop. What I said was, roughly, "Listen. You donors set this up. If you want it to succeed, you fund it right. Otherwise I'm out. This budget is not negotiable, because you're setting us up to fail. And if we fail, *you* will be held accountable for failing to do anything against the biggest epidemic in recent history." I actually shook him by his lapels. (David and I later became very good friends, by the way. He is now the senior UN coordinator for avian and human flu.) Before it got out of hand, Nils Kastberg, the Swedish diplomat who had headed the initial task force that set up UNAIDS in 1994, intervened to get us to simmer down, and ultimately the board gave us a mandate to develop a budget within an indicative range from US $120 to $140 million for the biennium 1996–1997.

It was lean, but we felt that we were on the cutting edge of UN reform. We were a taut little mammal in a world of brontosauruses.

We decided to launch UNAIDS at the UN in New York on World AIDS Day, December 1, 1995. Sally Cowal had ensured the participation of high-level diplomats, including Madeleine Albright, who was the US ambassador to the UN. The event was not a success. I was scheduled to make a speech in the ECOSOC chamber in the main UN building. We had invited all the delegations and a number of celebrities and activists. But we had failed to tell UN security that we were expecting outsiders, and many guests could not get past security on time. So we launched not with a bang but with a whimper.

By this time, over 20 million people were living with HIV globally. Perhaps the most serious epidemic known to humankind was now the focus of a staff of 100 people in a little office in Geneva.

Earlier that year, I had received a phone call from the private secretary of Albert the Second, king of the Belgians (and interestingly, not king of Belgium). He asked whether I would accept to be ennobled as a baron. This had definitely not ever featured in my life plan, and in fact I had mixed feelings about the persistence of these titles. But I recalled the saying about such honors—"one doesn't ask for them, but one doesn't turn them down"—and accepted; later, thinking about it, I found that I actually *was* honored. As my motto I chose "KEN UZELF: *Know yourself.*" But apparently I also needed a coat of arms. I wanted a red ribbon, symbol of the AIDS movement, in it. This led to some trouble with the Belgian Council of Nobility, as the red ribbon did not exist when the medieval rules of heraldry were established. But in the end they gave in. So now I have a coat of arms: an AIDS ribbon with two hands of solidarity and a pair of Nubian demoiselle cranes.

CHAPTER 17

Getting the Basics Right

F OR UNAIDS TO be able to deliver a credible message, we needed solid data on HIV; success stories; clear strategies about what to do against the epidemic; and a country presence. This, in addition to our efforts to start building a broad global constituency for the AIDS cause, was the agenda for our first couple of years.

As a scientist, I wanted to make sure that the facts about the occurrence and spread of HIV not only showed authorities and the media what the situation was in a given country and worldwide but also established a baseline against which our impact could be measured. WHO was previously responsible for numbers and epidemiological surveillance. What that meant in practice was basically that someone at WHO waited until the Ministry of Health filed a report, and then the WHO person typed it into a form: "Ah, 23 cases of AIDS in Romania." I had seen this essentially passive system and knew it was profoundly inaccurate, leading to massive underreporting, especially considering the deliberate, official denial of reality: "We don't have an AIDS problem *here*." Tardiness and poor standardization further sapped the data of any useful value.

I asked German epidemiologist Bernhard Schwartländer to set

up the system. Bernhard is a prince among epidemiologists, with an archetypical *grundlichkeit* (thoroughness), and his remarkable ability to bring people together turned out to be key to success. He designed a system in which every country's population was assessed and a sample size determined, so that, for example, 300 pregnant women (as a surrogate for the sexually active population) would be tested for HIV in a number of locations, in addition to samples of patients in STD clinics and other high-risk groups. We managed to obtain reports at standard times in a standard way, training people in almost every country to do the surveillance work, with quality-control checks on the data. It's not a perfect system but I'm aware of no disease where this was done at this scale.

We worked hand in hand with Daniel Tarantola, Jonathan Mann's right hand; he had moved to Harvard University, and they had started their own estimates of AIDS in the world. We also partnered with the US Bureau of the Census, which put together an impressive data bank on HIV. Finally, we asked the best epidemiologists in the world to independently review the methods and data, to make sure they were sound. The last thing we needed was to confuse the world with different and conflicting estimates of HIV!

Even though Bernhard's system was strong, getting the facts right took way longer than I ever expected. First there was the poor status of surveillance systems in many countries. Testing everybody in a country to find out the exact number of infected people is neither feasible nor affordable, so we had to rely on relatively small samples in the population, and then extrapolate to a country as a whole—just as opinion polls are done for people's voting intentions, for example. Estimating the spread of HIV was complicated because the virus is not distributed evenly across the population. Since it is sexually transmitted, it clusters in higher-risk groups. So representative samples of the so-called general population may not be useful; in many places HIV mainly affects gay men, or truck drivers, or drug users.

We also encountered political denial about HIV estimates, but it's hard to argue with vetted data and dead bodies. Countries like Russia, China, India, and South Africa at some point all accused UNAIDS of inflating figures. Russia, and in fact most former USSR countries (with the notable exception of Ukraine), simply did not want to deal with AIDS: at the time, the tidal wave of HIV that would swamp heroin users across the former USSR was still invisible and unreported, and they wanted to keep it that way. Even when Russia began to face an explosive HIV epidemic, in the late 1990s, it downplayed the problem.

China too wanted initially to control all information; and Chinese officials were reluctant to change their statistical systems to indulge our concept of scientifically established random sampling. The population is also so vast that any estimate is a huge challenge, with provinces of over 100 million people. Later, however, China became very open about its AIDS problem.

India has a long history of disputing the statistics of international organizations, and its politicians in the early 1990s were not yet open to discussing risks associated with prostitution, homosexuality, and other taboo subjects. As it turned out, our estimates were not solid enough, and in 2007, when better local data became available, we announced a major decrease in our estimated number of people with HIV in India. We also had big problems with South Africa's reports, especially after 2000, due to President Mbeki's denialist policies. Some European countries were sloppy about their contributions, too—surprisingly even more so than a few of the African countries. For example, as late as 2004, we received forms filled in with pencil from Austria.

Still, we checked and re-checked the data, to obtain some of the best global estimates on a single disease. I felt it was vital to be transparent and guided by the science, not by the imperatives of advocacy or communication, so when we had got the numbers wrong, we said so.

But numbers weren't enough. For UNAIDS to get its message across, we needed success stories, because to mobilize money and convince policy makers, it's not enough to demonstrate that something is a really bad problem. If you can't do something about it, and it's a hopeless case, then what's the point? As my old professor of social medicine in Ghent used to say, "a problem without a solution is not a problem." I started scouting for success stories back when I was at the Global Programme on AIDS. Then, Uganda and Thailand reported—basically, anecdotal evidence—that programs to shift people's sexual behavior were working. We saw this among gay men in some North American and European cities in the 1980s, but never in the developing world. So now I jumped on it.

Our data confirmed that the incidence of new HIV infections was declining slightly in both Uganda and Thailand—very different countries. In both countries, the key to this success was swift and early political action. In Uganda, President Yoweri Museveni had learned of the AIDS epidemic in 1986 from Cuban leader Fidel Castro, who helped him overthrow the previous Ugandan dictatorship. Museveni was a frank man—a former farmer and pastor, whose speeches were full of rural images and a very down-to-earth grasp of the world. He told me how shocked he had been the day Castro informed him that roughly one-third of the Ugandan soldiers sent to Cuba for training were positive for HIV. (At the time Cuba was testing everyone in the country and confining all HIV-positive individuals to camps.) To his credit, Museveni grasped the implications: he knew this might destroy both his army and his country. Unlike most African governments his administration acted quickly, with massive education campaigns through radio and traditional channels. The president's slogan was "zero grazing"—another cattle image: monogamy. This evolved into the "ABC" campaign: Abstain, Be Faithful, or use a Condom.

WHO's GPA and USAID provided strong logistic and financial support but the Ugandan response was inspired and led locally by AIDS pioneers such as Sam Okware, Elly Katabira, David Serwadda, Nelson Sewankambo, and David Opulo, as well as Noerine Kaleeba's TASO. It was the first country where AIDS became a subject that one could openly discuss in society at large. One evening I was having dinner with Ugandan friends when one of the attendees stood up before the end of the meal, saying, "Sorry to leave early, but I need my rest because of HIV." Nobody fell off their chair; we wished him good night, and the conversation continued where it had stopped. I thought, that's how it should become all over the world.

Nationwide, the prevalence of AIDS in Uganda peaked in 1992, by which time 31 percent of pregnant women tested positive. By 1996 it had fallen to less than 20 percent. (It is now just over 6 percent, though slowly rising again.)

In Thailand, Mechai Viravaidya, a former deputy minister of industry with a vivid personality and a contagious love for people, spearheaded a humorous and effective anti-AIDS campaign out of the office of Prime Minister Khun Anand Panyarachun, together with Werasit Sittitrai, who had joined our staff. Their program consisted of three major campaigns: 100 percent condom use during sexual encounters with prostitutes, a "respect for women" campaign, and a barrage of anti-AIDS messages that were aired every hour on TV and radio. Every school was required to teach AIDS education classes. Mechai also taught schoolchildren to blow up condoms like balloons, to reduce embarrassment; he even ran a chain of restaurants called Cabbages and Condoms. It got to the point where in Thailand a condom is known as a Mechai—surely the supreme tribute to good branding. In 2004 during the Bangkok AIDS Conference Mechai and I distributed condoms at a highway tollbooth. Every single driver, male and female, recognized Mechai, and nobody seemed offended.

Less spectacularly, but just as significantly, Thai Prime Minister Anand had moved responsibility for AIDS programs from the Ministry of Health to his own office. The Thai approach was about as pragmatic as possible, with its chief aim to keep sex (including the lucrative sex industry) safe. And the results were just as unequivocal: with nationwide tests on army recruits, their data were extremely precise, and they could trace a decline in HIV prevalence in specific parts of the country.

These two countries became our beacons of hope in a grim landscape. A little later we added Senegal, where low HIV prevalence was maintained, probably thanks to a powerful synergy of the political leadership of President Abdou Diouf, technical leadership by bright young Senegalese experts such as Ibrahim Ndoye and Souleymane Mboup, a solid fabric of society, and Muslim and Catholic leaders, who used their pulpits to spread HIV prevention messages.

So AIDS was a very bad problem, sure, but it now had the beginnings of a solution: committed leadership, well-funded programs for HIV prevention (there was no effective treatment when UNAIDS started), and grassroots activism and support. Uganda became a core part of our political and communications strategy, because (a) if Uganda could do this there was no reason why Zambia, or Cambodia or Guatemala couldn't achieve similar results; and (b) it was clearly worthwhile for Sweden, or Canada, to invest in such a strategy, because it promised to have real impact. We fondly imagined that Thailand, Uganda, and Senegal would soon be joined by other examples. But it was ten years before we could indicate over a dozen countries whose prevalence of HIV was falling.

I made Uganda the cornerstone of my speech at the first major international event for UNAIDS. The 11th International AIDS Conference, which took place in Vancouver in July 1996, was an important test of our influence in the broader (and highly critical) AIDS community, as well as with the world's media. By then this annual AIDS-research conference had morphed into a huge event, with 15,000 delegates and 2000 reporters. So it was a significant opportunity for me to publicize UNAIDS, and even though I had to overcome a high degree of shyness and fear when talking to big crowds—my natural tendency as a child was to sit in a corner with a book—I lobbied hard to obtain a slot for our unknown agency at the opening plenary. It was difficult. As past president of the International AIDS Society I thought it would be easy, but as it turned out some people felt I had switched sides when I went to work for the UN.

We presented our first attempts at standardized statistics. Over 33 million adults and children worldwide had been infected with HIV cumulatively. Over 90 percent of them lived in the developing world. In the past year alone, 3 million adults became infected: 8000 new infections per day. *Every day* over 6,500 adults were being newly infected in Africa; 800 in Southeast Asia; and 270 in the industrialized world. Partly because of these figures, Vancouver was the first international AIDS conference where the developing world was firmly on the agenda.

Most significantly, the Vancouver conference brought the AIDS community an extremely welcome shot of good news—a game changer that would completely change the life of people with HIV, as well as how the epidemic is perceived. A combination of three or more antiretroviral drugs, taken simultaneously, could significantly prolong life and delay the onset of AIDS symptoms in HIV-positive people. Known as highly active anti-retroviral therapy, HAART gave hope that seropositive people could live normal lives, with a near-normal life-span. I called Marie Laga, my successor in Antwerp, to share the news about this Copernican revolution for AIDS because she could not attend the conference; she was about to deliver and was more enthusiastic about the birth of her healthy boy Jef.

This treatment was incredibly expensive: up to US $20,000 per person per year. So although I was enthusiastic about the break-through, I was immediately concerned that the majority of people who needed it were in poor countries and simply could not afford the bill. Unacceptable. We needed to give patients in the develop-ing world access to HAART. Human rights—just simple justice—demanded it. Thus in my speech I called for "bold action on many fronts" to ensure access to antiretroviral treatment for people with HIV in developing countries. Many years passed before this dream became reality, however.

A next challenge was to unify the world's AIDS strategies, and in the first place those of UNAIDS' partner agencies in the UN. On some policy issues it was extremely hard to reach agreement. The prevention of mother-to-child transmission of HIV was a first and very difficult test case. In February 1998, the Thai Ministry of Public Health and the US Centers for Disease Control announced that a trial had shown that a short course of AZT could dramatically reduce the risk that pregnant women would pass on HIV to their newborns. Soon after, another trial indicated that single-dose nevirapin was also effective. This was, to me, absolutely terrific news, and I fondly imagined that a prevention regimen would be swiftly and universally adopted, since we finally had a classic medical intervention to save babies, free from all the controversies around prevention of sexual transmission of HIV. How wrong I was! I kept pushing UNICEF, as the UN agency responsible for the protection of children, to put the subject at the top of its agenda. But even today, nearly 15 years after the first scientific evidence came in, coverage for mother-to-child transmission prevention is still only 60 percent.

Slow action on mother-to-child transmission of HIV reflected partly the poor state of maternal and neonatal health services in many African countries. These clinics, I knew, were and are swamped with hundreds of women a day; typically, they can take your blood pressure and that's about it. But policy paralysis was also partly driven by a lack of leadership in international organizations, mainly due to the highly emotional controversy around HIV transmission through breast-feeding. There was no doubt that HIV can be transmitted by breast milk, but the research findings were sometimes conflicting; for example, some studies found that exclusive breast-feeding actually protected from HIV transmission. Above all, we knew that breast-feeding by HIV-negative mothers (the overwhelming majority of women) saved babies lives. UNICEF and others wanted to protect the progress made in promoting breast-feeding, which was always under threat from commercial pressures to sell baby formula. It is indeed true that in many areas, where clean water is not available, using baby formula can threaten children's health. But so can AIDS: very much so. The question was how to ensure that women with HIV have the option to use affordable and safe breast-milk alternatives, to protect their babies from both HIV and diarrhea, while at the same time making sure that all other women breast-feed. This created a terrible dilemma. It was clearly urgent to run studies comparing which policy would save more lives—breast-feeding (with the risk of HIV transmission) or bottle-feeding (with the risk of diarrhea). But unfortunately emotions took over the debate. I convened several meetings, but none of them reached agreement. For years UNICEF and WHO avoided dealing with the challenges, and even in 1998 WHO published a nutrition manual stating there is no good alternative to breast-feeding. Retrospectively, I think I should have reached out more to the breast-feeding lobby to bring them together with AIDS interest groups. The world is full of single-issue groups—just as we were a single-issue group around AIDS—and the psycho-politics of all this can lead to tunnel vision. Whatever the reasons, a lot of time and lives were wasted by indecision on a tragically important issue.

Controversy surrounding the means by which to prevent sexual transmission of HIV also continued to rage. The question moved from theoretical to empirical when we certified that new HIV infections were declining in Uganda. Knowing which prevention intervention had made a difference was important for other countries, and for concentrating our efforts. But even today, there are heated debates about what exactly caused this decline, with a few claiming that it simply reflects the natural history of HIV, which was bound to decline anyway when those at risk were all infected. (This position is not supported by the data, by the way.) Others claimed it was all because of condom use, but there were also arguments that attributed the success to sexual abstinence, or monogamy. Actually it was probably a combination of the three "ABC" interventions, plus the urgency of countrywide mobilization and openness in discussion; in HIV prevention, the *how* is as important as the *what*. However, some scientists and journalists continue to fuel the debate in a fairly obsessive search for the magic bullet in HIV prevention—the single thing that made all the difference.

I regularly got letters or e-mails along the lines of "Dear Dr. Piot, if *only* UNAIDS would _____ (fill in the latest fashion in HIV prevention), the epidemic would be brought under control." Some went further, accusing me of suppressing vital information. And on occasion researchers insisted that I was deliberately ignoring their own groundbreaking work. It takes a thick skin to be director of UNAIDS! But nuts and obsessives aside, I learned early on that anything with the word *only* does not work in AIDS: it is a combination of actions that has impact population-wide.

Stopping the spread of HIV in injecting drug users was no less controversial. HIV was spreading like a flash flood via shared needles in much of Eastern Europe and some parts of Asia. I had experience with it, having helped to set up the first needle exchange program in Belgium in the early nineties, before I moved to Geneva. It may seem counterintuitive to provide needles and syringes to drug users, but at UNAIDS we promoted needle exchange and methadone substitution programs, because there is very strong scientific evidence that both reduce transmission of HIV.

In the early years of UNAIDS, only a few European countries, plus Australia, Canada, and some US cities, were using this approach, but most countries opposed it, sometimes vehemently, as in Russia. For example, in 1998, US Secretary of Health and Human Services Donna Shalala tried—and failed—to fund "harm reduction programs" for injecting drug users; but they remained banned from federal aid until President Obama repealed them in 2010. (Meanwhile, a large number of states had supported such programs through independent funding.)

Addiction is a very complex and tragic issue. I admit that I have never been completely at ease with either purely repressive or totally liberal policies regarding addictive drugs. I had many confrontations with both sides. The AIDS community tends to be very liberal, and I had to disagree with some colleagues for whom using drugs was not a problem so long as the needles were clean. I always supported harm reduction techniques—which are scientifically proven to be effective—and the human rights of drug users, but to me, the loss of autonomy involved in addiction is a terrible thing.

Back in 1992, American researcher Don Francis and I were asked by the Swiss federal authorities to evaluate a needle exchange program in Zurich. (The Swiss still have no generalized paid maternity leave, but they have needle exchange and heroin distribution.) So we went to their "needle park"—a large garden near the Central Station—at around 4 P.M. It was full of people injecting drugs, and purchasing drugs, in plain view. I saw one woman shooting up in a jugular vein in front of her child, and men in expensive suits coming straight from the office to buy a dose. At a kiosk where I guess they used to sell ice cream, the city health department was giving out clean needles. Don and I were baffled. Epidemiologically, sure, the program worked: all kinds of infections, not just HIV, were on the decrease. But, my God, it was scary to see the collective insanity of addiction up close.

Later I regularly met with drug users, to try to de-emotionalize the issue and convince policy makers to adopt a rational approach—with very mixed success. When the UN Office on Drugs and Crime joined UNAIDS we had access to a political mechanism to promote harm reduction, but it was hard work to move them from a police approach to one of public health. I think that what matters is to continue the dialogue, search for solutions, speak up for the users and for policy change, and I keep hoping that one day science discovers an effective treatment for the various addictions. So I guess even I sometimes dream of a magic bullet.

ANOTHER VERY DIFFICULT question in our first, start-up year was how best to frame the AIDS epidemic. Did solving it require long-term social change? Public-health interventions? Economic development? UNDP was keen to consider the epidemic a problem of social, gender, and economic development; whereas Jonathan Mann saw it as a human-rights issue. Both these viewpoints clashed with the WHO and UNICEF culture of short-term technical solutions. And of course it's obvious that we cannot wait until everyone has escaped poverty and all women are equal to men before we bring AIDS under control. But it's also clear that the AIDS epidemic is determined by multiple social factors, and influencing these should help solve it.

Take the women in Zambia who sell fish. Some buy their fish on lakes in the northeastern part of the country, and sell it in the mining centers and capital city in the west. To keep the fish fresh and sellable during the journey, they need to store it in big refrigerators at the places where they stop overnight. Sex with the owner or manager of the fridges can bring the price down, but in a country with a very high HIV prevalence, it also places them at risk. So we arranged for the fisherwomen to collectively buy a refrigerator, and this eliminated the need for transactional sex. I liked this kind of very down-to-earth approach, which killed two birds with one stone: protecting women from HIV and providing them with a strong economic base. Again, it wasn't one or the other: we needed both short-term protection and a long-term solution.

WE NEEDED TO integrate all the different UN agencies, in every country, into a common approach to their AIDS programs. All of them—UNICEF with children, WHO with the health services, UNESCO with schools, UNFPA with family planning groups, the World Bank and UNDP with the Ministries of Finance—needed to be singing from one song sheet, with one strategic plan. This was Rob Moodie's job.

With a dose of humor, much meditation, and unlimited energy to motivate people, Rob's heroic efforts to establish UNAIDS at the country level were a continuous battle against bureaucracies and passive aggressiveness, in particular by WHO and UNDP. We had some very good candidates to become UNAIDS "Country Program Advisers" in key countries, but again, getting them into place was a seemingly never-ending uphill battle. We had prepared a shortlist of candidates even approved by partner agencies, but were still challenged. Candidates such as Heidi Larson—a PhD in anthropology who was working with the UN in Fiji and helping us on AIDS in the Asia region—was turned down by WHO and ministers of health in two countries because of not being a medical doctor or from the region. We began working on integrating programs through so-called interagency theme groups on HIV/AIDS in a number of countries. The various agencies slowly started to work together, from one budget, assisted by the Country Program Advisers whom we'd named. Over time they became Country Coordinators: this tiny semantic shift illustrated a much stronger position, because now they were *overseeing* the work. They became the driving force of UNAIDS, spearheading the AIDS response in several countries.

The UN resident coordinator—basically the UNDP country director, who traditionally represents the extended family of UN agencies—were the key people to make this happen. Where they were on our side, AIDS became a top issue for the whole of the UN in that country. That is what happened in Botswana, then the country with the highest HIV prevalence in the world: UN Resident Coordinator Debbie Landey, a Canadian, took the lead after I visited Gabarone in 1996. Together we advocated with Botswana's political leadership, which became one of the most engaged on AIDS. In 2005 Debbie became my deputy in UNAIDS.

We had to invest so much time on getting the UN's act together: endless months of theme groups, joint plans, meetings, meetings. A lot of ego and flag-planting—so many agencies that just wanted to be sure that the person on the photo was wearing their T-shirt. I disliked this posturing (and by the way always insisted that UNAIDS staff and cars *didn't* wear our logo). I told our staff: we have a hierarchy of values. Our first commitment is to defeat this epidemic. Our second is to people living with HIV and affected by it. Our third is to the UN system as a whole, because we may be dysfunctional, sure, but we're a family. And our fourth commitment is to this organization: UNAIDS. It seemed to me self-evident, but sometimes when I said it, it actually upset people.

In December 1996 we had a breakthrough in cooperation with the World Bank, which became a strong supporter after its initial reluctance. Its new president, Jim Wolfensohn, and the head of AIDS, Ethiopian immunologist Debrework Zewdie, were dynamite. UNICEF under its new leader Carol Bellamy, and UNFPA led by Dr. Nafis Sadik from Pakistan, also came on board gradually, but at the global level, the meetings I resented the most during the initial years of UNAIDS were those of the so-called Committee of Cosponsoring Organizations, which continued to feel like an avalanche of complaints and some more or less overt attacks. For example, even in October 1997, nearly three years after my appointment, Dr. Nakajima accused me of violating the UNAIDS memorandum of understanding, or of withholding money from developing countries. UNESCO supported him. This meeting was the first attended by the new UN secretary-general, Kofi Annan, and I was thrilled that he would be there, showing such strong interest in AIDS and support for our work. But it was also an embarrassing event exhibiting the dysfunctionality of the system, and I was furious that we had missed an opportunity to engage more with the secretary-general. In spite of this incident, Kofi Annan became the world's chief AIDS advocate, and without his support UNAIDS would not have been able to achieve what we did.

We were making progress in setting up the organization, but perhaps unavoidably this meant, to some extent, that we initially neglected action on the ground. The reality was also that there was a huge gap between what we were capable of doing versus what we wanted to do—in particular in terms of funding AIDS programs in the field. I was also trying to do too many things. This has been a trait of mine throughout my life, and I have had to learn to fight it.

CHAPTER 18

The Lesson of the Chameleon: Bringing Together the Brilliant Coalition

I N JULY 1998, the mood at the 12th International AIDS Conference, in Geneva, was very far from the euphoria of the previous conference in Vancouver in 1996, where HIV infection became a treatable disease. The time of scientific breakthroughs seemed over, the results of HIV vaccine research were disappointing, antiretroviral drugs had some serious possible side effects, and above all for us in UNAIDS, hardly anybody in the developing world had access to antiretroviral therapy—with the exception of Brazil where the government early on was providing such treatment free of charge. In addition, two-and-a-half years after our start, I felt we were going nowhere with UNAIDS: we had spent an enormous amount of energy in building the organization and fighting UN and donor agencies, but our impact on the actual epidemic was clearly negligible. I worried that I was not the right person to lead such a gigantic effort.

We were constantly under attack. Our critics were donors, but also—and more important, for me—AIDS activists and people living with HIV. *Science* magazine wrote that I had "the most impossible job in the world." I originally thought that within five years I could push

AIDS to the top of the UN's agenda and UNAIDS could then probably be absorbed into a reformed United Nations institution. Instead, I was in crisis. I needed advice.

So immediately after the Geneva conference, I convened another discreet brainstorming in Talloires, a tiny medieval town on Lake Annecy at driving distance from Geneva. I invited an unusual group of about 20 people, with about half working on AIDS and half outsiders. I wanted them to take a cold, hard look at what we were doing, and tell me frankly what they thought would make a difference against AIDS. The guest list included Bill Roedy, the president of MTV, whom I'd just met—a supercommunicator whose TV programs reached up to 800 million teenagers around the world; Larry Altman, the health reporter from the *New York Times*; Duff Gillespie from USAID and David Nabarro from the UK Department for International Development, two of our needling critics; and Helene Gayle, from the US CDC and a great supporter. I also invited Dr. Nkandu Luo, the Zambian minister of health, another constant critic. (I had offended many ministers of health by urging heads of state to take over AIDS leadership, thus taking away control over the AIDS budgets from their purview, so I needed to bring this constituency inside the tent.) Finally I invited several AIDS activists and people living with HIV, pharma executives, an adviser to President Museveni from Uganda, and Prasada Rao, who was trying hard to wake up India to the AIDS threat. The only colleagues from the UN system (besides some key UNAIDS staffers) were Daniel Tarantola, who was about to rejoin WHO, and Debrework Zewdie, who was rallying the World Bank to do more on AIDS.

As usual, I felt it is best to be open about the problems, and put everything on the table in the most honest possible way. So my opening speech was short and hard. I said I didn't see any progress, the epidemic was exploding, and I needed help.

Our debates were animated, with little agreement on anything, but they provided me with the ideas I needed to take UNAIDS to the next level. The conclusion was that UNAIDS was doing a reasonable job in terms of epidemiology and of formulating technical solutions, but we weren't enough in touch with the world of political power, where big decisions are made. I had begun to learn that in international politics there are only two things that count: the economy and security. As they say in France, the rest is just literature.

So we needed to influence ministers of finance. It's a bit like the joke about Murphy, who robbed a bank: when the policeman said, "Murphy, why did you rob the bank?" he answered, "That's where the money is." It's also where the power is in government—not with the minister of health.

We also needed the security establishment on our side; and although many people at that meeting were very skeptical about the UN there was one body they all took very seriously: the UN Security Council. That was key. Moreover, we needed to bring AIDS to other major political and financial platforms—G8 Summits, the World Economic Forum, and various regional bodies, particularly the Organization of African Unity and the Caribbean Community, as these were the most affected regions in the world.

Sometime before, my intuition told me that we had no chance to defeat this epidemic unless we pulled out of the "ghetto" of AIDS doctors, researchers, and activists, and built a broad coalition. Now at the retreat on Lake Annecy, I felt that we had the core strength that we needed. And while I complained about the difficulty of working in the hidebound UN system, nearly everyone else felt strongly that being part of the UN was a major strength. It gave UNAIDS legitimacy, potential access to top leaders, and a platform from which to deliver policy guidance—as long as I didn't become a prisoner of intra-UN coordination.

Our goal was to curb the soaring graph of HIV transmission within five years. While further building the organization and trying to lead UN efforts, I from then on mainly concentrated on the politics: on global diplomacy.

With Sally Cowal, Jim Sherry, and my new chief of staff, Julia Cleves—a brilliant Englishwoman who could write a speech in 30 minutes—we sketched out a more political approach to AIDS. As long as there was agreement on the ultimate goal, and some basics were respected—such as the principles of human rights—we could happily work with groups and people with whom we did not always see eye to eye. Some purists felt we sold out but our collaborative strategy ultimately saved millions of lives. More radical activism was useful—in fact, essential—but it was not our job.

We mapped out who our friends and our enemies were. Who could be convinced to join the coalition? Which people could leverage political and economic power? It swiftly became obvious that one essential person would be my boss Kofi Annan: we didn't just need him on board, we needed him to become the world's AIDS advocate. And to increase our leverage with other policy makers, I asked Bernhard Schwartländer and his team to begin working on two new areas of statistical analysis: more precise definition of the economic impact of AIDS, and also what level of financing would make a difference to the epidemic. Nobody had yet done this kind of investigation.

A few months later, in September 1998, Swissair Flight 111 from New York to Geneva crashed into the Atlantic Ocean near Nova Scotia. Jonathan Mann was on the plane with his wife, Mary Lou Clements, who was planning to attend a meeting on HIV vaccines. I asked Jonathan to come too, because I wanted to talk about his joining me in some capacity at UNAIDS. Jon was so great with ideas; as a spokesperson he was tireless, and I thought he could help with our new, high-visibility political strategy.

When Daniel Tarantola called me with the devastating news from Geneva airport—where he was waiting to pick up Jon and Mary Lou—I was speechless. It took a few hours before I realized that it was really true, and what a massive loss it was. It gave me an incredible sense of urgency: *I need to do so much before that happens to me too.*

A fine man named Michel Sidibé, who later became my successor, once taught me a lesson. We met in Uganda in 2000, where he was the UNICEF representative: he was chairing the interagency country Theme Group on AIDS. Michel was from Mali, had spent time in Zaire (now known as Congo), and he enjoyed life: we hit it off immediately. So we went out for dinner to Le Chateau, a steak restaurant in Kampala. And Michel told me a story.

At puberty, like most boys of his ethnic group, he went through initiation, so that he could learn to be an adult. He had to live alone with other boys his age and he was given a chameleon: for a week, he had to observe and think about this chameleon. After the allotted time, he returned to the elders and they told him about life and about the secrets of the ancestors. When they finished, they asked, "Tell us about the chameleon." So Michel said, "It changes color." "What else," they asked. He listed characteristics. This was a long, typically Malian story. But the conclusion was that just by observing a chameleon one can learn life's great lessons: First, a chameleon's head is completely still. It always faces the same direction. *Stick to your goal.* Second, the eyes are always moving, scanning the environment. *Always be prepared.* Third, the color changes in function of the environment. *Be flexible*, know how to adapt, but keep the head pointing straight ahead. If it moves you're an opportunist and you will fail. Fourth, a chameleon moves very deliberately. *Take one careful step at a time.* Fifth, the chameleon catches food by shooting out its tongue, and if it's too soon or too late it won't catch its prey—it will die. *Timing is everything.*

Michel and I ate a big steak together, became friends for life, and a few months afterward I asked him to join me in UNAIDS as head of all country operations.

The chameleon story doesn't tell you where to go, but it tells you to keep a balance between the need to change color and the need to stick to your guns. When I'm in a very complex situation, unsure how far to compromise and taking in everything around me, I ask, Does this fit with my strategic plan? The image of the chameleon is my guide.

THE PICTURE OF AIDS that was taking shape by the beginning of 1998 was much worse than anticipated, especially in sub-Saharan Africa. There was growing evidence of the economic impact of the epidemic. Productivity was declining and tax revenues plummeted in the worst affected countries, while pressures on health services increased. Orphans were a growing tragedy and cost to society. Women's vulnerability to HIV infection was clear. Our research revealed a shocking fact, not yet understood until then: in sub-

Saharan Africa, women under age twenty-five were more than twice as likely to be infected with HIV than young men of their age. In some regions, such as in western Kenyan, women were as much as six times more likely to be infected than their male peers, attributable to high vulnerability of young girls to HIV infection and to younger women becoming infected by older men, not by boys their age. In some countries in southern Africa, life expectancy at birth was falling to levels not seen in 50 years. In Botswana, the likelihood that a fifteen-year-old boy would become infected with HIV in his lifetime was a shocking 60 percent. What was the cost to a company, to a country, of numbers such as these? And how much would it cost to do something about it? We needed to understand the equation of lost productivity and the economic impact of sickness and death versus cost of treatment and prevention. Above all, we needed those figures to convince hard-nosed economists to finance the fight on AIDS to levels that would make a real difference.

In January 1998 I organized a seminar at the World Bank on the demographic impact of AIDS. We showed projections of the changes in population structures due to the epidemic. You could see what's called "the chimney effect." Suddenly the plump age curve of a normal society—which peaks at around age thirty and slowly tapers off as people grow old and die—shrank into a chimney, with maximum population at around age twenty. Moreover the overall population loss was huge. In several countries, life expectancy at birth began to drop back to levels not seen since the 1960s. AIDS wasn't just a health crisis: it was a development crisis that was damaging the future of entire societies. Those images had a big impact in the World Bank, because economists could look at them and immediately understand the age-specific impact on productive people. We were finally speaking their language.

You can't build a movement or a coalition by decree or by rational planning. It is a combination of trial and error, being there at the right time, and hard, hard work. I traveled frantically across the globe to convince policy makers to confront AIDS with the vigor it required. I was driven by outrage about the shameful inaction of those who controlled power and money, and by a great sense of urgency, as the number of people dying every day was growing, now more than 6300. It seemed that people dying from AIDS did not matter, and I wondered whether the reaction would have been different if this had been happening at such a scale in America or Europe.

The ultimate constituency of the AIDS movement is people living with HIV and those affected by HIV. UNAIDS needed to connect better with them, which was not easy, as they always—and mostly rightly—felt that we were not doing enough. Our relationship would always be complex, since we were an intergovernmental body accountable to governments. But often we did manage to work with HIV activists in a very complementary, and sometimes even well-coordinated, way.

After all, our agenda was the same—at least, that was how I saw it. However, my first attempts to engage with AIDS activists and groups of people living with HIV in the United States were sobering. At a meeting in 1996 with groups from all over the country at the American Red Cross in Washington DC, they told me that they needed all their energy to ensure access to treatment in the United States and to support American AIDS patients who had lost jobs and homes. They wished me good luck, but that was it.

I was disappointed, but at least they were honest. Most of the time people promised to help, but that was where it ended. One exception was Eric Sawyer, the tall, energetic cofounder of ActUp New York, whom I had met at the Paris AIDS summit in 1994: he was a rare, early convert to the global perspective on the epidemic.

The situation in Europe was different: antiretroviral therapy rapidly became part of the universal health care system, often free of charge to the patient. Hence there was less local activism about access to treatment. In France, very early on, the largest AIDS service organization, AIDES, began supporting groups in francophone Africa and in Eastern Europe. ActUp Paris was a very small group, but they had superb communication skills, were popular with the media, and vigorously fought nearly everybody, including us at UNAIDS. At one point ActUp activists invaded a meeting of our board and demanded universal access to treatment. Personal attacks were part of their style. One day they went too far, however, and alienated the French public.

I was participating in the Sidaction held in Paris TV studios—an annual major fund-raising event for AIDS—when the representative of ActUp shouted that France was *un pays de merde*, a shit-hole, and further insulted the people who were donating money over the phone. Donations collapsed, and the Sidaction never really recovered. I could understand the anger of activists as they faced complacency and handouts—we were all angry and frustrated—but it reminded me again how counterproductive and dangerous extremism can be. With friends like that, you don't need enemies.

One of the most moving encounters I had was in Kiev, Ukraine, in 1999 at the founding convention of the All Ukrainian Network of People with HIV. I was their special guest, and it was a closed meeting of about 200 infected people from all over Ukraine, which was going through an epidemic explosion of HIV infection. I entered the very cold room in a university building designed by communist architects, and it felt as though I could physically detect their energy, hope, and loneliness in a society that often violently rejected people with HIV. They were beautiful, sweet, intelligent young men and women—although actually most delegates and speakers were women, and indeed women are often the backbone of the AIDS response outside the Western world. I could not stop thinking about my daughter Sara, then of a similar age. These were not your stereotypical junkies; often they were highly educated and many had been infected through occasional and more-or-less experimental drug use.

I spent hours with them discussing their fears, their plans, and how we could help them. They were our raison d'être, and it seemed that my job was a cup of tea compared to what they were up against. Being united and taking a positive view of life was their force. In subsequent years, following many battles, they did make important changes to Ukraine—indeed, they were among the first of a series of grassroots democratic movements in the country. Following that meeting I went to the imposing presidential palace to see President Leonid Kuchma, whose daughter Elena Pinchuck ran a foundation active on AIDS. I transmitted the demands of the people I had just met, and we discussed a number of issues; later, Ukraine became an important voice on AIDS in the UN.

BRAZIL WAS AN early leader on AIDS issues. Its gay community had been badly hit by the epidemic early on. Following years of military dictatorship, there was a vibrant civil society in Brazil in the 1990s. The new constitution also stipulated that health was a right, which gave politicians and AIDS activists legal grounds for their demands. In addition, Brazilian society was open to very frank and pragmatic messages about HIV prevention, condoms, and sexuality; people seemed to have fewer hang-ups about these things than in many other countries.

The Brazilian AIDS Program turned Carnival around and used the enormously popular festival to spread HIV prevention messages and distribute millions of condoms. I attended rehearsals at the famous Mangheira Samba School in a crowded popular neighborhood of Rio de Janeiro in 1999. As the incredibly intoxicating carnival drums resounded and young and old sashayed and sambaed past dressed in the school's pink and green colors, people were debating how to make condom use more exciting and erotic. I was none too sure how to participate in the discussions.

I became a regular visitor to Brazil during my tenure at UNAIDS, together with my long-standing Brazilian colleagues Luiz Loures and Pedro Chequer. As well as being technically very competent—often the case with public health specialists in Brazil—both were also supreme political operators. Thus we spent quite a bit of time in the corridors of Brasilia, the unlikely, butterfly-shaped capital that was built in the fifties in the middle of the jungle.

In 1998, Brazil went through a major fiscal crisis, with enormous public debt and a devaluation of the national currency, the real. The International Monetary Fund also imposed drastic budget cuts as a condition for its assistance. And among the cuts being envisaged was the provision of antiretroviral therapy to AIDS patients. (Brazil was just about the only developing country that was offering this treatment on a large scale, and had started producing generic antiretroviral drugs to bring the price of treatment down.)

This would have been a death sentence for many currently receiving the treatment in Brazil. It would also have been a major setback internationally. I flew immediately to Brasilia. Actually, convincing President Fernando Henrique Cardoso and his Health Minister José Serra was not that difficult. Their commitment to the AIDS cause was profound. Cardoso and I gave a dramatic press conference at the Presidential Palace, confirming the country's commitment to treatment for AIDS patients.

This engagement continued under President Lula, who started a condom factory in the Amazon rainforest—the source of rubber. Lula was one of the most colorful characters among the many heads of state I met. During a meeting in his office in 2005 Lula embarrassed his minister of health by telling me: "My minister of health has said we should stop smoking, but the president likes his cigar. He says no sugar, but how can I drink coffee without sugar? No to alcohol— but the president likes his cachaça every evening. Are you now coming to tell me no more sex?" He then laughed loudly. Both presidents had instructed their diplomats to support UNAIDS and stand firm on access to HIV medicines in developing countries, including via generic medications. Brazil's ambassadors are extremely competent and could be very persistent when a multilateral organization did not stand up for the interests of poorer countries.

There is of course another side of Brazil, a country with some of the greatest inequities in the world. In 2002 I attended a meeting of the Inter American Development Bank in Fortaleza, in the northeast. I had learned how to talk to bankers and finance people in meetings, but socializing with them after the meetings was not always my cup of tea. So I walked around town and talked to people about their lives—difficult, but also full of joy and hope. While jogging along the beachfront in the morning, I saw children and adults digging into the garbage, and thought about the two kinds of people there are in this world: those who fill garbage bins with their castoffs, and those who empty them for their survival.

PEOPLE ALWAYS WANT to hear about my meetings with Fidel Castro, and it's true that he was a very unusual man. I went to Cuba a few times in the 1990s to attend conferences and meet with officials: Cuba had a small AIDS epidemic, mostly imported to the island by soldiers who were "assisting" with various African wars, but the authorities essentially imprisoned all HIV-positive people in sanatoriums, a policy that obviously violated their human rights, not to mention its impossible expense. In October 1999 I arrived in Havana for a meeting of all Latin American Ministers of Health with Luiz Loures, who was in charge of Latin America for UNAIDS, and Peggy McEvoy, the head of UNAIDS' Caribbean section. Peggy was an experienced American public health specialist who had grown up in Cuba in the McCarthy years, when her father, a scriptwriter, was banned from working in Hollywood. She spoke Spanish the Cuban way. Just as we were heading back to our rooms to sleep, exhausted from jet lag, I received a message: the *Commandante* wanted to see me.

It was about 9 P.M. when we arrived at the Presidential Palace in a torrential tropical storm. It is a mixture of Hispanic colonial baroque and modern buildings, with an amazing tropical fern and rock garden. After a short wait, Fidel arrived in olive-gray fatigues, a pair of old Adidas sneakers, and a cap. (By the way, it is impossible to call him Mr. Castro.) He was a surprisingly big man, his skin that of an elderly person but his posture vigorous, and he began talking—a flow of talk, almost uninterruptible—about the floods in several provinces. He seemed obsessed by figures, detailing the number of hectoliters of water per square meter that had fallen in each of the provinces. At some point I managed to say, "Excuse me, Commandante, we are in solidarity with your people suffering from the floods, but I'm here for AIDS."

"Hah! Yes, you're the AIDS guy." So he switched to a flow of questions about AIDS. How many cases in Jamaica, how many in Angola, what incidence, what prevalence. He led me into his office and asked what I drank, so I requested a glass of water. Absolutely unacceptable. So I asked for a mojito and the conversation continued. He wanted to know everything: which country had done best with the epidemic, and how, and why; and then me, my background, my experience in Africa, AIDS in Africa. There was an interpreter present, but Fidel's was the slow and highly articulated Spanish of a man used to speaking to crowds, so I could understand nearly everything, and he could pick up my English and French and rudimentary Spanish.

We discussed Cuba's policy of quarantining everyone who was HIV positive, and forcing tests on every one of their past sexual partners. I told him it was ineffective, as well as unfair, far too expensive, and all-around unworkable. He took it well. Then he broke off. "Aren't you hungry?" It was after midnight, but Fidel instructed his secretary to call in a vice-president, and some ministers—"Hah! There's this interesting guy in my office, come and meet him"—and within 45 minutes they had turned up, bleary eyed, and the door opened to the dining room. No sleep when you are in the Cuban government.

Peggy and Luis were still taking notes on table napkins about any discussions that seemed germane, but by now we had moved on to talking about global warming and the UN. Fidel made a windy statement about the imminent decline of capitalism. I said, "Come on, Fidel, don't give me that, capitalism isn't going to fall"—by this time almost all vestiges of diplomatic politesse had been shed.

Another long debate was certainly forthcoming, but by now my bladder was exploding. This can be tricky in a diplomatic setting: the protocol is never to evoke such lowly bodily functions. However, I said, "Fidel, donde està el baño?" and he quickly responded, "Hah! I'll go with you." So there was an unforgettable moment of striding behind Fidel Castro through the shadowy corridors of the Palacio de la Revolucion in Havana at two in the morning, past sleeping young soldiers in battledress with their guns propped up alongside them.

We bade each other adieu at about four in the morning, and although I was exhausted, I couldn't sleep. My meeting was at 9 A.M., so I showered and reviewed my speech, and managed to deliver it in my poor Spanish to the assembled Latin American ministers of health. In contrast to the director of the Pan American Health Organization, Sir George Alleyne, they were pretty hostile to UNAIDS, and indeed to the whole subject of AIDS, which was perceived as a homosexual problem and thus essentially deviant. Many also opposed condom promotion in their country.

But at around 11 A.M. there was a commotion at the door and who was there? The Commandante! Arriving unplanned, he was peering around, roaring, "Donde està Peter?" Fidel looked at me and said, "Hah. You didn't comb your hair. When did you get up?" Then he burst into a long, impromptu speech about AIDS—how important it was, and how the one guy who knew all about the epidemic and what to do about it was me. I think perhaps he had forgotten the name of UNAIDS, because he called it "el programa de Peter," which was pretty funny. It broke the ice with many ministers, because, even if most if not all in the room did not share the political views of the Commandante, they seemed to respect him—possibly because of Cuba's impressive track record in health and biomedical research.

After that I visited Cuba several times, and we set up a number of programs for technical cooperation and training. The epidemiology of HIV in the country was complex, with both heterosexual and homosexual transmission. One day I visited a school in Mazantas, a provincial capital. After a standard presentation on AIDS by ten-year-old children, one little girl stood up—in the presence of the provincial governor and the secretary of the Communist Party, both men—and said to me, "You know, Doctor, why we're having this problem of AIDS?"

I said no I didn't really, and I would very much like to hear her opinion of it. She said, "All the men here are bisexual!" Everybody roared with laughter.

I sometimes tried to discuss human rights issues with Fidel. During one of my trips, it was reported that 70 opponents had been jailed for up to 27 years, so I twice raised the issue. That did not go too well. Still, he remained very amenable to me personally, and to UNAIDS. At a South Summit in April 2000 Fidel told over 50 presidents that they should act against AIDS and that UNAIDS was the place to go for help. He introduced me to several African leaders, democrats and autocrats, including Robert Mugabe of Zimbabwe. And, incidentally, Cuba relaxed the sanatorium regulation. Nowadays, if a Cuban is found to be HIV positive, he or she is compelled to attend six months of training on safe sex practices.

ON JULY 13, 1999, Larry Altman of *The New York Times* published an interview of me in his weekly "Doctor's World." The title was "In Africa, a Deadly Silence About AIDS Is Lifting." Few people in the AIDS world believed me at the time, but from my numerous and intense country visits, I felt that something had started moving. The spread of HIV was slowing down—in just a few countries, sure, but I felt it had begun. And I felt a great part of this was attributable to leadership at various levels in those countries.

Nearly all leaders—most obviously in Africa, but also elsewhere—were guilty of very excessive delays and denial about the HIV epidemic. In Uganda, Yoweri Museveni, a robust, plain-speaking farmer-soldier, was one exception; another was Abdou Diouf, in Senegal, who corralled the Catholic Church and Islamic religious leaders into an active and intelligent prevention program. In Botswana, where by 2000 in excess of 30 percent of adults had tested positive for HIV, President Festus Mogae resolutely took personal leadership over the AIDS response. He was a soft-spoken former civil servant, democratically elected, and he held his whole cabinet accountable for what they were doing on AIDS. He was open to international partnerships, in particular with US institutions such as Harvard, the University of Pennsylvania, and the Centers for Disease Control. Mogae was not an easy man to convince, and he often asked numerous and probing questions, but once he felt that something was the right thing to do, he went for it. I remember a meeting with him in 2007, together with half his Cabinet and Tachi Yamada, then president of Global Health at the Bill & Melinda Gates Foundation, and Ann Veneman, the executive director of UNICEF. We presented the results of studies showing that male circumcision can reduce the risk of men acquiring HIV by 50 percent. This was a tough challenge for a country where men are not circumcised. We went over all the issues, and there was no conclusion at the end of the meeting, but male circumcision later became national policy. Equally important, over 85 percent of AIDS patients in Botswana now receive antiretroviral treatment. This is one of the highest rates in the world, better than in several high-income countries. The result of sound leadership, good management, and international collaboration.

In Rwanda, President Paul Kagame struck me as one of the most impressive people I've met: his intelligence was not showy but it was sharp and clear, and very strategic. I was one of the first high-ranking

UN officials to meet him in Kigali after the 1994 genocide. It was delicate, given the failure of the UN peacekeeping mission and the UN Security Council (along with all other world powers) to prevent and halt the genocide of around 800,000 people. Nonetheless, what had been scheduled as a 30-minute courtesy meeting went on for several hours.

Kagame received me in a sports shirt in his simple residence, which was heavily guarded by several circles of security. I asked for his strategic advice, and he asked a number of thoughtful questions before speaking up. We agreed to continue the process of jointly thinking things through, and he agreed to discuss AIDS issues with his colleagues in the region. His wife Janet, an elegant psychologist, became the driving force of the Organization of African First Ladies against HIV/AIDS; this group was active in several countries in the first decade of 2000, helping greatly to increase the visibility of the epidemic.

Kagame had put Dr. Agnes Binagwaho in charge of the Rwandan AIDS program. Agnes was an energetic pediatrician from the Rwandan diaspora in Europe, and she was a former student of mine, which made me very proud. She organized the AIDS response as a successful military operation, but with major involvement of community groups such as HIV-positive widows who had survived the genocide. I met with several of them: all had been raped during the genocide and probably became infected with HIV at that time. Many were also pregnant, and thus would be raising babies conceived by a rapist and killer, often the man who had killed their husband or older children. It created huge mental turmoil just to think about their situation. We made sure that they had access to antiretroviral drugs, and Jonathan Turgovnik—a photographer from *Newsweek* who was traveling with me through East Africa—since created a foundation to provide education for these often stigmatized children, and published a moving book *Intended Consequences: Rwandan Children Born of Rape*.

Rwanda was a haunting country, overshadowed by the horror of recent events. But I liked Kagame's crisp management style. Once Suma Chakrabarti, permanent secretary of the UK Department for International Development, and I attended a government retreat in the Akagera National Park where every cabinet minister had to give a PowerPoint presentation reporting on their department's performance against key indicators. In every ministry there was a chart with objectives, a timeline, and percentages achieved: it was very impressive by any standard.

Many other leaders in Africa refused to face the facts of AIDS, or hid behind moral arguments. I remember one time President Frederick Chiluba of Zambia—one of the most HIV-affected countries—actually pulled out a Bible from behind the desk he was sitting at and began reading aloud to me a passage that to him suggested that AIDS was punishment for "fornication." I think there was also uneasiness because of the Western discourse about AIDS: this was often perceived as very offensive, redolent of the common European fallacy of Africans' hypersexuality.

The more I thought about the reasons for the inaction of leaders facing an epidemic that was daily killing their most productive citizens, the more I thought, *Why would they?* Why *would* they care about AIDS if they didn't care about so many other forms of civic misery? I developed a quick technique for sizing up the potential of the heads of state that I encountered: the shoe or watch test. Kagame passed it: he wore a very technical watch, with all sorts of gadgets, but it wasn't an expensive one. In contrast, Gabon's Omar Bongo—who actually received people such as myself while he was seated in a thronelike chair on a raised dais—wore handmade crocodile shoes with elevator heels, and his watch was encrusted with diamonds. Another president actually traveled with his own portrait, which he displayed in every hotel room where he stayed. Their wives would change their complete set of jewelry at least once a day when on foreign trips. And I could go on with quite a list.

Meanwhile, we faced a special difficulty in South Africa. Early on, despite the proximity of the country to nations like Zaire where the numbers were disturbingly high, the profile of the epidemic in South Africa was like that in a European country: HIV was almost exclusively present among gay men. In 1990, prevalence in almost every area of the nation was less than 1 percent. Then around 1998, HIV exploded, with the same spectacular velocity as it had among gay men in San Francisco in the 1980s. In this case, however, the spread did not focus on one small community: it rolled evenly across the whole society, with the dramatic, uniform, apparently unstoppable force of a tsunami.

The root of South Africa's AIDS problem lies in apartheid, with its organization of labor that breaks up families all over southern Africa. Men working in the mines and in the cities were not allowed to bring their families; they lived separately from them for 11 months at a time in company hostels amidst other lonely men, now and then resorting to prostitution. Then came the *fall* of apartheid, which opened the gates to a surge of migration into South Africa, the wealthiest nation in a region hit by civil wars and drought. The end of homeland laws also freed people to migrate within the country.

But there were other factors too. High numbers of concomitant sexual partnerships may be a factor that contributes to the rapid spread of HIV; when you've just been infected with HIV your viremia level is particularly high, so if you are having sex with several people you are more likely to infect all of them. But there is no evidence that South Africans are more likely to have several simultaneous sexual partnerships than people in other nations. Lack of male circumcision? True, circumcised men are much less likely to become infected with HIV, and few men in South Africa are circumcised— but the same is true of most men in Europe, China, and other Asian countries. A particular sexual practice, such as anal sex? No evidence at all suggests it. Cofactors of untreated sexually transmitted diseases? A possibility, but one that exists in other societies where the epidemic has accelerated far less. A particular viral strain or genetic susceptibility? No evidence. Some posit that the key factor in southern Africa may have been gender relations: male dominance, sexual coercion. Others suggest it may be earlier sexual behavior, but in fact sex under the age of fifteen is not common among girls in southern Africa. More sex partners? Actually, worldwide surveys suggest that men and women in the United States have more sex partners in their lifetimes than Africans do.

My own feeling is that the disaster in southern Africa resulted from a mix of many factors. As in vector mathematics, where the resultant of a vector is the product of the cumulative impact of all the vectors, several seemingly small factors cumulatively created a multiple thrust, a perfect storm: a situation that we now call hyperendemic.

IT WAS NOT only developing countries that had to be brought out of denial about AIDS, and to be persuaded to pay for long-term treatment. Among the so-called donor countries, the Netherlands, Sweden, and Norway were very supportive of UNAIDS, and were actually among the very few countries that respected an international agreement that the wealthiest countries would give 0.7 percent of their Gross Domestic Product to international development. However, in the first few years of the new millennium they resisted the idea of spending development-aid money on antiretroviral treatment. They saw it as a bottomless pit, an unsustainable responsibility toward people on lifelong treatment, and also just too darn expensive given a per person price tag of $15,000 a year. France, led by President Jacques Chirac, made strong statements about the universal right to treatment, but was actually among the least generous countries in terms of development aid and therefore lacked credibility.

We knew the United States was key. It was both the most powerful and the richest nation in the world, and it set trends and framed the way other countries envisaged problems. President Bill Clinton had created an AIDS unit within the White House, led by Sandy Thurman, who tried hard to sensitize members of Congress and others about AIDS in Africa. During the final years of the Clinton administration, international funding gradually increased. However, USAID officials fought against earmarking congressional funds for AIDS work overseas, to protect their traditional agendas such as population control. Duff Gillespie, then a senior deputy assistant administrator at USAID, expressed the view of most international development professionals in the late 1990s when he wrote that in the absence of simple tools such as a vaccine, AIDS activities in the developing world would only "siphon off resources" from important aid programs, with limited or no impact on the epidemic.

In June 1998, Duff and David Nabarro from the United Kingdom sent me a fairly tough letter, on behalf of all the major donors, which was somewhere between a reprimand and a dose of stern advice on how to do better with UNAIDS. (Some of the criticism about our performance was entirely fair.) The letter concluded, *"funding for HIV/AIDS activities will not come easy in the next few years."* I blanched. But a year later, international AIDS funding for the first time exceeded $1 billion, and it continued to grow dramatically over the next decade.

Later that year, when I pressed a senior aid official in Washington to tell me why more was not being done about AIDS, his reply was, "But Peter, we did not plan for this." As if any of the millions of people who died from AIDS had planned for it! I was outraged by such a cold bureaucratic approach.

Predicting the future is always difficult, but all these people seemed dramatically out of touch with what was brewing in Africa, in civil society, and among their own politicians. Receiving that letter from Gillespie and Navarro was a difficult moment for me, but I thought of the chameleon, replied that we would improve our performance in a number of detailed ways, and went back to my mobilizing work—basically, working to prove that they were wrong. Soon after that Duff and David became allies for the AIDS cause.

Our efforts to reach out to media and reporters were starting to bear fruit. We had become the go-to place for information on the global epidemic, and our reports were becoming front-page news. Human-interest stories on a range of AIDS-related topics from orphans in Africa to the impact of AIDS on business started appearing on a regular basis in *The New York Times, Newsday, Newsweek, The Wall Street Journal, The Economist, USA Today, Le Monde, El País,* and others. I even made it to the Hall of Fame section of *Vanity Fair* in 2000. When *Washington Post* reporter Barton Gellman called me to say that he was planning to investigate how the world was responding to the AIDS crisis in Africa, I leapt at the opportunity to expose the appalling lack of action and offered total access to all our archives and my notes, except personal ones. Predictably, WHO refused such access. The result was a sweeping three-article series revealing that "most of those with power decided not to act," and that the response of aid agencies had been "demand management"—in other words, they had tried to minimize what should be done about AIDS by questioning the feasibility of both prevention and treatment. Gellman exposed what I suspected. Business was slowly waking up to the subject—albeit too slowly, just like everybody else. There had been some alert early-reactors, like Levi Strauss in San Francisco, but basically even companies doing business in heavily affected countries in Africa were slow to respond. As always, there were exceptions: even before UNAIDS I had done HIV prevention work with employees of Heineken breweries in Kinshasa, and in Zambia, Standard Chartered Bank had initiated a program to protect their employees. They were the pioneers, but we still needed to reach the heart of big business, companies that could help millions of employees protect themselves and that could also influence governments to do more.

The World Economic Forum in the Swiss Alpine village of Davos provided an ideal platform to get companies on board (and turned out later to be the perfect venue for negotiating price reductions for antiretroviral medicines). The Davos Forum is a very exclusive club, where you either pay a fortune to participate, which was not an option for UNAIDS, or you are invited as a key politician, academic, or thought-leader. Today there is almost always a strong contingent of heads of UN agencies, but that was not yet the case in 1997. My entry ticket to Davos was Nelson Mandela.

Through South Africa's then Minister of Health Nkosazana Zuma, who was also the chair of the UNAIDS board, Sally Cowal had managed to persuade President Mandela to attend the Davos Forum and deliver a plenary address on AIDS. It was Mandela's first speech on AIDS, and the Davos Congress Hall was too small to contain all those who wanted to hear the man who had become among the greatest icons of our time. He radiated a charisma I could physically feel. The other speakers at the session were Richard Sykes, CEO of GlaxoWellcome, the manufacturer of AZT, and me. There was a rather uncomfortable moment as we all sat together in the small green room, waiting to speak. Mandela's government was in the process of passing a new law to legalize imports of generic medications. The pharmaceutical industry—Sykes included—was heavily lobbying against the new law, and in fact went on to sue President Nelson

Mandela. (You don't have to be a PR genius to see what a very stupid move this was.)

The audience was blasé, but Mandela electrified them. He called for a global effort against AIDS and urged the business community to support it. I then called for the creation of a Global Business Council on AIDS, which was launched eight months later in Edinburgh at the Commonwealth Heads of State and Government Summit. Mandela was its patron, Richard Sykes its first president, but initially only a handful of companies participated. As Ben Plumley, then working at GlaxoWellcome and the council's first executive director, later said, "At the start, the business response was like getting blood out of a stone." It took a few more years for most major companies to see that their bottom line may be affected by absenteeism and death.

AT MARK'S CLUB, in London, in March 1998, over some smoked haddock and a superb Chateau Haut Brion, Bill Roedy—the president of MTV Networks International—and I hit it off. He was a very unusual business executive: a West Point and Harvard graduate, former commander of a nuclear missile unit, and friend of just about every rock star in the world. He had turned MTV into the first global communication network, with strong local roots across the world—with the exception of Africa. His channels regularly reached 800 million young people. The title of his autobiography, *How to Make Business Rock*, says it all.

Bill agreed on the spot to become a special UNAIDS ambassador—there were no clearance procedures then for this kind of honorary appointment—and we agreed that MTV would launch the "Staying Alive" initiative (now a foundation) to promote HIV prevention among young people. It was clear that if we wanted to reach young people, we needed to go through their channels, and clear too that journalists and communicators might save more lives than doctors, at least in terms of preventing new infections.

Organized religion was a final piece of the puzzle of the brilliant coalition I was hoping to shape. It was not my idea: I had seen so many churches and religious figures react judgmentally to the use of condoms, or brand people with HIV as sinners. However, Sally Cowal convinced me that all those who are part of the problem should be part of the solution, and she very sensibly pointed to religion's influence on billions of people. From my experience in interior Zaire I knew that outside major cities, religious organizations are often the only source of medical care and education: if we wanted to reach rural populations, we had to enroll them in our efforts.

In 1995 I made an eye-opening visit to the venerable monk at the Wat Pra Baht Nam Phu Temple near Chiang Mai in northern Thailand, a region where then about 8 percent pregnant women were HIV positive—the highest rate in Asia. The venerable monk was sitting on a dais surrounded by at least 50 small bags. These contained the unclaimed ashes of people who died from AIDS: their families had rejected them even after death. He explained that his temple was the only place in the area where people with AIDS could receive any care and support (this was before antiretroviral therapy) and that many were thrown out of their families' homes. Some were young women who had become infected with HIV while working in the brothels of Bangkok, often encouraged by their family to seek work in the capital—an extra source of income in this poor region.

That encounter had a profound impression on me, as did meeting Canon Gideon Byamugisha of the Anglican Church of Uganda, who was openly living with HIV. A priest with HIV—I thought that this must be one of the most stigmatized situations you can be in, and I felt for him. But he was utterly joyful, his big eyes full of vitality and a twinkle of laughter. He told me that his congregation had excluded AIDS patients, and how he had struggled to disclose his HIV status to his wife, his colleagues, and his congregation. But his bishop had asked him to head the Anglican Church's AIDS mission in Uganda. He surprisingly became a speaker on AIDS across Africa, and did a great deal to take the sting of stigma away from HIV in Christian communities and beyond.

A few weeks after that meeting I attended a health education session for young women in a Catholic mission in Côte d'Ivoire, near Yamoussoukro, the town where President Félix Houphouet-Boigny had at great public expense built the second-largest cathedral in the world at his birthplace. At some point, a drawing of a condom appeared on the flip chart, and I asked the (European) nun who was making the presentation, "Sister, are you promoting condoms?" She blushed, and replied, "Doctor, when I show this chart, I think as a woman"—meaning, I assumed, rather than as a devout Catholic nun.

I wondered what her superiors would think of this deviation from doctrine, and received an answer when I visited a Catholic hospital in Namibia in southern Africa. An array of condoms was available to all in a basket at the outpatient clinic. I asked the same question to the nun in charge: "Sister, are you promoting condoms?" Her answer was short: "Doctor Piot, Rome is a long way from Namibia." Away she went. It made me understand that even a religion with a hierarchical structure as apparently rigid as the Roman Catholic Church's is not in reality monolithic, but guided in its daily work by the variable styles of individual humans.

A former Dominican monk from Sweden, Kalle Almedal, who worked at UNAIDS, helped us establish an agreement with Caritas, the Catholic aid organization that is active on the ground in most countries. This was in 1996, a few years before most UN organizations started courting organized religious groups. Our project work with Caritas went smoothly, but some Catholic priests continued to preach against condoms in a fairly obsessive way, and Pope John Paul also spoke out firmly against them when visiting African countries.

To me, the Vatican's opposition to condoms was irresponsible and shocking. Nonetheless, we continued to work with members of the Church's hierarchy on the ground, and I met regularly with successive papal nuncios in Geneva—very reasonable men, whom I found both pragmatic and cultivated. Then one day in 2003, Cardinal Lopez Trujillo, head of the Pontifical Council of the Family, made a widely publicized statement that condoms could in no way prevent HIV: they had little holes through which the virus could penetrate. This was too much for me to tolerate. I called the papal nuncio in Geneva and expressed my dismay, saying that this was scientific nonsense and that I would publicly hold men like Trujillo accountable for people dying from AIDS. The nuncio was actually embarrassed, I think. We agreed that I should discuss the matter directly with the Vatican, where I had met twice with Archbishop Javier Lozano Barragan, the courteous head of the Pontifical Council for Health Pastoral Care. Somewhat the Vatican minister of health, he was an imposing man—a former teacher of Latin in his native Mexico—who reminded me of Francis Bacon's famous painting of Pope Innocent X.

Several weeks later the nuncio informed me that the Holy See had agreed to an appointment. I went to Rome with two objectives: I wanted to find more solid common ground between UNAIDS and the Church, and I wanted an armistice on the condom. I knew that Pope John Paul II would never promote condom use, and my inner chameleon told me that it was totally nonproductive to have our relationship dominated by this issue. But the Catholic clergy should at the least refrain from preaching against condoms, especially when such preaching involved misinformation.

I spent two fascinating days in the Vatican, walking from one cardinal's office to another through Renaissance and Baroque corridors festooned with cherubs, talking about AIDS. They were very well organized: by the time I saw someone, he had already received a briefing on my meeting with all his other colleagues. After a delicious lunch in a small trattoria in Trastevere Archbishop Lozano and I reached an agreement: UNAIDS had no competency in theological and moral matters, but, as he put it, the Church had no competency regarding "the quality of materials." In other words, the Church would refrain from statements about condoms and UNAIDS would refrain from criticizing the Church. This carefully worded verbal agreement saved, I think, many lives, and isn't the preservation of life the highest moral imperative of them all?

There is more than one pope in the world, and in 1997 in Cairo, I met Shenouda III, Pope of the Egyptian Coptic Church, together with Sally Cowal (who had to cover her hair with a big scarf). The Pope was accompanied by five bishops, who looked like clones of him: all six were wrapped in black, with long beards. All I could see of him under his vestments were his impressive nose and vivid eyes. I asked him to send a message to all churches to inform his flock about AIDS, and preach tolerance toward people living with HIV. He immediately accepted, but then in loud and heavily accented, but fluent, English pronounced, "Professor, AIDS is caused by illegal fornication."

His white beard nodded emphatically as he spoke and his sonorous, plummy voice lingered over every syllable: "*Forrr*nication. There are those who are born like that, and they should be treated, and there are those who do it for fun. And they should repent."

I glanced at Sally; we did not dare to look at each other or at the rest of the meeting. It was a silly, schoolboy reaction, for we then had a very interesting and open discussion about the nature of homosexuality. It was certainly not as bad as the conversation I had had the day before with Suzanne Mubarak, the First Lady of Egypt, who had told me that no tree could be high enough to hang "these homosexuals."

Our next appointment was with one of the most respected religious scholars in Sunni Islam, Sheikh Said Tantawy, the Imam of El Azhar Mosque. He seemed more like a professor than a cleric, in his office crowded with books. That too was a productive and essentially benign conversation, and as a result he too regularly talked about AIDS.

It can be very powerful when the whole religious leadership of a country comes together to send a message about openness and against discrimination of people living with HIV. That is what happened in 1999 in Addis Ababa, the capital of Ethiopia, following some meetings I had with Patriarch Abune Paulo of the Ethiopian Orthodox Church and President Negasso Gidada. It created a safe space for a few men with HIV to come out and give a face to AIDS in a country where the disease had been completely hidden, even though close to a million people were infected. Dawn of Hope, the first association of people living with HIV in Ethiopia, was born, and I was proud to have helped make it happen.

As so often, it was Archbishop Desmond Tutu from Cape Town who said it best, in an advertisement campaign on AIDS in South African newspapers: *Sex is a beautiful gift of God.* If only all his colleagues would think the same.

NOT EVERYTHING WE tried worked. In June 1998, I addressed the plenary session of the Organization of African Unity Summit in

Ouagadougou, the capital of Burkina Fasso, in West Africa. It was a rare privilege for a non-African and non–head of state, and I felt it reflected an increasing realization among Africans that bold action needed to be taken against the epidemic. I foresaw an international partnership that would bring together African governments and civil society, as well as donors and the UN, to mobilize money and action for HIV prevention and treatment.

But we did not succeed in mobilizing political commitments or the new money that was so badly needed. The partnership plan was, I think, too UN-focused; it gave African governments little sense that they "owned" the project. Also, at the time donor agencies were not ready to commit serious money to AIDS in Africa. *They* wanted to control the agenda, instead of UNAIDS, so they undermined the initiative in many subtle and not-so-subtle ways. They still didn't "get" that the epidemic was destroying their own programs for African development.

On the positive side, at their annual meeting in May 1999 in Addis Ababa, all the finance ministers of every African country discussed AIDS together for the first time. After I spoke about the epidemic's threat to economic development there was dead silence. I thought it was yet another moment of supreme denial—that, following this pause, everyone would manage to compose a straight face and go back to business as usual. But then the minister of finance of Benin took the floor, saying, "Yes, we have a problem, and it is high time we face reality." One after another the ministers spoke, sometimes referring to AIDS in their family or colleagues. That evening many joined me for a drink in the hotel, continuing the discussion, and asked how they could be of practical help.

The same year, the World Bank established an AIDS Campaign Team, ACT Africa, in the office of its vice president for Africa, with Debrework Zewdie as its head—another important development, as the bank wields great power in Africa. We also forced all the major aid agencies to discuss AIDS for the first time, among themselves, in London in April 1999, and again in December 1999—this time with African ministers, activists, and business leaders, at a meeting convened by UN Secretary-General Kofi Annan.

That meeting was a big gamble and it nearly cost me my job. I assured Annan's deputy, Louise Frechette, that there would be high-level participation at the meeting, and I concentrated my efforts on convincing Africans to be there. They came. But we then learned that, led by the United Kingdom and Sweden, the donors planned to take a passive-aggressive approach and send only junior staff. In desperation, Jim Sherry and I called upon some personal friends to break this de facto boycott by the donors. Sandy Thurman, Clinton's AIDS czar, and my compatriot from Antwerp, Eddy Boutmans (the Belgian state secretary for international development) changed their plans and arrived just in time to deliver strong messages of support. Annan was at his best, and the African participants made it clear then that they wanted to act on AIDS.

This, alongside Kofi Annan's newly visible commitment, signaled to the donors that they needed to get their act together. It also meant that Africa started slowly to take ownership of the AIDS issue. We had been the catalyst in this realization. But it had taken a long time—far too long—to get to this point.

By 1999 about 26 million adults and children were living with HIV, two thirds of them in Africa. More than 9000 new infections occurred every day, or over six every minute. More than one-fifth of those newly infected were young people aged fifteen to twenty-four. Some 5.9 million African children had been made orphans because of AIDS. In 16 African countries, 1 in 10 adults had the AIDS virus. And barely one-tenth of 1 percent of them were receiving life-saving antiretroviral treatment. Our annual report on the state of AIDS in the world suggested that in 1999 AIDS had become the first cause of death in sub-Saharan Africa. Out of nothing a few decades before, a virus had taken over all causes of ill health.

But by the turn of the millennium our "brilliant coalition" was taking shape in all its diversity and apparent chaos. What could the South African Chamber of Mines, Anglican Church, Communist Party, and trades unions have in common with the Treatment Action Campaign, Médecins Sans Frontières, and UNAIDS? A common goal: defeating the AIDS epidemic and caring for its victims. A powerful joint desire to be a force for change.

CHAPTER 19

The Tipping Point

T HE CHANGE OF century brought with it a sharp and sudden shift in the world's attitude to the epidemic. In the space of a year, it became an urgent, unavoidable subject for world leaders and organizations. I would like to think that this was partly because of our work at UNAIDS in "global health diplomacy" as it is sometimes called today—a mouthful of a term for what was an effort at combining science expertise with the tools of traditional diplomacy, where national and strategic interests are paramount, as well as a new form of transborder activism.

We succeeded in elevating AIDS to levels at which no health issue had ever been discussed before—to where the heavy lifting of international and national politics takes place. The key to this was indeed the UN Security Council, and the key to that was Richard Holbrooke: the tireless, acerbic, larger-than-life American diplomat who was the then the US ambassador to the United Nations. I had met him in a formal meeting at the US mission to the UN and was impressed, so when I learned that he planned to visit the Great Lakes region of Africa in November 1999, I asked his assistant for a detailed schedule.

I asked our staff to write up some short but powerful evaluations of the AIDS situation in Rwanda, Burundi, and Congo, and I made sure that they were in Holbrooke's background file. Then, in every town he visited, we alerted our UNAIDS country staff and local activist groups and people living with HIV to cross his path, ask him questions, show him the conditions in which they lived. That's what activists do—they heckle.

When Holbrooke got back to New York he gave a press conference, where he said, roughly, "Yes, the security situation is bad, but what's really killing people out there now is AIDS and we have to do something about it." He asked to see me, and when we met he said, "Peter, we're going to discuss this at the Security Council, because those guys have no clue what's really going on out there." Of course I knew that six months before Holbrooke too had not much of a clue, but I kept my mouth shut. Then he added, "To get it on the agenda I know what the hook should be: peacekeepers."

The Security Council is the locus of power in the UN. Anything discussed there can change lives. But its mandate is not infinite: ECOSOC normally oversees economics and social affairs. The Security Council's decisions are (in theory, at least) binding, and it makes decisions about war and peacekeeping. But as Holbrooke now knew, UN peacekeepers (currently 120,000 personnel) may catch, or transmit, HIV. His idea was to use this as a starting point to debate the national security implications of AIDS. Furthermore, since the United States would occupy the rotating presidency of the Security Council in January 2000, Holbrooke wanted AIDS in Africa to be the subject of the first Security Council meeting of the new millennium. It was brilliant.

To pull it off in a few weeks around Christmas was quite an effort. I assigned Ulf Kristoffersen, a Swedish former peacekeeper, and my adviser Jim Sherry to the job of working with Holbrooke's office to collate data and prepare for the meeting. Here went our Christmas break: I got confirmation mid-December that the session was on, we worked very hard when the diplomats at the UN were eating turkey or whatever back in their country, and we took everybody by surprise when they came back. All this was done in close consultation with

Louise Frechette, Kofi Annan's Canadian deputy secretary-general. She was a tough woman who at first seemed to protect Kofi Annan from engaging with what she may have seen as an irresponsible, NGO-type of entity that somehow made it into the UN system. Louise was razor sharp, a former deputy minister of defense with a good sense of humor; but once I had persuaded her that AIDS was not only important but actually had the beginning of a solution, she came on board with vigor, and made sure that I became effective in the minefields and labyrinths of multilateral politics. I owe her a lot.

US Vice President Al Gore chaired the debate on January 10, and said that AIDS was a threat to peace and security. Kofi Annan told the assembled dignitaries that the destructive impact of AIDS on Africa was equal to that of war. AIDS was causing socioeconomic crises that threatened political stability. I tried hard to focus on the speeches, but was somewhat distracted by the enormous painting hanging over Gore and Annan, a somber expressionistic work in dark colors with scenes as from the day of judgment. Very appropriate for the Security Council chamber, I thought, hoping that the country representatives might glance now and then to look at it when making their solemn decision about war.

Then it was my turn to speak, and I am often a nervous wreck before speeches, small and big. I stated the facts, redefining AIDS as a threat to development and stability—thus a new form of security threat—and asking that all peacekeeping operations have an HIV-prevention component (which the council voted in on July 18 as Resolution 1308, thanks to Holbrooke's tireless efforts).

The meeting had enormous impact. It highlighted the way AIDS swamps a country's health services; kills the active, productive elements of a population; and creates social and economic crises that can overwhelm and break a nation's political stability. Moreover, the very fact that it took place at all was in itself a breakthrough for us in terms of access. For years to come, presidents and prime ministers would tell me, "If AIDS was debated in the Security Council, this must a serious problem." Deep down I found this ridiculous, sure, but I quite literally heard that kind of reaction.

During the Security Council debate, the Ukrainian ambassador to the UN had suggested there be a Special Session of the UN General Assembly devoted exclusively to AIDS. Uniquely within the former Soviet bloc, Ukraine by this time was developing a relatively coherent approach to the epidemic, and I had visited the country twice to meet with its leadership and community groups. It was clearly paying off.

Ukraine's proposal for a Special Session of the General Assembly took everyone by surprise, and to be honest I had no immediate grasp of what it meant. I learned that to prepare for such an event is ordinarily a two-year project, involving regional preparatory conferences and premeetings that are basically very expensive and time-consuming talk shops. I thought that this would drain our energy and I wanted the shortest possible lead time. The first slot available was June 2001. (Another possibility was mid-September 2001, which would not have happened following the events of 9/11; and that too would have changed the course of the AIDS epidemic, for the Global Fund would probably not have been launched and much else would not have happened.)

A Special Session of the General Assembly would focus the minds of the diplomatic and political decision-makers of the entire planet. It was an opportunity we could not afford to miss: if we failed this, there would be no second chance to get AIDS on top of the world's agenda. So a few months later I sent UNAIDS Deputy Director Kathleen Cravero to New York full time to start hammering out the preparatory work. I had met New Yorker Kathleen in WHO while she was working with Mike Merson and later as UNICEF's representative in Uganda, where she was instrumental in the country's pioneering AIDS efforts. When she was head of the UN in Burundi she was nearly murdered while visiting a refugee camp in the midst of a civil war (two of her colleagues were killed execution style, but she escaped; it is still uncertain whether the assassins were rebels or government troops). Kathleen is a jewel in the crown of the international civil service; you can parachute her anywhere and she will do a superb job. She helped me to bring UNAIDS to another level, and when she felt I was stressed (actually most of the time) would find the joke that brought me back to life. Kathleen was the one who pulled off the Special Session for us. The protocol, the texts under debate—virtually everything was controversial, and nothing could be relied on to function smoothly.

The solemnity of the Security Council debate brought AIDS an entirely new stature in terms of the world's political agenda. It also startled the heads of our cosponsoring agencies at the UN. And UNAIDS became a subject of study when my daughter Sara told me a year later that she had to study my speech in her MSc class in international relations in London; it was presented as a first event at that level to broaden the concept of security beyond the absence of conflict.

Also, following the Security Council meeting, ministers of finance became far more interested in the economic losses due to AIDS. The media grew more attentive and that brought big corporations on board too. AIDS activists in developed countries started to focus more intently on the need to solve the problem in developing countries. AIDS started to touch a nerve among intelligence agencies, security agencies, religious leaders. The pieces began coming together.

BY 2000, OVER 4.3 million South Africans were living with HIV— the highest number in any country in the world. But because so many of these people had been recently affected, they weren't necessarily showing up yet as sick—or as fatalities. Still, it was clear to me that would be unavoidable.

Enormous amounts of time were being wasted, at the expense of hundreds of thousands of lives, because the top leadership failed to recognize that AIDS was an exceptional threat to the survival of the nation. South Africa was experiencing one of the fastest-growing epidemics in the world, and yet even after our meeting in Davos in February 1997, President Nelson Mandela didn't speak about AIDS in his own country until December 1, 1998, World AIDS Day, when I accompanied him to a military base in Kwazulu Natal, where in the presence of Zulu King Goodwill Zwelithini, he addressed the nation in a dramatic live televised address. Mandela said, "We admire the brave . . . who are with us today to say: We are the human face of AIDS—we are breaking the silence!" That day the most admired icon of our time also broke the silence for his nation.

When Thabo Mbeki succeeded him as president in 1999, I had high hopes for his leadership: this was clearly an extremely intelligent and articulate man of great integrity. But in March 2000, our director for southern and eastern Africa, El Hadj As Sy (he had joined me from ENDA Tiers Monde, a Senegalese NGO) alerted me that Mbeki seemed to have adopted some very highly unusual views on the epidemic. Basically, Mbeki had come under the influence of a molecular biologist from Berkeley, California, Peter Duesberg, whose profoundly erroneous theory was that AIDS stemmed from poverty and use of drugs (for recreational or medical purposes), while HIV either did not exist or was a harmless passenger virus. We had no idea to what extent these ideas had taken hold in Mbeki's mind, and I was sure that if I could only meet with him to discuss it, I could pull him back to reality as he seemed a man of reason.

As Sy obtained a meeting for me with Mbeki on a Saturday evening, March 31, 2000. I was in Nigeria, but because there was no direct flight that time I had to fly all the way back to Zurich to connect to South Africa, so by the time I arrived it was already about 8 P.M. As Sy drove me straight to State House, where I was greeted by Mbeki's wife Zanele, whom I knew from a group of African First Ladies against AIDS. She led me into her husband's study. A fire was burning in the fireplace, and Mbeki was smoking a pipe, with a glass of whisky beside him, wearing a woolly sweater. He was working with his speechwriter on a talk he was planning to give on the need for private investment in Africa at the Africa-Europe Summit in Cairo. It was a very British scene, a chilly autumn evening in these southern latitudes. He looked up and said, "Please have a seat," but there was no handshake, and kept on writing his speech. So I just sat there and at some point he thanked the speechwriter, who left. Then he passed me a Human Development report that the UN Development Programme publishes every year, and asked me to find some bits of data. Once he'd finished the speech, he looked up again and said, "So. What would you like to discuss."

I said I had come to find out how UNAIDS could better support South Africa in combating its very serious AIDS epidemic. I remembered his great speech at the conference of people living with HIV in Cape Town in 1995, but there was increasing concern about South Africa's response to the epidemic. I was coming to him as a scientist who had spent most of my career in Africa and as someone who admired the ANC's struggle against apartheid. I was up-front: I had heard rumors of alleged policy positions of his government that were in my view counterproductive.

Thabo Mbeki is a very courteous person, who I think probably rarely raises his voice, but he can be cold. His arguments were technical and detailed, but they were partial; there was always a nugget of some truth, possibly outdated, but with some evidence to it, but these nuggets were strung together into a completely skewed approach. He questioned the accuracy of data and the high degree of false positives that came up in HIV tests (this had been true, but was basically eliminated in more recently developed tests). I told him there was very strong evidence that HIV causes AIDS. He repeatedly made the point "But Koch's postulates have not been fulfilled." These were criteria that Robert Koch, the German discoverer of the tubercle bacillus in the nineteenth century, had developed to assess whether a microbe causes disease. The microbe must be present in every case of the disease; the disease must be reproduced when pure cultures of the microbe are inoculated into a healthy, susceptible host; and healthy people must not carry the microbe. Actually Koch's postulates *are* fulfilled with HIV; in any case, they are now obsolete with advances in microbiology and immunology, and the availability of far more sophisticated techniques. (Even in TB you have lots of healthy carriers: I myself test positive for the tubercle bacillus since I acquired an infection while working in the lab in Antwerp because of a dysfunctional protective hood.)

Mbeki continued. He claimed that a lot of so-called AIDS deaths were due in fact to tuberculosis, not HIV. So I explained about opportunistic infections. Then came a discussion about the impact of treatment, and the toxicity of AZT and nevirapin, the medication used to prevent mother-to-child transmission. Yes, indeed, AZT has side effects (so has aspirin; drugs can cause death, it's true). But there was no balancing intelligence, no weighing of the enormous benefits in lives saved versus mostly controllable side effects. He claimed that no one had actually seen the HIV virus, and I pointed out that I had seen it myself, under an electron microscope; but then he said that those were artifacts, and it's true that there are lots of artifacts under the electron microscope.

At every point Mbeki came up with arguments that were not insane, indeed all were based on some truth; but they were spurious. And his face and body language were inscrutable. I didn't know whether he was buying my arguments or not, because this was clearly a man who enjoyed debate, sipping his whisky. I had one too, though I rarely drink hard liquor, because I was rattled and exhausted; by this time it was after 11 P.M. and I had spent the last 24 hours in the air. Finally, he asked me to send him more information, and agreed to attend the international conference on AIDS in Durban that the International AIDS Society was planning, and mentioned that he would be putting together a panel to launch a national debate on AIDS and the cause of AIDS, at which he wanted "all points of view" to be present. Of course I agreed that UNAIDS should attend. And as I left he said, "Peter, don't you know, what the real problem is? Western pharmaceutical companies are trying to poison us Africans."

I was dumbfounded. It was close to midnight. I had a very late supper with Mrs. Zanele Mbeki, a simple goat stew with vegetables—these were people who passed the watch and shoe test—and I think I said barely more than a couple of words to her. I felt that I had failed. Mbeki had stressed time and again the need for an *African* response to what he felt was specifically an African problem. He saw AIDS in Africa as a wholly separate disease to whatever other mystery disease was affecting drug users and gay men in the West. And yet here he was, basing his argument on a lone American's unfounded theory. Mbeki was an intelligent, indeed coldly rational, man; and yet he was impervious to my reason. What could be the origin of this denialism? I had thought maybe it was economic—the cost of treatment—but after that evening I was convinced that could not be the case. Psychological, then. A blind spot—perhaps we all have one, but here, tragically, the president of the country most affected by AIDS had this specific blind spot: one that would harm enormous numbers of people. I wrote in my notebook: "I am devastated—this can have very negative consequences in Africa."

I immediately (and confidentially) alerted Kofi Annan and the heads of UN agencies working with us that we had what was potentially a major problem with South Africa's leadership. But Mbeki acted fast. This was clearly a very important issue for him. A few days later, on April 3, he sent a five-page letter to his colleagues all over the world and to the secretary-general of the UN. The tone was defiant and defensive, though he made some good points when stressing the need for Africa to find its own way of confronting AIDS, as its epidemic and societies are so different from the West's. He said that a "simple superimposition of Western experience" would "constitute a criminal betrayal of our responsibility to our own people." Very strong words. He compared criticism of the bizarre claims of AIDS revisionists (such as Duesberg) to "heretics" being "burnt at the stake" and observed that "Not long ago, in our own country, people were killed, tortured, imprisoned and prohibited from being quoted in private and public because the established authority believed that their views were dangerous and discredited." He continued, "We are now being asked to do precisely the same thing that the racist apartheid tyranny we opposed did, because, it is said, there exists a scientific view that is supported by the majority, against which dissent is prohibited . . . The days may not be far off when we will, once again, see books burnt and their authors immolated by fire."

Years later, when the dust had settled over the dark Mbeki years for AIDS, and President Zuma had put the AIDS response on the right track. Professor Malegapuru Makgoba, the eminent immunologist who was head of South Africa's Medical Research Council and now vice chancellor of the University of Kwazulu Natal in Durban, shared with me another, private, letter on AIDS he had received from Ngoako Ramathodi, the premier of Limpopo province, and thought to reflect President Mbeki's views. The 22-page letter dedicated a few pages to me: "one of the contributors to the criminal cruel and insulting mythology about AIDS and Africa was none other than the Belgian Professor Piot." The author compared me to a "European *sangoma* (witch doctor) in Africa," and implied my attitude stemmed from a colonial approach originating in Belgium's colonization of Congo. It had become very personal and ugly.

The following month there was a two-day meeting of a South African "Presidential AIDS Panel" to debate the cause of HIV, with Senegalese Awa Coll-Seck participating on behalf of UNAIDS. It essentially gave equal time to real science and to denialist quackery, only muddying the waters. For years, Mbeki's active opposition to antiretroviral treatment was a formidable headache for me and an obstacle to a much needed emergency response to AIDS in southern Africa. The whole South African diplomatic corps was enrolled in this crusade, personified by Mbeki's Minister of Health Manto Tshabalala-Msimang. At every international meeting they made sure to distinguish the virus and syndrome as separate, unrelated afflictions—HIV *and* AIDS—rather than grouping them as "HIV/AIDS." Language and symbols mattered for Mbeki, and he succeeded in imposing his semantics: the AIDS community started to use the same terminology, not realizing what it actually meant. Regardless, very few African leaders had the interest and guts to stand against Mbeki, even if in private most disagreed with him, and the Western powers needed the new South Africa for stability on the continent. So I knew that I could not count on our usual allies because of macropolitics.

But the net result of these "higher politics" was more dead bodies. In November 2008 the *Journal of Acquired Immune Deficiency Syndromes* published a Harvard study that estimated that 365,000 people died because South Africa did not provide antiretroviral treatment to pregnant women and other AIDS patients in the eight years of Mbeki's presidency. To this should be added deaths in countries in the region that slowed down their AIDS response because of Mbeki. This failure also did him a lot of harm politically. He had been seen as a shining leader in Africa but in the end, when he resigned in September 2008, he was widely contested, and the scandal of his mismanagement of his country's most dramatic health problem was an important element in that loss of reputation.

Thabo Mbeki was not alone in adopting conspiracy theories. In June 2000, in Geneva, his colleague Sam Nujoma, president of neighboring Namibia, deviated from his keynote speech for the annual conference of the International Labour Organization, which under Juan Somavia's leadership later became the eighth cosponsoring agency of UNAIDS. In front of nearly all the ministers of labor of the world, as well as business and union leaders, Nujoma suddenly put his speech aside and stated that AIDS is a man-made disease. He continued, "States that produced chemical weapons to kill other nations are known—they are probably here, and they have the responsibility to clean up this AIDS mess." I was sitting next to the rostrum, and nearly fell off my chair. This was not as sophisticated as Mbeki's views, but I suspected that the aging Nujoma said loudly what many secretly thought. In my speech, which followed his, I set the record straight, and over lunch I tried to convince him that besides the absurdity of the conspiracy, the technology was not there yet to create a new virus. He clearly did not believe me.

THAT YEAR, FOR the first time, the International AIDS Conference took place in a developing country: Durban, South Africa's biggest port, was the host city. Mbeki would speak at the opening ceremony, as would I, and we had agreed that then we would fly together to Togo for the summit of the Organization of African Unity. But when Mbeki arrived at the huge Kingsmead cricket stadium where the opening ceremony had started in a chilly sea breeze, his chief of party said there would be no space for me in Mbeki's plane, and that he would speak before me and then leave. It seemed as if he didn't want to hear my speech.

The first speaker at the opening ceremony was a very young boy living with HIV I had met during a previous visit to Johannesburg, Nkozi Johnson, who gave a very moving speech that left many people in tears. (He died a year later, aged twelve.) Then came Mbeki, who started reading page after page, verbatim, of an old WHO report on poverty and health: his message was, "*This* is Africa's problem: it's poverty." Which is indeed a crucial problem in Africa, but he did not say much about AIDS. It wasn't just disappointing, it was chilling. The audience was silent, disgusted, I thought, at what was a collective insult and provocation. And when his speech ended all eyes turned to me.

I was angry but I could not afford to burn all bridges. I started by saying loud and clear that HIV causes AIDS. Applause—the audience's outrage and frustration came out. I spoke about the need to do more, to offer treatment, but my main message was a universal one: I felt strongly that we should not let Mbeki's ideas hijack the conference, the movement. What I said was: "This is the time to move from the M word to the B word. We need billions, not millions, to fight AIDS in this world. We can't fight an epidemic with peanuts." I was convinced that we had no chance to defeat this epidemic and save the lives of the millions already infected with a small incremental increase of the current resources (then about $300 million for Africa). We needed a qualitative leap forward. Some donors did not forgive me, and already during the conference an aid official called me to say that someone in my position should not make this kind of irresponsible statement and that the money was not there: I should stop dreaming.

But perhaps the most vivid voice at the conference was that of the Treatment Action Campaign. TAC opened the conference with a massive march for access to treatment, and ended it by kicking off a "defiance campaign" to import generic fluconazole, made in India, to South Africa. (A treatment for fungal infection, one of the most common among the opportunistic infections in AIDS patients, generic fluconazole was much cheaper than its brand-name equivalent of Pfizer's, but generics were still not permitted in the country.) Founded late—at the end of 1998—to campaign for access to affordable treatment for all people with HIV in South Africa, TAC was in my opinion the smartest AIDS activist group of all, worldwide. They combined three strategies: street demonstrations and civil disobedience; a broad alliance with churches, the Communist party, business leaders, academics, the Chamber of Mines, and just about everyone else, including some people in the ANC; and legal tactics to enormous effect. South Africa, in contrast to many other African countries, enjoyed the rule of law and a functioning and independent legal system. And TAC's constant lawsuits ultimately forced Mbeki's government to provide nevirapin to prevent mother-to-child transmission.

By this time TAC had become a mass movement, with thousands of totally devoted members, and Zackie Achmat was its mastermind. Zackie was in the first place a genius political strategist and organizer, hardened by the struggle against apartheid and by his campaigning for gay rights; moreover, he was clever, quirky, and articulate. By refusing to accept antiretroviral treatment for himself until it could be made available to all, he used his own body as a billboard for TAC's campaign. I sought Zackie's advice at crucial moments for UNAIDS, even if TAC also put constant pressure on us to do more. During the years of ineffective government action, UNAIDS funded TAC directly, which annoyed the government, and we also helped them to raise funds from others, by facilitating a tour of North America.

South Africa's health minister Manto Tshabalala-Msimang went into overdrive at the conference, trying to control all the messages, attacking the 5000 scientists who had signed a declaration affirming unambiguously that HIV causes AIDS, questioning Mbeki's position on this, questioning the effectiveness of treatment in general and of methods to prevent mother-to-child transmission of HIV. I had several very tense meetings with her, and at one point she even threatened to take away the citizenship of Hoosen M. "Jerry" Coovadia—a remarkable professor of pediatrics in Durban, a long-standing antiapartheid supporter, and co-chair of the conference. (Of course a minister of health has no legal power over citizenship.) In no other country had AIDS become so political and confrontational, and this situation continued for another five years.

The conference ended on a real high: rumor was that former President Mandela would close the conference, and so he did. Over 10,000 participants chanted "Nelson Mandela!" when he entered, doing the Madiba walk to the music of Hugh Masekela. Mandela called upon the world to join forces to provide HIV treatment, and though he stopped short of criticizing his successor, he saved the honor of South African politicians.

The Durban conference was where the debate on access to treatment in developing counties really got out into the open, though still basically limited to the global AIDS community. At that time, besides groups such as Médecins Sans Frontières, only France and Brazil and UNAIDS were backing such treatment in the developing world. Neither WHO nor any major aid agency was on board in this fight.

But Mbeki's inexplicable notions about HIV and the AIDS epidemic had continuing repercussions throughout the region. He became a real militant of his own ideas, trying (without much success) to convince other African heads of state of his position, particularly through his minister of health, who insisted on treating AIDS with beetroot, garlic, and more or less fraudulent "medications." A few years before Mbeki resigned, in 2008, the country's AIDS policies improved very swiftly. But it was so late, following such a horrible waste.

In September we had another defining moment. The largest-ever gathering of 160 heads of state and government, at the first UN General Assembly of the millennium in New York, agreed on 10 goals to make the world a better place by accelerating action on very concrete issues, including poverty, hunger, maternal deaths, and child mortality. Millennium development goal number six was "Combat HIV/AIDS, malaria and other diseases," with a target for 2015: "Halt, and begin to reverse, the spread of HIV/AIDS."

Placing this among the 10 millennium goals had entailed yet another diplomatic battle with our sister agencies. Rumor had it that only malaria would be included—AIDS would be left out. So I went to see a phlegmatic and humorous Canadian scholar John Ruggie, who worked in a small office on the 38th floor of UN Headquarters, next to the deputy secretary-general. I introduced myself, gave all the arguments why there should be an AIDS goal, and told him I would not leave his office until he had agreed to include AIDS! He was a bit startled, as I doubt that such activist tactics are common on the well-protected 38th floor. But fortunately John was sympathetic; the head of the UN Development Programme, Mark Malloch Brown, was totally on our side; and it did not take much to convince Kofi Annan that AIDS must be on the list.

From then on, the politics of AIDS switched gears. The year 2001 was the tipping point in the fight against the epidemic. At the beginning of the year I brought many key UNAIDS staffers to a retreat. I kicked it off by saying, "From now on, think *big*. It's time for breakthroughs. Our job now is to ensure AIDS is on the top political agenda in all regions of the world within two years. We need money to increase exponentially. By 2005 we should start seeing a 25 percent decline in HIV prevalence in Africa." Our job was crystal clear.

While Kathleen Cravero was working 24/7 on what seemed like the impossible task of pulling off an AIDS session of the UN General Assembly in five months, I went around the world seeking support for a strong commitment of top leaders, and to ask for their participation at the event in New York in June. No country is too small to take care of its citizens, I argued, and to play an international role.

Caribbean countries were increasingly affected by HIV; following the early heterosexual epidemic in Haiti, HIV was spreading rapidly throughout the very mobile region, which hosts millions of tourists. Thanks to smooth collaboration with the brilliant Sir George Alleyne, an eloquent scholar from Barbados who headed the Pan American Health Organization, I was invited to the CARECOM Summit in Port of Spain, Barbados, on February 15, 2001. Prime Ministers Owen Arthur from Barbados, Denzil Douglas from St. Kitts and Nevis, George Alleyne, Yolanda Simon (founder of the Caribbean Regional Network of People living with HIV/AIDS), and I launched PANCAP: the Pan-Caribbean Partnership against HIV/ AIDS. Collaboration among countries is crucial in a region with many small island states, few of which have the capacity to address a complex issue such as AIDS, and where there is very high mobility among the islands. At the summit, all prime ministers pledged to combat AIDS in their country and they agreed on a joint strategy for the UN summit in June, emphasizing the need to offer access to antiretroviral treatment. So the Caribbean was the first region to put AIDS top on its agenda, and we had a determined ally.

After the opening ceremony, Prime Minister Arthur invited me to a private lunch with his 12 colleagues and George Alleyne, a rare privilege. Standing in the hilly tropical garden overlooking the deep-blue Caribbean Sea, I discussed with Arthur how I could raise the issue of the "antibuggery" laws that made homosexuality illegal throughout the Caribbean. I did not want to embarrass my host, but he agreed that I could raise the issue. Most of the assembled prime ministers seemed to know each other from law school at the University of the West Indies—a unique regional university with campuses on several islands—and much of the conversation was about common acquaintances, people I did not know: this was really a personal community, as much as a political and economic one. When the discussion turned to one of the hot topics of the summit—the creation of a Caribbean High Court—I felt that my moment had arrived.

What I said was, roughly, "I commend you on establishing your own highest judicial body, so that your people and lawyers no longer have to go to London to plead their appeals. Perhaps this is also the time to abolish another obsolete law from the days of Queen Victoria. The antibuggery laws are a major obstacle to effective HIV prevention. They drive people underground and make it very difficult to reach them." An uncomfortable silence followed. Owen Arthur broke the ice and said that whereas he disapproved of homosexuality, "Peter has a point, and perhaps we should reconsider." A lively discussion ensued, but no conclusive agreement. I continued to raise the question at many subsequent visits, but as of today these laws are still active in the Caribbean, where homophobia can be strong.

In April 2001 we saw another major milestone: a special summit on AIDS, tuberculosis, and other infectious diseases (the latter a diplomatic concession to South Africa) was organized by the Organization of African Unity in Abuja, Nigeria. President Olusegun Obasanjo was the host. I had met him in Davos at the World Economic Forum and asked him, as the president of the OAU for that year, to convene his colleagues at a summit to say, loud and clear, that Africa has an AIDS problem and is ready to confront it. This was not only important for the peoples of Africa, but also because donor after donor told me that Africans never raised the question of AIDS, and therefore it must not be an important issue deserving of funds.

Kofi Annan and almost 50 African heads of state, as well as former US President Bill Clinton, who is very popular in Nigeria (in Abuja the road between the airport and town is named for him) attended the summit. That was very important: just about every head of state of Africa was talking about AIDS (and a little about TB) for two days. It was also one of the most chaotic summit meetings I've ever seen, with President Obasanjo even intervening to clear the security at the entrance of the conference center, and the official dinner starting after 11 P.M.—though the waiting was amply rewarded by seeing Bill Clinton dance to Nigerian *high life* music. I've often reflected that I'm lucky to have started my career as an organizer in Zaire, because everything else—except Nigeria—has felt easy.

One by one, African presidents broke the silence about AIDS. It was wonderful, even if I knew that the distance between words and action can be a long one. But is it not one of the basic principles of psychoanalysis that before we take action, we need to be able to name the problem? Thus the assembled heads of state adopted a declaration that stated, "AIDS is a state of emergency in the continent." They pledged to make the fight against AIDS "the highest priority issue in our national development plans" and to "take personal responsibility and provide leadership for the activities of national AIDS commissions." That was truly vital, because it dissipated the thick cloud of denial about AIDS that had shrouded attempts to grapple with the problem in Africa.

The meeting also "resolved to enact and utilize appropriate legislation and international trade regulations to ensure the availability of drugs at affordable prices and technologies for treatment, care and prevention of AIDS and other infectious diseases." Every country also made a solemn commitment to spend 15 percent of its gross domestic product on health issues, and specifically AIDS. (By 2010, only Botswana, Burkina Faso, Malawi, Niger, Rwanda, and Zambia had honored this commitment.) I always pushed for ambitious goals, but I tried also to avoid totally unrealistic ones, which can in fact be demoralizing instead of inspirational.

Kofi Annan was the keynote speaker in Abuja, and he was magnificent. We had worked hard with his speechwriter, and provided as much intelligence and data as possible. UNAIDS had estimated that we needed roughly $7 to $10 billion to stop the epidemic and Annan called for just that—a global, multibillion-dollar fund to be set up to halt and reverse the spread of AIDS in Africa. Annan called it a "war chest." It would become the Global Fund to Fight AIDS, Tuberculosis, and Malaria, a completely new kind of public-private partnership.

The $7- to 10-billion figure did not come out of the blue. It was based on a study that Bernhard Schwartländer and colleagues (in UNAIDS and other institutions) had published in *Science*, which for the first time had established an estimate of what it would cost to turn around the epidemic and provide treatment to a majority of patients. (Importantly, they specified that one-third of these resources could come from domestic resources of the developing countries, and two-thirds from international resources—a fact often ignored by activists and journalists, who only remembered the $10 billion figure, and presented it as if all the money had to come from high-income countries.) The estimate was a breakthrough that framed the funding discussions at the UN Special Session in June, as well as many other meetings.

Annan's speech at Abuja was a key part of our strategy of building momentum toward the special session in June. It was also the first time I was formally part of the UN secretary-general's official delegation. This is a highly efficient self-contained unit that operates 24 hours a day, with Kofi Annan continuing to handle the political crises of the moment wherever he may be in the world. My respect for him, already high, increased considerably.

The closing session of the summit was surreal. For protocol reasons, it fell to Moammar Kadhafi to deliver the vote of thanks in the hot and overcrowded conference hall. What is normally a brief formality turned into a 50-minute tirade against the "great Satan" (America) that had fabricated this virus to wipe out Africa. This man was not a drunk in a bar, but head of an oil-rich state, among the most senior of Africa's leaders. I found it profoundly upsetting that I and over 40 presidents had to listen to this insulting nonsense. After a while, Clinton and many Western delegates walked out in protest—rightly so. But I must say that Kadhafi was a great showman, speaking softly, almost in a whisper, and then crescendo with fervor, dominating the audience in his sunglasses and long brown Bedouin robe. Still, it was remarkable that the diplomatic niceties should dictate that such a clearly disturbed man could demand the attention of the leaders of an entire continent.

A few weeks later, in May, during a visit to Washington by Nigeria's President Obasanjo, US President George W. Bush hosted an event at the White House where he pledged $200 million for a global AIDS fund. Annan, also in attendance, donated the $100,000 prize for the Philadelphia Liberty Medal that he would soon receive. This was extraordinary: multimillion-dollar pledges to something that did not even exist yet. But the wind had changed: there was now a robust determination to come to grips with AIDS.

With the UN summit in June looming large, we were in nearly daily contact with two formidable women, Deputy Secretary-General Louise Frechette and Marta Mauras, her chief of staff, and received regular advice from Kofi Annan at critical moments. Kathleen Cravero, Jim Sherry, As Sy—who I had asked to move from South Africa to New York to lead our office—and many others did not sleep much during the first half of 2001. I went to New York every few weeks, and fell in love with one of the greatest cities in the world.

While there was generally strong support for a major effort on AIDS, there were also major disagreements on what to do and how to do it. After some initial skirmishes about secondary issues, basically four thorny topics remained: mentioning homosexuality, drug use, and prostitution in the declaration; access to antiretroviral treatment and associated intellectual property issues; a financial commitment; and participation of AIDS activists. We had to de-mine them one by one. Contrary to a common belief, political decisions in the United Nations are not made by the organizations or the secretary-general but by the 192 member states, which have divergent and often mutually exclusive interests to defend. UNAIDS could only provide technical advice and logistic support.

The president of the General Assembly, then the Finnish diplomat Harri Holkeri (the function rotates annually), had appointed two "facilitators"—ambassadors who would lead negotiations behind the scenes. We were very lucky with his choices: Ambassador Penny Wensley from Australia and Ambassador Ibrahim Ka from Senegal. I knew Penny from Geneva, where she was the Australian ambassador to the United Nations and an early and firm supporter of the AIDS cause. A hardworking and multilingual perfectionist, she was one of the most respected ambassadors in New York and worked tirelessly to forge consensus on a strong declaration in June.

Another, even more formidable, force intervened: "civil society," the accepted term for all sorts of AIDS activists and interest groups. They too wanted to influence the negotiations. Many diplomats were disturbed by these intruders, with their poor manners and constant demands for more. But I was adamant that they had the right to speak up, and though we might have disagreed—sometimes quite strongly— I did feel that we shared a language. Besides, I'd read the UN charter, drafted by Eleonor Roosevelt: "We the people . . ." These *were* "the people." Such involvement of nonstate actors is now increasingly common in international forums. It represents a new form of democracy outside the formal national and international institutions, with no obvious leader, often transnational and connected by rapid communication. UNAIDS made it possible for them to be in the room; once again, AIDS was exceptional, a trailblazer.

Again, Kofi Annan came to our aid. He personally phoned heads of state and urged them to attend. Every time he met a head of state or government, or ambassador, he would talk about AIDS and he always made time to see me. On another, much later occasion, in the midst of the Iraq crisis, when I entered his office I could feel the strain coming off him. I said, "Secretary-General, I won't take any more of your time—I know you have important things to deal with." But Annan responded, "More people are dying of AIDS today than they are in any war." He shared with Nelson Mandela that precious quality that consists in giving you the impression of caring, of pure concentration on your issue and on you as a person: you might only see him for a half hour, but that half hour was completely yours.

Also, in terms of working within the UN system, Annan was an operator of the highest order. But he was also a very demanding boss, with far less patience than his soft voice and gentle manners express, and cut in no time to the heart of a problem.

There was an irresolvable clash of cultures over even mentioning homosexuality in the special session's closing declaration. Some countries, led by Egypt on behalf of the Organization of Islamic States—and supported by just about all African and Asian members states—stated that they could not agree to include the keywords *men who have sex with men, sex workers, or injecting drug users* in the text, as that would imply an acceptance of behaviors that were and are against the law in their countries. I spent hours debating with them, trying vainly to convince them that stating facts of life and important realities of the AIDS epidemic by no means implies approval. This went beyond my diplomatic skills, and poor Penny and Kathleen had to listen with me for hours to homophobic statements very difficult to tolerate.

Eventually the leaders agreed on the compromise term "vulnerable populations," a phrase that became code for the three groups that still today cannot be named in UN documents. I have often reflected on why many otherwise reasonable people become so irrationally passionate about sexual orientation. Is it because they are confused about their own sexuality? Hard to believe, but it seems to me this is the crux of it. Certainly the issue of homosexuality nearly derailed the opening of the august session. Even at the last second it wasn't certain that the Special Session would even begin at its scheduled time in June. UNAIDS had proposed among a few hundred other NGOs that the International Gay and Lesbian Human Rights Commission attend a round-table debate as an observer (not even a formal participant). But many countries objected, and Egypt and a few others threatened to walk out. I felt it was a matter of principle that the people most affected by the epidemic should not be excluded from discussion.

The European Union (then without recent members such as Malta and Poland, which supported Egypt's position) spoke up in favor of the commission's inclusion, and eventually Canada insisted on a plenary vote in the UN Assembly, which had never had to pronounce on such a loaded social issue. So the opening of the special session was postponed for an unprecedented vote on the admission as observer of one NGO—in reality, a vote on gay rights. It was very tight: we won by one vote. I am not convinced that the outcome of such a vote would be positive today.

Sadly, no compromise was reached on another crucial issue: access to antiretroviral treatment. Ten years later this is particularly hard to understand. The "Rio" group (Latin American countries led by Chile and Brazil), the Caribbean, France, and Luxemburg proposed a target of providing treatment to the millions of people with HIV who would otherwise die. But these countries were a small minority, and despite eloquent and well-organized efforts by the Rio group, and several sessions until well after midnight (the only limiting factor being that at 2 A.M. the interpreters went home), the Europeans—led by the United Kingdom and supported by the United States—and even African nations (led by South Africa) blocked any meaningful reference to a treatment goal, or to lower prices for HIV medication. The donors were scared about the cost. It was shameful, and I felt powerless in the face of their resistance. Worse, some AIDS activists held me responsible for this failure, and one even tried to attack me physically.

Surprisingly, the donor countries gave in on a target of $7 billion in funding by 2005, which was ironic, given that it included money for the treatment they had opposed in their negotiations on the declaration. So I was reassured. The other way around would have been far more problematic: a commitment to access to treatment without money would have made progress impossible. So I kept my mouth shut.

During the three hectic days of the special session in June 2001, the red AIDS ribbon was displayed every night on the UN building in New York. Even this had been hard to arrange, with multiple authorizations from departments I had never heard of. When our time and my patience ran out, I called in Louise Frechette, who agreed in 10 seconds that it was a great idea, and photos of this symbol zipped around the world: my contribution to monumental art. We also made sure that AIDS was visible in New York City, a town that had a serious HIV problem, from posters on buses, to church services, and red ribbons everywhere.

Meanwhile, in the austere General Assembly hall, 46 heads of state and government and high-level representatives of countries in the world, along with—a first—a South African woman living with HIV—gave one five-minute speech after the other. But we still had no agreement on the concluding declaration! When it was my turn to speak, I took a deep breath and went to the green marble rostrum I had so often seen on TV, from which just about every world leader since World War II has spoken. I looked into the mighty hall and said, "Two paths lead from this General Assembly Special Session. Two possible futures. One path simply continues from where we are today: an epidemic that we are fighting, but that is gradually defeating us. But there is another. The path out of the Special Session must be one of commitment to stop this epidemic. To go on until no one living with HIV is stigmatized, excluded, shut out; until all our young people know how to protect themselves from infection; until no infant is born infected with HIV. To go on until children orphaned by AIDS have the same prospects as any other children; until antiretroviral therapy is essential care for anyone living with HIV."

Was it an impossible dream? I was already thinking of the follow-up, and how to make sure that the closing declaration would not be meaningless. The negotiations about its wording were at a standstill, but I used the opportunity to meet with an endless succession of presidents, prime ministers, and delegations, overwhelmed by the effort of ensuring that I would be in the right cubicle with the right country at the right time. As ever, Marie-Odile Emond, my executive assistant, had it all under control, as she would for many years stoically organize my life with devotion and an exceptional eye for detail, regardless of crisis. Without her, I could never have done this or many other tasks. The most remarkable meeting was with the delegation from "Somalia": for the first time the three autonomous parts of what once was Somalia had decided to do something together—even though AIDS was definitely not the number one priority amid their never-ending civil war and famine.

Finally, Wensley and Ka, with Cravero on their side, hammered out an agreement on detailed, quantified targets for the fight against the epidemic. At 4 A.M. on the third and final day of the special session, we managed to reach a declaration that was acceptable to all. It was vague on homosexuality and worldwide access to treatment, but strong on every other issue, calling, most notably, for the creation of a "Global Health Fund." It set up a global road map, including the need to establish national AIDS commissions under the direct oversight of the president or prime minister, elevating AIDS to the level of real policy; quantified and dated targets for funding and reduction of the number of new HIV infections; and directions for nondiscrimination, condom promotion, and prevention programs. The "Declaration of Commitment on HIV/AIDS" became a benchmark for global action. World leaders became accountable to a clear set of commitments that they endorsed. Extensive media coverage on a scale unprecedented for an AIDS event contributed to raising awareness globally. Leaders could no longer claim that they did not know about the exceptional magnitude of the AIDS crisis or what needed to be done to stop it.

Retrospectively, 2001 was truly the tipping point in terms of politics, incubating the funding that was soon massively released. But I remained frustrated by our extremely slow progress in terms of making the various UN agencies work together. (There were seven, after the UN Office for Drugs and Crime joined.) There was great support at the top of the agencies, from people such as Jim Wolfensohn of the World Bank, Carol Bellamy of UNICEF, Nafis Sadik of UNFPA, and Mark Malloch Brown, the future deputy secretary-general. And on the ground there were good examples of synergies. But midlevel management remained entrenched in old habits and constantly increasing jealousy of our achievements at UNAIDS. I knew we should not let ourselves be deterred from our mission by such bad behavior, but it was at the very least a sad waste of resources.

CHAPTER 20

The Price of Life

F ROM THE EARLIEST days of the epidemic, patients and doctors
alike were desperate to find effective treatments that could stave
off the prospect of a swift and inevitable death from AIDS.
And as always in times of suffering and war, some try to capitalize
on the despair of people. Bogus treatments were promoted in many
countries, particularly before antiretroviral therapy was widely available, sometimes with very high-level support from unscrupulous or
deluded government officials. Unwillingly I got involved in many
such cases, and had to speak up against scientific fraud and politically
connected commercial interests.

Back in 1987, the Zairean government summoned Robin Ryder, the
director of Projet SIDA, and me to a press conference that announced
to the world that two African researchers had found a cure for AIDS,
claiming that the virus had been cleared from patients' bodies and
they had even become HIV antibody negative. (This did not make
sense biologically.) In honor of the presidents of the researchers'
countries of origin, an Egyptian surgeon and a Zairean hematologist,
the "cure" was called MM1 for Mobutu Mubarak Number 1. We
were pressured to endorse this medicine but never had access to its

composition, nor to a vial of the pricey substance. Meanwhile desperate patients traveled far, some even from the United States, for this supposedly miraculous, but entirely bogus, treatment. At Mobutu's request the African Development Bank gave Lurhuma, the "cure-finding" hematologist from the University of Kinshasa, millions of dollars, so for a while we at Projet SIDA kept a low profile in Kinshasa, for we had no treatment to offer.

There was a similar story in Kenya: during one of my visits in January 1990 to Nairobi, the Ministry of Health asked me to attend a press conference where Dr. Davy Koech from the Kenya Medical Research Institute (KEMRI)—a well-respected organization—announced at a press conference that "Kemron," a low dosage of interferon alfa, cured patients with HIV. Again, some allegedly even tested HIV antibody negative after treatment. No details were given about the trial design, and there was no control group to assess whether the treatment was better than a placebo. (Though championed as an African invention, it actually originated in Texas, in the lab of a doctor named Joseph Cummins.)

Again, the "treatment" attracted patients from all over the world, who at great cost did *not* get better and certainly were not cured of HIV infection. Dr. Koech had high-level political support, and because there may have been some biological basis for the treatment with interferon alfa, very expensive trials were funded, including by WHO. In 1998 Ugandan AIDS researcher Elly Katabira independently demonstrated that Kemron was not better than placebo.

South Africa had its own quack remedies, with political support coming from President Mbeki. While still deputy president in 1997, he arranged a meeting of the full cabinet with cardiovascular researchers from Pretoria who claimed that "Virodene PO58," presented as an African discovery, could cure AIDS. Not only was their scientific evidence not credible but also the researchers had performed human trials without ethical approval. Virodene contained dimethylformamide, a toxic industrial solvent. The subsequent chairs of the South African Medicines Control Council, Peter Folb and Helen Rees, courageously refused to bow to political pressure and refused to approve human trials. (Rees did not even waver after receiving death threats.) They were supported by the prestigious head of the Medical Research Council, Professor Malegapuru Makgoba. Despite this, the investigators, with support of the South African Government, conducted trials in the Tanzanian army as late as 2000. The South African government also supported claims by German physician Matthias Rath that his nutritional supplements could treat AIDS. At a press conference in Johannesburg in 2005 I had to denounce these claims, because they were putting people's lives at risk.

In 2007 Gambia's President Yahya Jammeh went even further by claiming that he personally could cure AIDS, asthma, and hypertension with natural herbs. Jammeh actively promoted his medicine as an alternative to antiretroviral therapy. (It is ironic that Gambia hosts the prestigious Medical Research Council laboratories, which have made major contributions to African health.) Jammeh even expelled the UN Resident Coordinator Fadzai Gwaradzimba, who had expressed doubts about the cure. African scientists, led by Professor Souleymane Mboup from neighboring Dakar, reacted strongly in an open letter denouncing these practices.

THE LAUNCH OF UNAIDS in 1996 coincided with the discovery of antiretroviral treatment, but five years later we had made little progress. AIDS remained a death sentence in the developing world. The odds were against us, and in the 1990s it was impossible to conceive that a brand-new proprietary drug—moreover, a totally new class of drugs—would be made available to the poorest of the world: people who don't even have access to basic care. There was just no precedent to build on, and yet we had no choice but to do everything possible to bring antiretroviral treatment where the needs were greatest: in the first place, Africa. We could not wait for normal market mechanisms to operate.

The obstacles were formidable and plural. Where did the resistance stem from? Not (yet) from the virus, but from institutions and experts; and there was as yet no dialogue that brought together all relevant parties. At first, long lists of why HIV treatment is not feasible in the developing world came from those who should have been at the forefront of the fight against AIDS. They were of course right that particularly in Africa, health services were in bad shape and health spending was very low, but by focusing on the obstacles, they entered into a state of intellectual and conceptual paralysis. Even WHO refused to include antiretrovirals on the list of essential drugs until 2002.

Development economists were as adamant as public health experts. As late as May 1998 World Bank economist Bill McGreevy wrote in a memo (as quoted by Barton Gellman in the *Washington Post*) "the brutal fact was that those who could pay for Africa's AIDS therapy—the pharmaceutical industry by way of price cuts, and rich-country taxpayers by way of foreign aid—are very unlikely to be persuaded to do so." Indeed, why *would* politicians commit taxpayers' money to poor Africans, drug users, or prostitutes? Among politicians, President Jacques Chirac of France was a lonely voice calling for access to HIV treatment in Africa, which he did in Abidjan in December 1997—alienating other wealthy countries, for France's actual commitment was limited to words until the creation of the Global Fund in 2002.

Thus international development agencies refused to support our calls for widespread access to HIV treatment. Here as well, there was a reasonable argument that it is risky to commit public funds from rich countries to provide lifelong treatment for a disease in another country, with ethically no possibility of pulling out (unlike most other forms of development assistance). In addition, the pharmaceutical industry had a very real interest in maintaining the high price of this new family of medications, as well as concerns that the development of resistance, due to inappropriate use of the drugs, would make their medications ineffective. Justifiable or not, intellectual property is the foundation of the industry's business model. We had to deal with the big pharmaceutical companies, because for several years there were no real generic alternatives for these new medicines.

Many ministers of health in Africa were ambivalent about HIV treatment. On the one hand they were confronted with a growing burden of patients and hospital costs because of AIDS, and they could have put cheap drugs to good use. But their budgets weren't even sufficient to deal with all the other health problems in their populations, and they were concerned that they couldn't deliver on promises for HIV treatment. In addition, South African Health Minister Dr. Tshabalala-Msimang argued loud and long to her colleagues in the region that antiretrovirals were toxic and didn't really treat AIDS at all—just as she did in front of the South African Parliament in Cape Town, when she claimed, with no proof whatsoever, that nevirapin had killed several women.

Activists such as Médecins Sans Frontières and the US Health Gap were great allies for UNAIDS, with their campaigns for universal access to HIV treatment. But at the same time, their extreme position regarding intellectual property rights—which they rejected —alienated industry and many governments, making a dialogue very difficult.

I did my own analysis. Working in Africa, I had seen how difficult it can be to administer even short-term, seemingly simple health services. I thought about what it would take to bring successful HIV treatment to people in Africa. Here's what I came up with: First, we needed to make HIV testing more available and accessible. Before they can be treated, people need to know that they're infected and people shouldn't have to fear that if they test positive they will lose their jobs or social network. (Years before, in Nairobi, Marleen Temmerman and I encountered numerous pregnant women who were beaten by their husbands, or even expelled from the house, when they announced that they were HIV positive.) Second, we needed affordable, accessible medical and laboratory services on the ground to assess what stage of disease people have attained and ensure follow-up care. Third, we needed access to affordable, usable drugs. Fourth, we needed to help patients take their medication correctly. In those days it was essential for effective performance of the antiretroviral medication for the dozen or so pills to be taken exactly on time; people walked around New York with alarm clocks. In any case, I was convinced that we needed a public health approach to HIV treatment with uniform regimens—not only to ensure adherence to treatment, but also to reduce the risk of resistance development.

Many people argued that for that timing reason alone, antiretroviral treatment would never work in Africa. There's a comment on the subject by Andrew Natsios, the administrator of USAID: "Many people in Africa have never seen a clock or a watch their entire lives. If you say, 'One o'clock in the afternoon,' they do not know what you are talking about." Many people—public health specialists at WHO and staff of international development agencies—seemed to make lists of every single obstacle they could think of, and their conclusion was always that this was a nonstarter. The lists were reasonable then and, sadly, still are reasonable. But today 7 million people *are* receiving antiretroviral treatment, and it is keeping them alive.

I thought, well, fixing the health systems across Africa is probably more than UNAIDS can handle right now. And promoting more testing, when the drugs weren't available, simply wouldn't work: there was no incentive. So my conclusion was that we needed to get the price of the drugs down before we worked on the rest.

I became fairly obsessed by it. Basically every day I asked myself, how can we bring the price of antiretroviral treatment down? I had no experience in this, but there were already some examples of vaccines that had been made available to some countries via UNICEF at far lower prices than in the West. Moreover, I knew that if I bought almost any medication in a French pharmacy it would cost less than in Switzerland, even if the manufacturer was Swiss, because the French negotiated the price down. And when you take an airplane the person beside you may have paid one-third of the price of your ticket. So differential pricing wasn't that unusual; we just hadn't approached the problem in this way before.

There was one successful example: Merck had a lucrative drug, Ivermectin, originally developed for treating parasites in animals. But when Ivermectin was later shown to cure river blindness in humans, Merck provided it free for distribution in West Africa, where huge areas of fertile land infested with the infective agent, black fly, were available for farming. Could that be a model? I talked with some of the people who had been involved, like Dr. Ebrahim Samba of the WHO, but no. Why would a company freely distribute a recently developed, very expensive medication for lifelong treatment when it needed return on its investment? Merck's Ivermectin had no human use in the developed world, but that wasn't the case for antiretroviral medications. In addition, in the case of AIDS, we were talking about ultimately over 30 million people in low- and middle-income countries who would require treatment for life, not a short course as is the case for river blindness. The challenge in AIDS was simply far too big for such an approach; we needed affordable drugs, and given the level of poverty, the funding capacity of developing countries, and the scale of the problem, that meant very drastic price reductions: even a 50 percent price reduction on $10,000 was still out of reach for most countries in the world.

Back in 1991 Dr. Nakajima, the head of the World Health Organization, had convened meetings in Geneva with 18 pharmaceutical industry executives to discuss access to medicines to treat HIV and opportunistic infections. They led nowhere, as industry basically refused to discuss prices, saying they needed the income to fund R&D, and that in any case health services in Africa were not equipped for complex treatments. At a meeting in 1992 the pharmaceutical industry even objected to the use of the word "affordable" in text. There was hostility on both sides, with WHO also not able to come up with any funding, and the talks ended in 1993.

This was also the time when the Clinton administration was promoting *greater* patent protection worldwide, with Vice President Al Gore advocating the pharmaceutical industry's lawsuit against Nelson Mandela over generic drugs; the World Trade Organization was launched in 1995, and its new agreement on Trade Related Intellectual Property Rights prohibited developing countries from producing or purchasing generics.

I decided to follow several paths to bring HIV treatment where it was needed most. The first one was to demonstrate that it is feasible to provide antiretroviral therapy to people in poor countries, to silence the skeptics with facts. The second was to negotiate lower prices. And the third, simultaneous with the others, was activism to put public pressure on industry, funders, and health ministers, because morally, I knew our case was very powerful.

First, though, I needed to get the governors of UNAIDS on board, because without the board's agreement I couldn't legally spend money on the question of access to antiretroviral treatment.

In December 1996 I moved their board meeting from Geneva to Nairobi. Before we started business they spent two days visiting the slums to look at AIDS projects: I wanted them to see the urgency of the problem, and the human side, which you can't capture in white papers. I wanted them to see, too, that ordinary Kenyans were organizing themselves to confront AIDS. Some diplomats had tears in their eyes. Still, despite their personal empathy, board members from most donor countries were reluctant to endorse action by UNAIDS to promote access to treatment, whereas the NGO representatives lobbied hard in favor.

So I said, "Let's go for a study. Just a pilot project—just to look at feasibility." If we could prove that the medication could be properly administered and utilized in developing countries, then, I felt, the moral case for action would be almost unassailable. The board agreed. We called it the Drug Access Initiative, and worked with Uganda, Vietnam, Chile, and Côte d'Ivoire. With the help of Brian Elliott, an Irish former pharmaceutical manager with unparalleled experience in Africa, Awa Coll-Seck sent people to all four countries to set up the projects, which were all very different. For example, in Uganda we actually had to provide $150,000 to set up a company called Medical Access Ltd. to import antiretrovirals, because the pharma companies had no confidence in the Ugandan central pharmaceutical body. (The company is still thriving.) It all went very slowly, as there was no precedent to follow, and at the same time we had to convince pharmaceutical companies to lower their prices.

Under growing pressure from public opinion, which was starting to question the high profit margins for pharmaceuticals, Richard Sykes, the tough CEO of GlaxoWellcome (a company which by then produced two antiretrovirals), was the first to agree to some modest price reduction early in 1997, apparently taking his own managers by surprise. Finally, in December 1997 Dr. Peter Mugyenyi, a good-humored army doctor in Kampala who doesn't take no for an answer, began treating his first patient at the Kampala "Joint Clinical Research Center," where he saw patients in tents.

We were getting a 40 percent discount on the antiretrovirals for the Drug Access Initiative: they were costing $7200 per person per year. It was still stratospherically expensive for any developing nation: a start, but not a solution. But UNAIDS had started Africa's first antiretroviral treatment program, together with a program in Congo Brazzaville assisted by the French Red Cross and later followed by numerous NGOs, in particular Médecins Sans Frontières.

At an AIDS conference in Abidjan, Côte d'Ivoire, in December 1997, President Jacques Chirac of France proposed an international fund to provide antiretroviral drugs in Africa. At a dinner over a grilled "poulet bicyclette" (as free-range chickens are called in Cote d'Ivoire) with Dr. Bernard Kouchner, the popular founder of Médecins Sans Frontières and passionate spokesperson for humanitarian causes, we discussed how this "International Therapeutic Solidarity Fund" announced by Chirac would function. But unfortunately France did not provide adequate funding, and other donors, apart from tiny Luxembourg, rejected the whole enterprise, which was way ahead of its time.

I intensified discussions with senior people in the pharmaceutical industry, at first via Ben Plumley, who was head of a program at GlaxoWellcome called Positive Action, which was trying to establish better relations with activist groups by, among other things, giving them grants. These were not easy discussions. Pharma executives were very suspicious about the UN, and concerned that we would undermine their patents. It was also not easy to get their attention. At the turn of the century over 90 percent of antiretroviral sales were from just five Western countries, and Africa was terra incognita for them. But I needed to work it out. No company was producing all three drugs necessary to treat HIV infection, so I wanted to put GlaxoWellcome in a room with people from Merck, which also had an antiretroviral drug and had been under heavy attack in the United States from activists because of its high price, and Bristol-Meyers Squibb. (There were no generic medications then: this was 1997/1998.) But because of antitrust law the companies didn't want to be in same room with each other to discuss price. I don't have a legal mind, but I always supposed that antitrust laws exist to prevent upward price fixing, not what we were trying to achieve, which was *lower* prices.

In the meantime I went several times to Brazil, which by 1998 had begun producing generic antiretrovirals at Farmanguinhos, a state-owned company in Rio de Janeiro. When I first visited them, it was clear that they were struggling with international standards of pharmaceutical manufacturing, but they soon solved these problems. The experience of Brazil's AIDS treatment with locally produced generics then folded into the body of evidence that argued for differential pricing of brand-name drugs, as our negotiations progressed.

WHO explicitly did not want to be associated with our efforts. The experts at WHO's Program on Essential Drugs thought it was foolish to introduce high-tech medication in developing countries when they were struggling to distribute basic drugs for malaria. And the drug manufacturers still solidly opposed the proposal for differential pricing. They claimed this was above all because compliance with treatment would be inadequate, and that might generate resistance. But they were also concerned that if they provided the drugs at discount in Africa, they might be re-exported, and then pop up at low cost in the United States and Europe, undermining their business.

By the end of 1998, the first results of our four pilot programs for antiretroviral treatment in developing countries were beginning to come in. We had them very rigorously evaluated by independent agencies: the US Centers for Disease Control and the French National Agency for AIDS Research. The conclusion was that compliance in the developing world could in many cases actually be *better* than in Europe and North America. People, even in Africa, absolutely could read watches and they could very clearly see that the drugs were keeping them alive, so they were strongly motivated to adhere to the protocols. With minimal investment in refurbishing local health systems and training medical personnel, even very sophisticated treatment could be made to work and was saving lives. The real problems were money—no donor wanted to fund—and logistics; in Côte d'Ivoire in particular frequent stock-outs lead to very dangerous treatment interruptions for patients. (I received alarming phone calls from angry AIDS activists from Abidjan at all times of the day to have me fix this.) All this meant that in the first year only 4000 patients benefited from the initiative.

These pilot projects whisked away what had been the main argument of the pharmaceutical companies and donors: that there was no point in bringing down the price of treatment, because compliance was impossible. From that point on, their only arguments were economic, thus exposing a certain amount of what was perceived by many people as greed.

Then in 1999 small quantities of the first *generic* versions of antiretrovirals were imported into Uganda and Côte d'Ivoire from the Indian company CIPLA and Spanish Combino Pharma. Yusuf Hamied, the agent provocateur of the Indian generics industry, popped up on the world scene. Hamied is the white-haired CEO and main owner of CIPLA, a company in Mumbai founded by his father. Thanks to Indian patent law, he and others were able to build a solid pharmaceutical production capacity, imitating medicines still under patent, which would have been illegal in other countries. CIPLA is now the largest supplier of antiretrovirals in the world. (I saw their products in the remotest areas of Africa.) The appearance of these Indian companies was a game-changer for widespread HIV treatment. However, I also learned that simplistic views about the "good" generic producers and the "bad" propriety-based companies were wrong. The companies just employed different business models, and by definition generics would not exist without the originals.

This combination of activism and media attention, pressure from the UN, demonstration that HIV treatment was feasible in Africa, and the appearance of competition from good-quality generics, created a climate amenable to serious negotiations with the drug companies. I was struck by the ignorance of many of these executives about the developing world. I understood why—these were small markets for them—but I thought it was vital to our cause that we put an end to it. So we suggested trips, meetings with patients, tours of some of the better projects in Africa. Ken Weg, the president of Bristol-Myers Squibb, was I think particularly affected by this experience, as was Ray Gilmartin of Merck: I could feel that they were both struggling with the ethics of the situation, though some of the other pharma men were entirely impervious to any argument outside profit and shareholders.

The new head of the World Health Organization, Dr. Gro Harlem Brundtland, helped me with these talks, a major and very welcome shift in WHO's position. And Kofi Annan became very proactive. He took on AIDS as a personal cause and went far beyond his "terms of reference," if I may dip into UN-speak. He convened several meetings with pharmaceutical CEOs, the first one in Amsterdam in April 2001 and then in New York, followed by a private dinner at his residence. Preparing these meetings was my job, together with my UNAIDS colleagues. It was nerve-wracking, as the companies had patent and antitrust lawyers and experienced public affairs people, and we had none of that kind of support. At some moment of the Amsterdam meeting a lawyer even interrupted Annan, invoking antitrust law. I found that a key tactic was to get the CEOs to the table on their own, they then seemed more open to dialogue and could make unorthodox decisions.

UNAIDS came under quite a lot of attack during this process, which took a number of years. In 1999, when generic companies began to enter the market in a more significant way, some activists criticized UNAIDS for engaging only with the big pharmaceutical companies. I freely admit that we initially did have concerns about introducing generic drugs into the process. Their manufacturing was not always up to international standards, and the legal framework for using them was still shaky at best. Groups like Médecins Sans Frontières, Health GAP, and Jamie Love's Knowledge Ecology International—which argued that patent rights make medicines more expensive, are therefore evil, and should be eliminated—had some valid points in an ideal world, but they were not dealing with the urgency of reality, nor with the fact that we would need new HIV drugs when the older ones lost their effectiveness, which was more or less unavoidable.

We needed to put aside differences for the common purpose of defeating AIDS *right now*, and so long as they agreed with some basic principles then any groups, from religious groups to industry leaders and the most passionate activists, were welcome, indeed needed, at the table. So if ActUp didn't want to sit down with Evil Big Pharma, so be it, but Big Pharma was still invited, and we would continue to also deal with ActUp. (Perhaps that sounds opportunistic, but I remembered what Deng Xiao Ping said when he opened China up for capitalism: "No matter whether the cat is white or black, so long as it catches mice." I wanted results.) And, actually, I do think that intellectual property is fundamentally needed as an incentive for innovation—although you can argue that its use for public goods like drugs and vaccines requires a clause that permits access by the poor. So on this point, which was very controversial at the time, I split somewhat from the AIDS activist movement. This was just another example where the chameleon came in: I needed to keep my eyes fixed on the goal, which was maximal access to treatment, ASAP.

What I proposed to industry was a new social contract: in return for reasonable profits in high-income markets and a monopoly on new products (in other words, functioning patents), the pharmaceutical industry would invest in R&D for much-needed new medication, and provide new essential drugs immediately at cost (plus a small margin) to developing countries, instead of waiting for their patents to expire. I felt strongly that the poor should not pay for innovations that benefit the whole world.

I became a regular participant of the annual World Economic Forum in Davos and became deputy chair for global health under Mark Foster, a brilliant executive of Accenture, who introduced me to numerous health care executives. Gro Brundtland and I took advantage of the opportunity to directly make our case for lower prices at the forum in January 2000. Gro, a former prime minister of Norway, was a highly respected figure in Davos circles. We saw many pharmaceutical executives. One meeting was in a snowed-in mountain hotel with Merck CEO Ray Gilmartin, accompanied by Vice President Jeff Sturchio, who was a central figure in our ongoing negotiations. David Nabarro, who had been instrumental in setting up UNAIDS and was Brundtland's chief of staff, and Ben Plumley, ex-Glaxco staff and who was now working with me, also attended the meeting. We were hopeful, because of Merck's history with river blindness elimination in West Africa. Gro and I made our usual points, and basically Gilmartin told us that his shareholders would never accept an agreement to give the company's expensive new medication away at cost. While the Merck team disappeared in the snow, Gro and I looked at

each other, and said "another waste of our time." But we were determined to continue with our campaign; too many lives were at stake.

A few weeks later, Ray Gilmartin flew especially to Geneva to
meet with Brundtland. At the same time, Ken Weg from Bristol-
Myers Squibb called both of us. They both had the same proposal.
They were ready to discuss prices and how to deliver the drugs in
low-income countries. Our meetings in Davos paid off after all.

The companies wanted assurances against re-exportation of the
cheaper medicines to high-income markets, and some guaranteed
financing. My position was that we should base our notion of a fair
price on the prices that Brazilian, and now also Thai, manufacturers
were proposing for their generics, because they provided an indication
of the actual cost of manufacturing the medication. Meanwhile, the
IFPMA in Geneva, which represented the proprietary pharmaceutical industry, tried to undermine the process through very hard-line
public statements on intellectual property and against tiered pricing.
Industry was clearly no longer united, and that was an opportunity.

We worked very hard, in an exceptional joint effort with WHO,
where Jonathan Mann's old right arm Daniel Tarantola led the effort
with Ben Plumley and my chief of staff, Julia Cleves. In mid-2000,
our negotiations with the drug companies finally began to bear
fruit. Five companies (Boehringer Ingelheim, Bristol-Myers Squibb,
Hofman-La Roche, GlaxoWellcome, and Merck) agreed to quite significant cuts in the price of HIV drugs for regions severely affected
by the AIDS epidemic. We launched the Accelerating Access Initiative in May 2000, not alone as in 1997 with the Drug Access Initiative, but this time with WHO, UNICEF, the UN Population Fund
UNFPA, and the World Bank. It was a paradigm shift, although the
drugs, even priced at $1200 per patient per year—a 90 percent reduc-
tion from the price asked in Europe—remained excessively expensive
for most developing countries.

The deal got major media coverage worldwide, and the expectations were so high it was frightening. Our big gap remained the
absence of a funding mechanism: even with the price discounted,
someone still had to pay. My bet was that with drastically reduced
prices, we could now convince donors to pay for treatment. I learned

once more that no good deed remains unpunished. At the World Health Assembly in Geneva, the same month of May 2000, the African ministers of health, led by the always confrontational South African Minister Manto Tshabalala-Msimang, rejected the initiative and objected that we had not consulted them—as if we could have negotiated price reductions with 45 ministers in the room. We clearly had a major communication challenge on our hands. I was double-gutted when Bernard Pécoul of Médecins Sans Frontières compared the project to "an elephant giving birth to a mouse."

The immediate impact was disappointing. In the absence of international funding the uptake was poor. Senegal, and then Uganda and Rwanda were the first countries to use the mechanism. Access to treatment improved very rapidly in Senegal, but the country did not have as many people in need of treatment as the other two. We had made a mistake in accepting that the final price negotiations had to happen country by country, as industry wanted to keep control over the sensitive cost structure of their drugs. I sent battle-scarred staff members such as Julian Fleet, Jos Perriens (who had worked with me in Kinshasa), and Badara Sam to assist interested countries, and we shared very informally all the confidential price information we could get, so that people negotiating in country X would know what country Y was paying, a major asset in bargaining.

The European Commission then moved in with its own initiative, driven by Lieve Fransen, the Belgian epidemiologist who had worked with me in Kenya and Antwerp. We worked with them toward a very unusual round table in September 2000, which brought the Big Pharma CEOs together in a room with Yusuf Hamied and other generics manufacturers. Generics were no longer taboo. I was amazed that the chair of the European Commission, Romani Prodi, was present throughout this unprecedented half-day meeting; he was accompanied by several of his commissioners, including Pascal Lamy, a remarkable representative of French Cartesian thinking and one of the sharpest brains I have met, who later became head of the World Trade Organization. All companies present agreed to the call for differential pricing, asking only for better predictability of demand for their drugs in order to plan production, guarantees against re-exportation of the cheaper drugs into high-income markets, and price protection in high-income countries. If European countries were to ask for the same price reductions as developing countries, then clearly the whole deal would collapse.

Despite all these meetings, I also continued to travel across the world to mobilize support and money. Still too few patients in Africa had access to treatment. We set up a system with WHO and Médecins Sans Frontières to monitor the price of antiretroviral drugs globally. It was a very worthwhile, but also very frustrating, exercise: in general there is not much openness about prices from either side of the transaction. We constantly had to intervene. For example, in December 2000, Glaxo attempted to block access to generic drugs in Ghana, even though the price of CIPLA's generic was only slightly lower than Glaxo's medication: $1.74 per day versus $2. In some low- and middle-income countries, in particular in Central America, the Middle East and Eastern Europe, prices for HIV drugs were even higher than in the United States often because of the middlemen. Thus in Uganda we found that in 2001 a drug called Sequinavir cost 17 percent more than in the United States. And there was still the pending lawsuit by pharmaceutical companies against the government of South Africa's imports of generics. As long as that was not resolved, we could not be confident that they were committed to affordable treatment in developing countries.

Kofi Annan started pushing the companies to accept a settlement with the South African government, as he believed this was a global obstacle. Some pharma CEOs also understood that the court case was doing more damage to their reputation than any benefit it could ever hope to gain them. Jean-Pierre Garnier, the new CEO of the now-merged GlaxoSmithKline, broke ranks with other companies, and in February 2001 the pharmaceutical industry withdrew its complaint. It was a major victory for both the South African government and for the AIDS movement. The Treatment Action Campaign was jubilant. And the power relations in health care shifted slightly.

For me it was one box to tick off, one headache less, and more time to devote to AIDS advocacy. The climate in the pharmaceutical industry was changing at various levels. Later that year, Professor Rolf Krebs, chairman of German Boehringer Ingelheim, told me he had canceled corporate donations to the arts and to culture, and had moved it all to AIDS. Then in January 2001, India's CIPLA generic pharmaceutical company announced that it would sell a generic first-line antiretroviral treatment for $350 a year per patient, a dramatic cut in price. Yusuf Hamied was becoming a major player, even if his prices did also greatly vary from country to country, depending on their market and negotiation power—thus Combivir cost between $95 and $195 depending on the country. After that big move, the market did its own work, forcing the price down. By February 2001, a year of treatment cost around $400 in Uganda, and by July around $300: less than $1 a day. More than ever, the real gap was the funding gap.

International legal obstacles and uncertainties in terms of patent rights began to weaken. In 2001, at their conference in Doha, Qatar, the member states of the World Trade Organization agreed on the right of poor countries to issue "compulsory licenses" to override pharmaceutical patents in public health emergencies such as AIDS. This gave poor countries the legal right to produce low-cost generic drugs, provided they compensated the patent holder. In 2003 low-income countries lacking manufacturing capacity received an additional waiver to import generics from abroad. We were very involved in these breakthroughs through our American human rights lawyer Julian Fleet, whose legendary patience got him through the often Byzantine discussions—I could not have done it. His main task was to provide up-to-date technical information to delegations from developing countries, who didn't have the expertise in their administrations.

But the United States, Europe, and Japan tried afterward to circumvent these favorable multilateral agreements by imposing bilateral free-trade accords, which often extended patents beyond what was agreed internationally, in negotiations that did not involve public health officials and where the developing country understandably concentrated on its main export industries rather than pharmaceutical imports. Our impact on those negotiations was very limited, and I am concerned that in the future, progress made in access to affordable treatment may be jeopardized by these bilateral treaties.

From then on, there was progress on many fronts. In 2002 antiretroviral drugs were finally accepted on WHO's essential drugs list—a prerequisite for some countries to use them in the public sector. The Clinton Foundation ingeniously shaved off costs throughout the production process of antiretrovirals, announcing further price reductions with generic producers, and then on pediatric formulations as well. Fixed-dose combinations of three drugs in one pill were launched on the market by Indian generic manufacturers, improving drastically both quality of life and treatment adherence: from 10 to 15 pills a day, patients could now take just 2.

Yet most donors remained very reluctant to fund lifelong HIV treatment in developing countries. In October, I was invited to meet all main aid donors in the Netherlands, which was reconsidering its position, for a discussion on HIV treatment. They were still using the same arguments, and the Canadian International Development Agency even distributed a strategy document on AIDS that hardly mentioned treatment at all. Some of the discussions were almost completely detached from reality: some really believed that we had a choice between HIV prevention and treatment, in countries where every day hundreds of people were dying from AIDS—over 8000 every day worldwide in 2002. However, over a drink, most aid officials told me they felt personally very uncomfortable about their country's official positions and asked for help to change them. So I went on a tour of Europe, Canada, and Japan to meet with ministers of international development, to garner support for HIV treatment. With the notable exception of the United Kingdom, most were open to breaking the taboo of funding chronic treatment in developing countries.

The real breakthrough came only when the Global Fund to Fight AIDS, Tuberculosis and Malaria was launched in 2002. It accelerated dramatically when, in January 2003, President Bush asked Congress to approve an Emergency Plan for AIDS Relief, with a goal of offering 2 million people antiretroviral therapy. These were game-changers.

Today the cost of antiretroviral treatment has fallen from $14,000 to less than $100 per person per year. In 2000, fewer than 200,000 people in the developing world were on antiretroviral treatment—most of them in Brazil; in 2011, there were about 7 million. In 2000, barely 0.1 percent of African people with AIDS received treatment; today it is about 40 percent.

Mortality from AIDS has declined dramatically in just about every country. By any measure this is spectacular progress, unparalleled in international development. It's not a perfect situation: half of all people with HIV are still without access to treatment; as a result, in 2010, 1.8 million died who could have been saved. But the world's commitment to universal access to antiretroviral treatments has been the most sweeping international commitment to global public health in the modern era. It changed the way the pharmaceutical industry is doing business: today, when a new antiretroviral treatment is launched, it comes immediately with lower prices for developing countries, instead of a tiered pricing system coming delayed and reluctantly, under pressure. An economist would say that with AIDS, new medicines, still under patent, are no longer considered just private goods for wealthy individuals or countries, but have become "merit" goods available to everyone.

What is clear is that AIDS changed the landscape for health in the developing world. My own contribution was only one among many, but very often each step of progress happened under the UNAIDS platform. The question that haunts me until today is whether we could have done it earlier, faster.

CHAPTER 21

A War Chest for AIDS

W E NOW HAD political leadership, more or less affordable drugs, and programs on the ground—but still no real money. On April 26, 2001, in Abuja, Nigeria, in front of nearly all Africa's presidents, Kofi Annan put it sharply: "The war on AIDS will not be won without a war chest." Back when UNAIDS began, about $200 million were spent on AIDS in developing countries, and by the turn of the century it was still below $1 billion. There's no way that you can stop such a complex epidemic worldwide with that kind of money.

We simply had not been bold enough in our thinking: there was no precedent for a sudden and long-term billion-dollar financial commitment in international health, and the donor governments kept hammering that the money wasn't there. I was constantly reminded of the letter I had received from all donors on June 10, 1998, which concluded with the warning "that funding for HIV/AIDS activities will not come easy in the next few years." But they had not grasped at least four major factors: the swelling influence of the AIDS movement; the catastrophic impact of AIDS deaths in parts of Africa, which led to calls for help from more and more African leaders; the declining price of HIV treatment; and the growth of official development assistance after years of decline.

The donors' strategy of "demand containment" was slowly disintegrating; they just didn't know it yet. In 1993, when Michael Merson, then director of WHO's AIDS program, called for $2.5 billion per year to prevent half of all new infections, people were shocked. But the figure didn't include the cost of treatment, as there was no treatment for AIDS in 1993. While preparing for the AIDS Summit at the UN in 2001, we refined the estimates and came to a figure of closer to $10 billion, assuming the price of treatment would continue to decline. Because the world's economy was in a growth phase in the late 1990s, these had not been impossible demands—a bigger pie meant that we did not have to take away money for AIDS from other important issues. In fund-raising it is essential that you are clear what the "ask" is; now it was very clear, but very daunting.

There was another important, perhaps decisive, factor that tilted the balance in favor of massive AIDS funding: policy makers felt we now had a solution even if objectively it was not. The "Lazarus" effect of antiretroviral therapy, which brought life back to the dying, made for spectacular and poignant human stories, and also could be relatively easily measured and quantified. In contrast to what academics may think, policy decisions are not always driven purely by metrics and evidence. I met on one occasion with the board of directors of South African mine giant Anglo American, at their headquarters in Johannesburg. I had been lobbying them to offer HIV treatment to their employees, since the government was not providing it. Their head of medical services, Brian Brink— a soft-spoken physician who later played an important role at the Global Fund—was a strong supporter, and it was an easy meeting: I barely had to make the case at all. The CEO and chair of the board announced their decision to provide antiretroviral therapy to all staff who needed it. The only difficult questions were what to do with their families, many of whom were infected with HIV, and what would happen when the miners' contracts ended and they returned to countries without such treatment. When I asked whether I could see the economic analysis of how they had come to this important decision, Tony Trahar, the CEO, told me that they had tried to embark on one, but it was too complicated. Simply, they felt this was the right thing to do, because AIDS was affecting their workforce (and their bottom line—AIDS increased the cost of producing an ounce of gold by 70 Rand). But they would monitor carefully the program's impact and cost.

Here was a sophisticated company with some 100,000 employees, and it had made a decision—a sound one—in the absence of detailed economic analysis. In contrast, donor agencies constantly pushed me to provide economic justification of why HIV treatment should be considered cost-effective on the scale of a whole country, and even the planet.

My frustration mounted. I knew that treatment alone would not stop the epidemic. But without major funding for treatment, the real solution—prevention campaigns—would, I thought, be a nonstarter in communities with massive mortality from AIDS.

US CONGRESS REPRESENTATIVES Barbara Lee (Democrat) and Jim Leach (Republican) attempted to create a special fund for AIDS and TB in 2000. My policy adviser Jim Sherry worked hard with congressional staffers to provide technical underpinning for the proposed legislation. The bill proposed to create a special fund in the World Bank to channel money to developing countries. There was no better mechanism at the time, and I thought that as a matter of principle we should use existing institutions rather than create yet another international agency. The bill was passed, but then died a quiet death, mostly because of opposition from the US Treasury Department.

David Nabarro of the UK Department for International Development was the first one to propose a "ring-fenced" fund associated with UNAIDS, which basically would pay for drugs and condoms. However, I knew that in practice we would not be *able* to operate transfers of huge amounts of money with any degree of efficacy, as we were dependent on the administrative systems of WHO and UNDP. These were slow, bound up in red tape. I also knew that the Bush administration and US Congress were not fans of the UN, and feared that it was unlikely they would accept a massive new UN fund. Except for Mark Malloch Brown, the politically very astute head of the UN Development Program, the other cosponsoring agencies were keen on a UN fund.

Luckily, Kofi Annan and his deputy Louise Frechette shared my view. Louise had an even darker view of UN efficiency than I did, and Annan felt that no US Congress would vote for billions of dollars in new funding for anything to do with the UN. So while still negotiating lower antiretroviral drug prices, we started an assertive campaign for a special financing mechanism for AIDS in 2001.

By early 2001 there were a number of proposals by various donors to set up special multilateral funds for AIDS, for malaria, for tuberculosis, and for other infectious diseases in developing countries. (It was quite chaotic, and the developing countries most affected by these diseases were not at the table, not even consulted.) We could also build on a commitment made by the G8—the eight richest nations—in Japan, in 2000, that they would work on a fund for infectious diseases in developing countries. However, around March 2001 we all reached agreement that it would be nonsense to create multiple funds. We would all work together toward the creation of a single fund—though WHO announced at a meeting of donors and UN agencies in London in April that it "did not endorse UN consensus on this," causing consternation among participants. It was only after Annan and Brundtland met at the African AIDS summit in Abuja a week later that WHO joined our ranks, and after that worked very closely with UNAIDS throughout the process. Lieve Fransen from the European Commission started playing a convening role. The same month Kofi Annan raised the need to create a global fund for AIDS with President George W. Bush, who was supportive, but asked for a strategy and clearly stated deliverables.

From then on things accelerated dramatically, and what had seemed a naïve dream suddenly became a real possibility. During the special session of the General Assembly in June 2001 we lobbied hard, and every country signed off on a paragraph calling for a special fund. This gave it universal legitimacy, and we now had a mandate to move forward with the creation of a special mechanism that would move large amounts of money, fast.

I had no time to enjoy the success of the June AIDS summit in New York, or for any rest. First I had to get my budget through the UNAIDS board—always a week of great stress—and we then had to start immediately with preparations to create the fund. We could not afford to lose time; without even being able to imagine the unimaginable September 11 attacks, I was always concerned that the political winds would turn away from us. I had discussed our agenda with Kofi Annan, whom I represented in the negotiations. We fully accepted that the new fund would be independent from the UN. It would focus on AIDS, have a small secretariat, and include on its board developing countries, the private sector, and nongovernmental organizations—not only donor countries. It would provide additional resources, and not simply subtract money from other health or development issues. And it would itself not implement programs, but work with existing institutions.

Starting in Brussels in July 2001, a series of long meetings of a working group tried to figure out the best solution. I put Jim Sherry and Julia Cleves on the challenge. Julia worked closely with her husband Andrew Cassells, who was representing WHO—an unusual stress-test for a wonderful couple. The negotiations were very tense, as the interests and political views among countries diverged widely. But the major donor countries and the European Commission agreed on one thing: they were on a war path against the UN. I often had to swallow my pride, as when France proposed to replace UNAIDS by a pharmaceutical company representative, or the United Kingdom expressed "regrets that UNAIDS was not withdrawing from the working group" and blamed us for increasing the size of the group.

Bill Steiger tried to remove UNAIDS and WHO from the working group completely. He was a Bush protégé representing the United States and he micromanaged the US international health relations from his position as the director of the Office of Global Health Affairs, including by vetting all US scientists and public health experts who attended WHO meetings as advisers. Bill was a sharp man, who went through the details of all the papers before a meeting, and although he could socially be very likable, he was ferocious in his never-ending attacks on the UN and WHO. I did agree, though, with his insistence on strict accountability regarding the special fund's finances.

Going over my detailed notes of these meetings, I am amazed that serious diplomats could come up with some of the scenarios we considered. There was a proposal that the Rockefeller Foundation distribute the funds; I doubt whether anyone had bothered to ask the foundation whether it would even consider this. Outside the official meeting room, the pressure on us from AIDS activists was intense. The main controversies were whether the fund should be independent or be hosted by the World Bank, where it should be based, who should head it up, which health problems it would finance in addition to AIDS, which countries could benefit, whether it would only pay for commodities such as drugs and condoms or also for actual programs, who would decide where the money would go, and much, much more.

But we managed to hammer out a completely new organization in record time for this kind of international enterprise. (I'm sure a few PhD theses will come out of it.) In January 2002, the Global Fund to Fight AIDS, Tuberculosis, and Malaria was launched in Geneva under the aegis of Dr. Chrispus Kyonga, the Ugandan minister of health, whom Kofi Annan had asked to chair. It fell to me to tell the South African minister of health, who had been running for this honorary position, that she had not been selected. Needless to say this did not help our already parlous relationship, but that's how it goes the world over: the boss offers the job, and people like me bring the bad news.

Uniquely for a multilateral organization, the Global Fund board seated three NGO representatives with full voting rights—moving communities of people living with HIV from activists to decision makers—as well as representatives from the private sector. Together with the World Bank and WHO, UNAIDS was a nonvoting *ex officio* member of the board, to avoid conflicts of interest. Thus for the next seven years I served on the board of this fascinating institution. Countries received funding only after approval by a national committee whose members came from government, business, NGOs, activist organizations, and academia. This bottom-up approach was a breakthrough. Many countries had no democratic tradition of civil society dialogue with governments. I believe that in some countries the AIDS response contributed to greater democracy and transparency, via the Global Fund's "Country Coordination Mechanisms" and UNAIDS' campaigns for the involvement of people living with HIV.

At a board meeting at Columbia University in New York in April 2002, Richard Feachem, a British global health professor at the University of California at San Francisco, was elected as the first executive director of the Global Fund—despite his earlier opposition to HIV treatment in the developing world on the grounds of cost-effectiveness. The able US candidate George Moore, a former ambassador to the United Nation in Geneva, was hamstrung by the lack of diplomatic experience of the US delegation. The United Kingdom, the European Commission, and the NGOs campaigned aggressively for Feachem, whose experience at the World Bank proved very valuable in setting up the systems of the fund.

The world was shifting. UNAIDS had developed enormous credibility in a short space of time, and AIDS had surged to the top of the world agenda, despite the terrible events of September 2001 and the new preoccupation with terrorism. One of the fund's first decisions was to fund generic drugs. Our strategy of establishing a dedicated funding mechanism to boost financing for AIDS had worked, but we were at risk of becoming the victim of our success. Paradoxically, the establishment of the Global Fund meant that UNAIDS was no longer the only game in town, and it meant, too, that we did not control the money. Many of our staff felt threatened, and some media and Geneva diplomats predicted (once more) the end of UNAIDS. Developing countries courted the Global Fund, and donors asked me probing questions about our added value.

The UNAIDS staff had grown to over 600 people, with offices in over 60 countries. I told them that our job was to assist countries to prepare strong proposals for financing from the Global Fund, and then to assist with the actual implementation. In every country, we were the paramount group of HIV experts. The fund had the money—and that job can be a headache—but we were the global guardian of AIDS policies, we evaluated the impact of programs on the ground, and it fell to us to do the still much-needed political work of high-level advocacy. So I reoriented our work in that sense, and after some hesitation, the donors continued to support us.

Still, it was not always easy to maintain a good relationship between UNAIDS and the Global Fund. Initially the fund was fairly arrogant and rejected anything that had been done before; I imagine we may have been a little like this in the early days of UNAIDS vis-à-vis WHO. Perhaps UNAIDS was also too protective of its turf. Sometimes a small and silly incident created serious tension. In 2004, at the enormous International AIDS Conference in Bangkok, I lost a folder of documents. (This is a great failing of mine; when I was a child my mother would tell me I would lose my head next.) The folder, which I had placed beside a sink in the men's room, contained a confidential note from me to Kofi Annan about the latest Global Fund board meeting. My notes tend to be fairly clinical, and perhaps too forthright for diplomatic reporting, but what is the point of over-sanitized reports where everything must be read between the lines? Thus I had discussed in my memo some difficult discussions about the fund's performance and accountability. Within 30 minutes, my note appeared in the media center, which always loves a good controversy. The fund felt that I was undermining them, and the relationship became a bit strained for a while, until Feachem and I had lunch in my favorite Japanese restaurant in Geneva. Another storm in a teacup, but poor Achmat Dangor, my new director for advocacy and communications—working at his first international AIDS conference, always chaotic—had to manage the damage and handle the press.

Since then I have been careful what to take to the men's room, but I have not changed my style of reporting. Achmat is one of South Africa's great writers, and one of my favorite novels is his *Bitter Fruit*, which, thrillingly, was shortlisted for the Man Booker Prize in 2004 while he was working at UNAIDS. He was unflappable, soft-spoken, and thoughtful. He understood domestic and international politics, having played a part in the antiapartheid struggle, and is now CEO of the Nelson Mandela Foundation in Johannesburg.

The international AIDS conferences continued to swell both in their attendance and political influence. The 18th conference in Barcelona, Spain, in July 2002, attracted 17,000 participants, and for the first time, heads of state and senior politicians attended. The general mood was upbeat. Barcelona is one of my favorite Mediterranean towns, with its eccentric architecture, warm people, and tapas bars. However, my attendance got off on the wrong foot as the police had intercepted e-mail messages with death threats to me, and I could only walk around with a bodyguard.

Wanting to push the momentum further, I gave quite a militant speech at the opening ceremony before the assembled luminaries. I said, "Let us bring forward the day when leaders who keep their promises on AIDS are rewarded—and those who don't, lose their jobs. That's not negotiable!" In the corridors that week, people shouted at me "Not negotiable!" but some took it very personally—as I thought they should. After activists prevented US Secretary of Health and Human Services Tommy Thompson from giving his speech, he blamed it on me, grossly overestimating my influence on AIDS activists, who occasionally would heckle me as well. Then the activists grew upset with me because I was quoted in *The New York Times* as saying I disapproved of their heckling of Thompson; I feel strongly that we should not censor people even if we disagree with their opinions.

It was important not to break up the broad coalition in the fight against AIDS. We still needed to mobilize money, and you don't do that by yelling at the people who control the purse. Barcelona was also the moment when Bill Clinton emerged as a major player on AIDS, with announcements of further price reductions of antiretrovirals brokered through his foundation, and high-visibility events with his acquaintances. The other Bill, my friend Bill Roedy, organized an MTV debate with young people that gave Clinton an opportunity to display his unique popular charm, bringing the AIDS message to a few hundred million teenagers worldwide.

In a far more intimate event, Clinton's former AIDS czar Sandy Thurman organized a breakfast attended by Mandela and his wife Graca Machel (the only woman who has been married to two presidents); President Jorge Sampaio from Portugal, a thoughtful intellectual who was the only European head of state at the AIDS Special Session in 2001; President Paul Kagame, the master strategist of

Rwanda; and Inder Kumar Gujral, the eighty-three-year-old former prime minister of India. We discussed how to engage more top
leaders in the fight against AIDS and how to boost financing for the
Global Fund. The coalition was broadening into spheres never before
attained by a health issue.

Then something took me completely by surprise. On August 23,
2002, I had a regular working lunch with Gro Harlem Brundtland
to discuss our collaboration. Later that Friday afternoon (a classic
time to bring out difficult news) Gro stunned her staff and the public
health community by announcing that she would not seek a second
term as director-general of WHO. She had not made the slightest
allusion to this in our meeting a few hours earlier. In five years' time
she had already built a lasting legacy at WHO. Her Commission on
Macroeconomics and Health showed that investing in health is good
for economic growth—until then, the conventional wisdom had held
that the opposite is true—and most important, she had negotiated the
Framework Convention for Tobacco Control, a binding treaty that
commits signatory governments to take action against the biggest
killer of our time. Nonetheless, Gro had not been able to turn around
the hidebound culture of WHO or improve the quality of its work in
developing countries; to do that would have required another term of
five years.

Brundtland's resignation was alarming. We had developed a constructive working relationship of mutual support, even if we did not
agree on everything. She surrounded herself with capable experts, but
I knew that the WHO bureaucracy still largely perceived UNAIDS
as an interloper, and I feared that her successor might direct the
agency to return to the constant harassment of the previous regime.
People from outside UNAIDS started suggesting that I run for the
WHO director-general position, saying that it would be the best way
to ensure that WHO would play its part in AIDS, and finally operate
in harmony with the rest of the UN system But I was initially not
interested as I felt that there was still so much to do against AIDS.

I truly did not care about the power or prestige of the WHO job,
but I wanted the position to go to someone competent and caring for
health in the poorest populations, as well as a genuine collaborator on

AIDS. Too often the executives of international organizations were not chosen on merit alone but as a result of international power relations leading to some real horse trading. Of course I understood that international politics has to play a role. Votes are traded for geopolitical support, for development aid, or, even worse, for plain corruption. Paradoxically what seems the least democratic, an appointment by the UN secretary-general, has often led to better leaders (and certainly more women) in the UN system than elections, which is the rule in so-called specialized agencies such as the World Health Organization.

One of the main candidates to succeed Brundtland was Pascoal Mocumbi, the prime minister of Mozambique, a medical doctor with a decent record of government, and also, incidentally, a friend of mine. From the beginning Mocumbi was the front-runner, and the world-leading medical journal *The Lancet* was subtly campaigning for him; many said it was "Africa's turn" to lead WHO. I went to see the young Belgian Prime Minister Guy Verhofstadt for advice, because if I were to run I would need my own country's support first (only candidates nominated by their country are eligible). Verhofstadt was terrific. Belgium would support me, he said, but there would be no deals, no kickbacks, and no buying influence. I was proud of my country and officially became a candidate.

Then Julio Frenk, minister of health of Mexico decided to run. He had been one of Brundtland's assistant directors-general and was also a good friend of mine, and honestly he might have been the best choice. But at the last minute Dr. Jong Wook Lee stepped up, a South Korean who had been working at WHO for 20 years.

After my own board meeting early December in Lisbon, I took leave from UNAIDS, put together a campaign team, and traveled nonstop to lobby nearly all 32 members of the WHO executive board who would vote at the end of January 2003. These were probably the most exhausting eight weeks in my life, and on Christmas day in Cairo, Egypt, I almost fainted from fatigue. Election campaigns are an endurance test as much as a strategy challenge, and also a test for resisting conflicting pressures and not losing your integrity. Issues like abortion, patent rights, the interests of the food industry, and the power of WHO's regional offices were regularly raised but hardly any country asked for a vision on how to strengthen WHO in a changing world.

It took seven rounds of secret ballots to elect a new director-general. During the voting rounds I was sitting in my office filling in overdue health insurance and other forms to do something useful. After each round of voting, one ambassador in the closed room of the executive board called me, in Spanish, to report the (confidential) results of the latest ballot. After the vote was twice deadlocked between Lee and me, I lost the job when one country switched sides, according to diplomats present in the room, following an intervention from the US representative. The position went to J. W. Lee, whose Foreign Ministry had been aggressively lobbying board members. Remembering Kofi Annan's advice from 1994—"don't bleed"—I was the first one to congratulate Lee in front of the South Korean TV cameras. I was too exhausted to feel sorry for myself, and invited all my supporters to a big party at my home. Later Lee and I developed a habit of having dinner together nearly every other month when we were in Geneva, and we would drink Tignanello from Tuscany and he would tell me how South Korea had negotiated the votes. The dinner bill was always left for me to pay.

Obviously I was disappointed, but retrospectively, I would have to say that failing to get the director-general position was not a bad thing for my life. Paradoxically it strengthened my political standing, because I lost by one vote, and everyone in the UN system and in diplomatic circles knew that I had been a completely clean candidate. They saw the support I had in developing countries: it seemed that every African country on the board except Eritrea voted for me, even though there was an African candidate, Mocumbi, who was an honorable man. Losing the election also put my ego back in the right place.

After the vote I flew to Nepal for a gathering of UNICEF staff and young people from Asia with Carol Bellamy, the workaholic New Yorker who as head of UNICEF had become a great ally. While in Kathmandu I sat down (on the floor with my legs crossed, and could hardly get up after an hour) to talk with 25 prostitutes who were members of a group called WATCH. They told me about the hardship

328 of their lives, and daily violence from their customers, the police, and

of their lives, and daily violence from their customers, the police, and their husbands. It was very moving and a sobering antidote against the intoxication of an election campaign. Then I did something I had always wanted to do: I went to the beautiful colonial town of Antigua in Guatemala for a fortnight of total immersion in Spanish, and learned about the history and suffering of indigenous people of the region. It was my consolation prize.

IN THE MIDST of this process, President George W. Bush's request for $15 billion for AIDS relief, made during his State of the Union address on January 28, 2003, took nearly everyone by surprise. Few people, including in his own party, had anticipated such a bold and truly game-changing step from a conservative president on what had always been seen as a "liberal" issue. I realized that *something* was cooking. I appointed Michael Iskowitz, a most unlikely but very agile operator, to be the UNAIDS representative in Washington. Iskowitz was a gay man with a ponytail who had been a staffer for Ted Kennedy and a series of other Democrats in Congress. (I developed profound respect for congressional staffers: they are the people who write the questions for the ferocious congressional hearings, for example, and they often have deep knowledge of a surprising range of issues. Iskowitz was one such.) In addition to his encyclopedic intelligence, Iskowitz also had very solid links to a number of Republican senators. Just one example: he had convinced conservative Jesse Helms from North Carolina to cosponsor legislation to fund the fight against AIDS in Africa, and he had convinced Senator Orrin Hatch from Utah to support the UNAIDS contribution in the Senate.

We had been working very closely for some time with Anthony Fauci, my old cosponsor from Projet SIDA, who was the head of the National Institute for Allergy and Infectious Diseases in Bethesda. Mainly we provided data on the epidemic and on funding needs. (Our investment in statistical expertise was paying off.) By the end of 2002 Fauci's requests for more information were starting to come in thick and fast, so I grew convinced that something big was in the air, and I learned later that our data were instrumental in setting the level of the new US effort. Political Washington was starting to engage in a big way: Bill Frist—a cardiac surgeon who became the Senate majority leader—and Senator John Kerry launched a high-powered AIDS Task Force at the Center for Strategic and International Studies in Washington, of which I was a member. AIDS became (and still is) a rare bipartisan issue in US politics.

The day before President Bush's State of the Union address, Iskowitz called me and said, "There'll be a big announcement tomorrow and we need to be sure we're ready to catch the ball." Then came the announcement: the creation of a President's Emergency Plan for AIDS Relief (PEPFAR), a five-year, $15 billion initiative to combat AIDS around the world. Ten billion of this was completely new funding, beyond the United States' existing commitment. It was the largest health initiative ever launched by one country to address a disease, and it blew me away: not only the sum of money, but the fact that over half of it was earmarked for *treatment*. PEPFAR's goals for 2010 were to provide antiretroviral treatment to 2 million people with AIDS in poor countries; to prevent 7 million new infections; and to support care for 10 million people (the "2-7-10" goals).

This was a complete reversal of the US policy that had dismissed any prospect for treatment of AIDS in developing countries. I was flooded with a sense of relief and joy. I knew that we were finally in business: the brilliant coalition had done its work, for here was Kofi Annan's war chest for AIDS. So on the very same day that I lost the election at WHO, the war on AIDS was propelled to an unprecedented level by President Bush. That mattered far more than a prestigious job for me.

In much of the AIDS world, PEPFAR was greeted with suspicion and criticism. It was another example of tunnel vision; to many activists and Europeans it seemed that everything George W. Bush did necessarily had to be bad. On a personal level I was not in favor of Bush's policies in several areas, but on this I felt he was exactly right. I had certainly preferred the United States joining a multilateral effort, the Global Fund, but I had learned enough about American politics to understand that this was not an option in US Congress. And in the end, increased US funding for global AIDS would greatly benefit the Global Fund, of which the United States is by far the single largest financier. The role of evangelical Christians such as Bush's chief speech writer Michael Gerson and Rick Warren of the Saddleback Church in California in the launch of PEPFAR had been important, and through his then deputy chief of staff, later chief of staff, Joshua Bolton, the new program had quasi-direct access to the president—a precious lever in the brutal jungle of Washington. So to the dismay of some of my friends, I welcomed the PEPFAR initiative and instructed Iskowitz to do everything he could to ensure we teamed up with the new initiative.

Randy Tobias, a former CEO of Eli Lilly, was named to head PEPFAR, and during a lunch in Washington we immediately found common ground—perhaps natural between a down-to-earth Midwesterner and a man from the Flemish fields. Tobias had made a fortune in the communications and pharma industries—a Republican who wanted to give something back to the world. He didn't know much about AIDS, but he knew business. He had been all over the globe and had direct access to the White House. But again, there was suspicion all around. He was said to be just another symbol of how Bush's programs were sold out to industry, were just operations to funnel money to the big pharmaceutical companies, and so on. But AIDS needed that money, and we developed a very strong alliance between UNAIDS and PEPFAR, which continued under Eric Goosby, the dynamic head of PEPFAR under the Obama administration.

We soon found out that in terms of interagency rivalries Tobias and I had similar challenges, but the big difference was that he controlled the money, and had real administrative and political authority. He rolled out his mega program in record time, by a bottom-up, decentralized approach to much of the planning and implementation in priority countries. Initially, PEPFAR's activities were mostly implemented through American nongovernmental organizations and universities, for whom PEPFAR became a major source of revenue—sometimes I believe at the expense of the core mission of a university. However, as so often, the US Congress micromanaged many aspects of the initiative, leading to inefficiencies and ideological priorities.

Over a dinner in Paris, where both of us were attending a moderately interesting conference, Mark Dybul and I had a first session of a still-ongoing series of picking each other's brains about how to end the epidemic. Mark was Tobias's deputy, and when Randy resigned in 2006 he became the US global AIDS coordinator at the age of forty-three—and the first openly gay man with the rank of assistant secretary of state. He had an unusual combination of scientific and political intellect, artistic and spiritual sensitivity, and a street fighter's guts. We became firm comrades in arms, and I was very upset when one day after Obama's inauguration in January 2009 Mark was fired, despite being asked initially to stay on by the transition team. He was the victim of intolerance, blamed for previous US congressional policies that were not necessarily his.

At times it was difficult: to start with, PEPFAR did not fund generic drugs, thereby not only wasting taxpayers' money but also causing treatment chaos in countries. For example, in Tanzania, all US-funded programs had at one point a different prescription for antiretrovirals than programs funded from other quarters, since the latter opted for the cheaper, generic drugs. This changed gradually after 2004, when the US government accepted to buy generic antiretrovirals from anywhere in the world as long as they were approved by the Food and Drug Administration, even if they were not marketed in the United States. Once more AIDS rewrote the rules of the game, this time by bypassing the Buy American Act of 1933 and domestic pharmaceutical policies.

On other issues, the government and Congress turned out to be highly inflexible, ignoring scientific evidence. Randy and I "agreed to disagree" on them: a ban on federal funding for needle and syringe exchange programs (going back to the Clinton years); the antiprostitution loyalty oath, and abstinence-only promotion as one-third of all HIV prevention funding, despite evidence that it is not only ineffective but actually actively counterproductive. (Research in the United States found that teens trained in "abstinence only" tend to have sex a little later than their counterparts, but when they do have sex, they more rarely use condoms and actually have more sex partners.) Although President Bush had exempted PEPFAR from the "global gag rule" on abortion and family planning, there remained confusion in the field, and many of the faith-based organizations who became major beneficiaries of PEPFAR funding only promoted abstinence and fidelity, whereas it was key to offer a spectrum of options to prevent the sexual transmission of HIV (called "combination prevention"). Very few developing countries turned down the conditions associated with US funding; Brazil is the only one I am aware of. Paradoxically, at the same time, the US government was also the world's largest provider of condoms!

While I kept criticizing these counterproductive policies in interviews, speeches, and in meetings with legislators, we managed to work around our scientific and ideological disagreements, brokering bespoke funding arrangements so that PEPFAR could fund programs that it approved of, while other donors, such as the Dutch, the British, and the Nordics, picked up programs in more controversial sectors. This kind of cherry-picking by donors can be very dangerous, because the unpopular pieces can get left out, but the UNAIDS country coordinators handled the job very well, developing rational overall country plans with very few funding gaps.

Above all, PEPFAR threw its funding massively to the work of making antiretrovirals widely available, saving millions of lives. And it led the way for other countries to step up funding too, because in multiple ways, the United States still set the world agenda. Thus in July 2003 Tony Blair pledged £1.5 billion (then approximately $3 billion), the first one to follow Bush.

In September 2003, Richard Feachem from the Global Fund and I joined the new WHO Director-General J. W. Lee to launch "3 by 5," his flagship initiative to provide antiretroviral treatment to 3 million people in developing countries by 2005. Gro Brundtland, Lee's predecessor, first suggested this initiative in 2002 at the AIDS conference in Barcelona, but WHO did not follow through until Jim Kim, Lee's creative American adviser and Paolo Teixeira, the Brazilian director for AIDS, turned it into an energizing campaign which was not without risks, as it nearly undermined the launch of the President's Emergency plan for AIDS Relief by giving the impression there was no longer a need for an American effort. Even if the money was elsewhere (with the United States and the Global Fund), "3 by 5" put pressure on both donors and ministries of health in developing countries, none of whom liked the challenge. For a brief period, WHO became again very active on AIDS treatment, which was very welcome, but it often went alone and was again duplicating work that other agencies were better placed to do. It seems institutions never learn.

Four years later, 3 million people with HIV were on treatment. The "3 by 5" initiative was not reached in time, but the target played its role, and did better than many other initiatives such as WHO's 1978 goal of "Health for all by the year 2000."

MY RELATIONSHIP WITH donor countries was a complex one. Some were reform-minded, and some were true allies. However, I felt that my primary loyalty should be to the most vulnerable populations and the countries most affected by the epidemic—all developing countries, most of them in Africa. So whenever I had to choose, I chose for them, not for the donors' interests; this was most acute in the unnecessarily long debate about access to HIV treatment.

UNAIDS had no guaranteed budget from the UN, every cent had to be earned year after year. This is fair enough, as it was performance based, but it also meant I had to spend about one-third of my time on fund-raising, when I needed all my energy to fight AIDS. Also, to some extent we had started off on the wrong foot. Some donors saw the creation of UNAIDS as an opportunity to reduce their contributions, compared to what they used to give to WHO's old Global Programme on AIDS. With some donors, in particular the United States and the United Kingdom it was tough love: the UK Department for International Development was politically a great supporter—in particular when Hilary Benn was secretary of state—but at the same time constantly invented new performance targets, demanded one report after the other, and was obsessed with "global architecture" and evidence for "value for money," desperately trying to quantify coordination. Their interventions at times came close to torture, but some of that was constructive, as it forced us to sharpen our focus on accountability. And in the early days of UNAIDS our US-based funding came from USAID, which treated us like any other contractor, a competitor for American nongovernmental organizations. This improved greatly when US funding came from PEPFAR.

The challenge in the United States was micromanagement of the federal budget by Congress, to a degree far beyond anything I have seen in any other country. So I had to spend a lot of time meeting with members of Congress and their staff, trying to convince them that we were worth the investment. Less than a year after our creation, the Government Accountability Office, the investigative arm of US Congress, issued a report on UNAIDS, saying we had not delivered: it was a tough moment when I had to appear at a congressional hearing, but at the end of the day everybody agreed that such conclusions were premature and that you can't stop the AIDS epidemic in a year.

But I preferred by far the tough love of the United Kingdom and the United States to the lip service of some other countries who were long on words, but short on cash. France, a G8 member, was only our 17th largest donor, way behind Luxembourg, and was always pushing to recruit French nationals. (France did become a major donor to the Global Fund—when French national Michel Kazatchkine became its second executive director.) Italy was probably the worst at making promises, but often not paying at all. While I was a candidate for WHO, Italian officials unashamedly gave me the CVs of five fairly junior Italians for recruitment as a condition for their vote for me.

Each country required a specific approach in function of their political and societal culture. Thus in my annual meetings with my favorite donors, the Dutch (consistently the largest donor to UNAIDS) and the Nordic countries, I had to put all our problems on the table like some kind of confession (they knew anyway), explain almost penitently what I would do to improve our performance, set some goals. After a very direct discussion, they announced their contribution, and paid promptly. Trying to spin-doctor problems or be too diplomatic was counterproductive in their culture. In contrast, I learned not to show any problems in other places such as Washington, as that would have been interpreted as weakness. Throughout, I called on my inner chameleon: Adopt protective coloring; look from side to side; but keep your head pointing toward the real goal.

CHAPTER 22

An Unfinished Agenda

B Y 2004 WE had figured out the politics, the money, and the in-country programs, and we knew what to do, but thousands of people were still dying and thousands became newly infected every day, even if the spread of HIV had started to slow down. We had to move from a start-up to a large-scale operation. The key challenges for the next five years of UNAIDS were *to make the money work* for people on the ground, ensure sustainability of funding and activities, and overcome some difficult issues, from HIV prevention among injecting drug users to AIDS-related human rights violations.

With literally thousands of small and a substantial number of big players in the fight against AIDS, developing countries faced transaction costs, duplication of efforts, conflicting policies, and gaps in essential activities. Their small number of officials had to receive sometimes hundred of missions from donors and the multilateral system per year, who all wanted to meet with a cabinet minister, even if it was a junior delegation. This was not unique to the AIDS field, but the sudden influx of AIDS funding exacerbated this burden on governments, particularly those in Africa that had the weakest capacity. All this happened in spite of clear agreements among donors at conferences in Monterey in 2002 and Paris in 2004 to harmonize their procedures and in-country work. When I started receiving a growing number of complaints from Africa I knew it was time to step in—desperately needed resources for HIV treatment and prevention were being wasted and further lives lost.

I asked Sigrun Mogedal to document what was going on, and to propose some solutions. Sigrun was a seasoned and highly respected international development expert, who had been state secretary for international development in her native Norway. She was personally also very active in the AIDS activities of the Lutheran Church, and I liked her no-nonsense approach with people and institutions. After extensive consultations with various actors in Africa and in donor capitals, Sigrun sent me a report in September 2003. It was a sharp analysis but the report had too many recommendations; I put it down a few times, until a few weeks later I read it again, trying to distill the essential action points to improve international support for AIDS. Suddenly I saw them: One national AIDS strategy developed with all partners; one national coordinating authority; and one system for monitoring and evaluation of activities (as every donor imposed its own system and indicators on countries). I had just seen an exhibition of Chinese propaganda posters, and wrote on top of the paper "Three Ones!" This became a simple concept to bring some order and greater efficiency in the AIDS response in developing countries. The Three Ones were endorsed by all donors and a number of developing countries at a meeting cochaired by Randy Tobias from the United States, Hilary Benn from the United Kingdom, and myself, on April 23, 2004, in Washington in the margins of the World Bank/International Monetary Fund Spring meetings—a powerful gathering of treasury and economics officials. AIDS started to influence international development practice, paradoxically by having generated both new types of distinct funding mechanisms (PEPFAR and the Global Fund), and new ways of working together. The principles were straightforward, but progress on it was slow, due to a combination of weak governance capacity in some African countries and legal conditionalities in many donor countries.

By 2005 HIV treatment and prevention programs were well under

way, and there were over 1 million people on HIV treatment in low-
and middle-income countries. This was serious progress, but we still
had a long way to go; frustration took a front seat. The UK government was keen to push through stronger donor coordination and
impose a division of labor among the various UN cosponsoring agencies of UNAIDS—not a bad idea, but not something one can fix in
one meeting or impose from outside, as I had learned the hard way.
We also agreed with Gareth Thomas, the UK parliamentary under
secretary of state for international development, and AIDS activist
Robin Gorna, his AIDS director, to use the "Three Ones" platform
to agree on a financial framework for international AIDS funding.
What should have been a routine and fairly technical event turned out
to be a nightmare with some of the worst behavior I have seen from
UN staff, donors, and activists. What was the problem? UNAIDS
had refined the estimates of what was needed to confront AIDS, and
for the first time I had asked to do two things: remove elements not
directly related to AIDS such as caring for all the orphans in the
world and paying for medical infrastructure and staff development;
and prepare different scenarios to take into account a gradual building up of implementation capacity in countries instead of assuming
that developing countries can offer full coverage of all necessary services and interventions—basically good planning practice. When in
addition I said that we must improve how we were using AIDS money
because resources are not infinite, all hell broke loose. I was attacked
by colleagues in the UN for sabotaging fund-raising for their particular interest, by the Global Fund for undermining their resource
mobilization events, by activists for minimizing resource needs and
suggesting that we try to spend money better, by donors for inflating funding needs and for not keeping UN agencies under control.
For once I had succeeded in upsetting nearly everybody, and poor
Achmat Dangor, Jim Sherry, and Ben Plumley worked day and night
with Robin Gorna to repair the damage and try to reach consensus.

In the running up to the meeting called "Making the Money
Work" in London on March 9, 2005, I regularly received mass hate
e-mails from American AIDS activists, the nicest being titled "Peter
Piot Puppet of the Donors"—even if we called for a near doubling

of AIDS funding by 2007 to about $14 billion, up from $8 billion available in 2005 (the actual sum spent in 2007 was $10 billion). In those days there was simply zero tolerance among some for anything other than advocating for more money, and while non-AIDS interest groups claimed that AIDS got too much money, they lobbied hard to get their issue included in AIDS budgets—often with success. For months trust among UNAIDS cosponsors evaporated. It was not possible for me to have a conversation with some of our cosponsors that wasn't immediately leaked to activists, who then put everything on the Internet, making the development of a consensus very difficult. The lines between scientific evidence, professional institutional loyalty, and activism blurred. In the end we did not have to give in on the technical foundation of our work, and I was glad we had launched the discussion about optimizing, not only mobilizing resources. I still failed to understand what provoked the violent reactions but they clearly illustrated the passion of those working on AIDS, and the difficulty in international relations for an evidence-informed and transparent dialogue. It was also striking that the whole debate was among people and institutions from the the north; those directly concerned were not involved—they were doing the work. I often fantasized about the following experiment: a team of junior African economists goes to London or Washington, and tells the government what they must do to reduce public debt or to reform health care. There would be a general outcry all over the media and in Congress and Parliament, but isn't that what happens every day in low-income countries?

In many developing countries there was and is a major crisis in terms of the health workforce. This was a serious obstacle to providing HIV treatment. I saw this acutely during a visit to Malawi in 2004 with Suma Chakrabarti, the permanent secretary of the UK Department for International Development. Suma was a remarkable man in many respects, very young to be permanent secretary, and committed to reforming international development policies and UN reform. We had met for the first time in Moscow, where I had challenged him to get personally involved in the AIDS response, and we had agreed to regularly travel together, which was a feast for the brain. On every trip I learned something from him. After witnessing firsthand the dramatic shortage and emigration of doctors and nurses in Malawi, we mobilized the government and all donors, to launch that same year a $273 million "Emergency Human Resource Relief Programme" for six years, which has now resulted in an increase in doctors and nurses in the country. This agenda required urgent attention, but few countries had a systematic approach to it, as did Ethiopia whose minister of health, Dr. Tedros Adhanom, one of the most dynamic ministers in Africa, embarked on massive medical and paramedical training programs, often with AIDS money.

I felt we should do more in this area, so I tried to support various initiatives to strengthen the health workforce. Because it takes decades to train sufficient doctors and nurses (and retain them in the country), task shifting, wherein medical tasks are performed by people with less advanced education but trained to perform a limited set of specific tasks, was an obvious way to go. Research in Uganda showed that specially trained assistants performed as well as full professionals when it came to follow-up HIV treatment. Sadly, though, I discovered that the people working on AIDS and those working on health service strengthening often don't see eye to eye. In March 2008 at a conference on "Human Resources for Health" in Kampala, Uganda, when I called for a genuine partnership between our two movements, I was booed by about a quarter of the audience. I was startled, but understood that we needed to communicate better with each other.

MAKING THE UN system work together was the hardest part of my job, and where I did not feel we had made enough progress. The institutional construction of UNAIDS was based on the goodwill of every agency to work together, a few semibinding mechanisms such as channeling global funds, a division of labor among agencies, and joint reviews of each others' global activities. To a certain extent it worked, and certainly far better than any other interagency collaboration in the UN system. However, the nature of the various agencies is so different, with a bank, technical and normative agencies, and operational organizations, that a uniform approach is a major challenge. Each agency needs to raise funds to survive, which creates competition among them and drives their often aggressive communication work. In theory this could be easily resolved if donor countries put their money where their mouth is, but in practice they were often speaking with a forked tongue: in the UNAIDS board they stressed how essential a uniform UN response to AIDS was, but then at the next board meeting of WHO they pushed WHO to pursue the full range of AIDS activities, when other agencies might be better placed. Furthermore, after having put pressure on country offices of UN organizations to agree on a joint plan of action with a division of labor (which usually took many months to pull off), donors funded activities outside such agreed frameworks. These behaviors obviously reflected how national administrations were organized in very separate boxes with little communication among them—just as the UN system. An additional challenge for us was that careers depended on promoting your own organization, not on how well you contributed to an overall UN effort. The UNAIDS partnership meant that every component had to give up a bit of power to ultimately have greater impact together.

But the struggle was not only one of power. Colleagues throughout the UN and the World Bank who were living with HIV could not be open about their condition for fear of being discriminated against or stigmatized—and in fact they often were. WHO, the guardian of health in the world, passed several resolutions condemning HIV-related discrimination but refused to apply to itself what it told the rest of the world to do (it took years to convince them to allow hiring people with HIV). In some country offices confidential access to antiretroviral therapy was also difficult. Kofi Annan met a few times with the UN+ group—an interest and support group of colleagues living with HIV throughout the UN system—as did his successor Ban Ki-moon. The latter turned out to be a strong supporter of UNAIDS, but in the beginning was more at ease in diplomatic circles than with the rich plethora of characters that make up the AIDS movement. I wanted the new secretary-general to understand what AIDS meant for people's lives, so at the very beginning of his term I organized a first meeting with UN+ members, all living with

HIV. I had briefed my new boss about the sensitivities around being HIV positive in our system, and I had had a dry run with the positive staff urging them to be concise and strategic in their demands with the secretary-general. Everything was under control, I thought, when we gathered in the august wooden-paneled secretary-general's meeting room. But then Ban Ki-moon slowly looked around and said: "But you don't look ill . . . you look so healthy . . ." You could have heard a pin drop. People stared at me for a signal as to what to say. I thought, disaster!, and was already thinking how to handle the fallout with AIDS activists, but Ban went on, this time saying, "it is shocking how you are discriminated, please tell me what I can do." By the end of the meeting we did hear the daily big and small problems of living with HIV in the UN, and Ban Ki-moon announced that he would send a message to all UN staff, saying that this was one of the most important meetings of his life and that he does not tolerate discrimination in the workplace. And so he did the same day. In the end I actually preferred a man who spoke from his heart, rather than from his briefing notes, even if in the most non–politically correct way. On another occasion, at the launch of the report of a high-powered commission on AIDS in Asia that the UNAIDS Asia Director Prasada Rao had delivered with his usual efficiency, Ban Ki-moon called for the decriminalization of homosexuality and prostitution in front of all Asian ambassadors to the UN in New York. Sitting next to him. I had held my breath wondering whether he would support the recommendations of the commission, but he delivered without hesitation to an astonished audience.

HIGH TURNOVER OF staff in WHO was another challenge, as each new director of their AIDS program had a different view of priorities and how to work with us. And, in the first 14 years of UNAIDS' existence, WHO had no fewer than nine directors of its AIDS program.

These were also very difficult times for the UN and for multilateralism in general. Relations with the United States were at an all-time low because of the war in Iraq, and before that the food-for-oil scandal, which considerably weakened Kofi Annan and the UN system as a whole. Despite the extreme stress that he was under, Annan kept a keen interest in the AIDS response, and relentlessly lobbied for the cause, ably assisted by his chief of staff and then Deputy Secretary-General Mark Malloch Brown, who was equally supportive. In December 2005 Annan sent a very unusual note to all UN country teams, directing them "to establish a joint UN team on AIDS . . . with one joint programme of support." In other words, Annan was directing UN country teams to do what UNAIDS was supposed to establish, and to become a flagship example for his efforts to "Deliver as One," as the UN reform report was titled. In UN terms this was a bold move, as formally the secretary-general has no authority over specialized agencies. Several commentators went on to depict UNAIDS as a "success story." To the outside world, we at UNAIDS were an "example" of UN reform and joint action. This was nice to hear, but I felt we still had a very long way to go in this area.

NOT EVERYTHING WENT as smoothly as it looked from a distance. If prevention of sexual transmission of HIV was fraught with emotions, moral judgment, and heated academic debates, it was nothing compared to the passion and the inability to think rationally when it came to drug use. The combination of heroin and HIV epidemics was perhaps my greatest policy challenge. One place where we failed to inspire an adequate response to the epidemic was the former Soviet Union. In late nineties it was becoming obvious that there was an explosion of HIV in Russia, driven by the use of heroin. This was something we had not anticipated in any of our epidemiologic scenarios—a gross underestimation. But while courageous epidemiologists such as the soft-spoken Vadim Pokrovsky, head of the Russian AIDS Center, whom I had met during a brief visit in 1988 to Moscow, published one alarming paper after the other, the Russian government was implacably opposed to the reality being revealed. So as usual, I decided to go into the lion's den. In the end of November 1998 I went to Moscow to launch our annual report on the global state of AIDS for World AIDS Day, which is celebrated on December 1 every year since 1988. This was of great interest for national and international media, and close to midnight at the end of an exhausting day I gave my last live interview for the French TV station Antenne2. It was my scariest interview ever: I was sitting on the slippery ice-cold ledge of an open window on the eleventh floor of the Russia Hotel near the Red Square so that French TV viewers could see the Kremlin in the background. I had a serious fear of heights, and had a really hard time concentrating on the camera, but I smiled when I thought how my life might end falling on the heads of a group of prostitutes and body-guards with automatic guns who were laughing loudly underneath the entrance of the hotel. It took many skills to be executive director of UNAIDS. In any case, our efforts paid off, and for the first time worldwide media picked up the rampant spread of HIV in the countries of the former Soviet Union.

I actually liked Moscow with its history, museums, and metro, and even more the Russians themselves. They were very cultivated and warm people with a great sense of humor mixed with a some special form of *weltschmerz* and a sense of not being understood by the rest of the world, even if I definitely could not follow the vodka toasts at the numerous banquets I had to attend (dinners with all 12 ministers of health of the Community of Independent States—all former Soviet republics—were the greatest challenge, as my toast could only come after all the countries had made theirs). However, in spite of my love for the classic Russian authors and some solid friendships, relations with the government were always very tense.

We mostly interacted with the chief sanitary physician of the Russian Federation, Gennady Onishchenko, who was a very old-Soviet style man of my age with a GI haircut. Talking with him was like talking to a wall. Russia was a very homophobic society, and as for drug users, the authorities seemed not even to understand why we cared whether they lived or died. I attended preparatory meetings for the Eastern European AIDS conferences between 2005 and 2008 with Onishchenko publicly bullying NGOs and gays. The UNAIDS representative at the time, Bertil Lindblad, an experienced Swedish diplomat, was highly respected locally and helped me considerably with the UN Special Session on AIDS. He was fluent in Russian and had built a vast network of both influential Russians and civil society activists—as I expected him to do. Bertil lived in one of the huge landmark "wedding cake" buildings from the Stalin area, and hosted dinners for me so that I could hear versions of the AIDS situation in Russia other than just the party line. The AIDS activists were very courageous young men and women, who operated in a system with little tolerance for dissident views and were always short of money.

The old Soviet Union had had a decent public health system and sanitary infrastructure, combined with a huge and often coercive surveillance system for infectious diseases, but after the fall of the wall there was a sudden cessation of funding of the public health sector, the rise of a brutal free market economy, and a general collapse of traditional social norms. Epidemics of all kinds were bursting forth in the 1990s: not just AIDS, but also diphtheria, hepatitis, typhoid, and sexually transmitted infections. Except for some isolated cases of HIV, nearly always imported from abroad, in 1988 during the Soviet Union era about 250 children had been infected with HIV by their doctors and nurses, mostly because of reuse of unsterilized syringes and catheters at a hospital in Elista, Kalmykia. Some of the infants even transmitted HIV to their mothers while breast-feeding, probably through a cracked nipple. There were other, smaller outbreaks of the same kind elsewhere. In April 1998, I visited an institution just outside St. Petersburg for HIV-positive children, many of whom had been infected by faulty medical treatment: they were essentially abandoned. They had arrived undernourished at the hospital, and nurses and children begged for my help, but what could I do? It was an incredibly depressing experience that would haunt me. I think the authorities were so secretive about this partly because it was such an indictment of the Russian medical system.

The hospital spread of HIV among children was tragic, but the scale of the AIDS epidemic among adults went out of control at the turn of the century. By 2005 around 1 million people or just over 1 percent of the adult population was infected with HIV, even if the Russian authorities rejected the UNAIDS estimates (they only accepted a number based on the officially registered cases of around 300,000). It was a young epidemic, and an epidemic among the young: 80 percent of HIV-positive people were under twenty-nine years of age, and 40 percent were women. Initially, the overwhelming majority of people with HIV were injecting drug users. So, addiction and social breakdown were at the heart of the epidemic in Russia and other ex-Soviet countries, such as the Baltic States and Ukraine. However, many of the mainly young people who became infected through sharing contaminated needles and syringes were not classic drug users, and it was not just heroin coming from Afghanistan (introduced by Afghan war veterans). More often these were occasional weekend users, sharing locally produced ordinary opiates such as *kompott* among friends, which made the spread of HIV even more difficult to control: harm reduction approaches like needle and syringe exchange and substitution treatment for opioid use are less likely to work for occasional users.

There was a whole corps of physicians in Russia known as *narcologists*, who specialized in addiction treatment—not to the mega epidemics of alcohol or cigarettes, but to opiates—and these people were a huge obstacle to any rational approach to dealing with drugs— meaning a combined approach of education to prevent people from using drugs, treatment for addiction, repression of drug trade, access to clean needles and syringes, and oral substitution therapy with methadone and other substances. Their approach was basically to put the junkie in a cold room and often beat him, and if he resisted in any way, to then confine him in a straitjacket: I am barely exaggerating. There was no medical treatment at all, and the Russian government up to this day subscribes full-heartedly to this approach, although a punitive-only approach to drug addiction only drives drug users underground. The narcologists were particularly adamant in their opposition to gradual treatment of addiction through the use of methadone, which has been the cornerstone of opioid dependency treatment in the United States since the early fifties. By delivering orally an addictive substance, methadone, that doesn't give the "high" of recreational drugs but does remove the craving, methadone facilitates the beginnings of a dialogue with addicts, so you can start the difficult process of treatment and resocialization. It also keeps them away from injections that transmit infections that will kill them and others. In particular, Russian prisons were an absolute incubator of disease, through overcrowding, rape, and shared needles. (It wasn't just AIDS: there was also tuberculosis, one piggybacking on the weak immune system created by the other. Exacerbating the problem, much of the TB was drug-resistant.)

Russia is one of the countries I visited the most, but without much impact. I knew Russia's leaders were sensitive about demography. The population had been in decline since the fall of the Soviet Union, despite immigration, because of low birth rates and very high mortality, especially among men. This affected the quality of the armed services, productivity of industry, and the future of the nation from just about every point of view. Even with a modest 1.1 percent prevalence rate of HIV, AIDS would exacerbate demographic decline in Russia much more than in an African country with much higher HIV prevalence but an annual population growth of 2 to 3 percent. I thought this could be my entry point for a breakthrough in our discussions with Russian officials, but it never happened. In contrast to nearly all other countries where I asked for this, I never managed to meet the then head of state, President Vladimir Putin, but I am not sure whether it would have made a difference. In democracies, where there's a responsive system of governance, there's no real need to meet the top man, but I had learned that in more authoritarian traditions the state leader has a massive impact even on fairly minor things. However in 2006 in the running up to the G8 Summit in St. Petersburg—the first ever in Russia—I met the then First Deputy Prime Minister Dmitri Anatolyevich Medvedev, who would become Putin's successor as president. Medvedev listened carefully, recognized that the country had an AIDS problem, and announced that the State Council Presidium had just decided to establish a national coordinating authority on AIDS—a breakthrough—but also confirmed the government's opposition to methadone as "non-scientific." This was very disappointing, but I didn't give up, and continued to advocate for better and more humane HIV prevention, working closely with media figures Vadim Pokrovsky and Russian speaker Michel Kazatchkine, the new French head of the Global Fund, and with groups such as AIDS InfoShare, Médecins sans Frontières, Open Health Institute, and even with the Russian Orthodox Church. During an audience with Patriarch Alexy II, I agreed to support a training program on AIDS for priests, as the

Church was increasingly filling a moral and ideological vacuum after the fall of communism. I also went on media-covered street visits to see HIV prevention work with sex workers and injecting drug users—their living conditions, personal misery, and constant harassment by the police were horrific. Sadly, none of the visits made a difference for official policy, although they did for local initiatives. However, by then Russia was providing antiretroviral treatment to people with AIDS, but basically only to "good citizens," and often at a cost above that in the West, probably because of the involvement of several middlemen.

At the end of a conference of G8 health ministers in Moscow in April 2006, J. W. Lee, director-general of WHO, and I were sharing a laugh in the hotel lobby about the absurdly choreographed meeting. This was the last time I had some social time with J.W., who was in good spirits, though looking extremely tired. He unexpectedly died on May 22, 2006, from subdural hematoma, just before the start of the annual World Health Assembly meeting. Even though competitors for the election of his position, we had developed a good relationship, and I was sad. (As so many told me afterward, I also thought of the extreme stress of this kind of position.) The irony of history was that I ended up sitting next to a chatty Margaret Chan on the flight back home from Moscow to Geneva. We had met a decade earlier in Hong Kong where she was director of health, and she was now in charge of pandemic influenza at WHO, which badly needed an entrepreneurial woman such as Margaret. Even during Lee's funeral service I was approached by several countries to run again for the position, which I found shocking. I quickly decided that this time I would not run: I had no confidence in the electoral process of WHO and felt there were at least two excellent candidates in Julio Frenk and Margaret Chan. (Chan won, becoming the first Chinese to head up a specialized agency of the United Nations.)

Russia's western neighbor, Ukraine is the country most severely affected by HIV in Europe, with half a million people or 1.5 percent of all adults being HIV positive—more than France, Germany, and the United Kingdom combined. At the turn of the century, Ukraine had the most progressive AIDS policies in Eastern Europe, with drug substitution officially allowed since 2003. I visited its historic capital Kiev several times to ensure that the politically unstable country would continue its more open AIDS activities, each time nearly starting from zero with the new minister of health. I was also focused on narrowing the gap between national policies and local practices— despite clear national policies to the contrary, intimidation and even prosecution of HIV prevention workers by the police had started again in cities like Odessa, where over half of all injecting drug users are HIV positive. Each visit was closely prepared by Anna Shakarishvili, the Georgian UNAIDS representative, with people like Vladimir Zhovtyak and Natalia Leonchuk from the All-Ukrainian Network of People Living with HIV at whose founding conference I spoke, and with the International HIV/AIDS Alliance from Brighton, United Kingdom, which was the main foreign supporter of AIDS programs. As always I did not limit myself to official meetings, but also roamed through the huge apartment complexes in Kiev's suburbs in freezing-cold temperatures to observe needle and syringe exchange programs managed by former drug users. The clients for these clean needles were not what people may expect as junkies, but included a working woman walking her dog, a man with groceries on his bicycle, and other people you cross all the time on the street. These encounters were a precious source of information for my interaction with officials. My last visit to Kiev was in 2008 with Crown Princess Mette-Marit of Norway, who was a very active UNAIDS ambassador, as was Crown Princess Mathilde of Belgium—my favorite princesses because they were smart and combined great class with genuine human empathy while remaining down to earth and approachable, though traveling with them involved numerous security and protocol constraints. They were great allies to bring the AIDS message to the public and indirectly to decision makers across Europe. I was always amazed by the princess effect on people.

WHEREAS MOST HIV infections in India are due to sexual transmission, in the Northeastern states injecting drug use was the driver. In the states adjacent to Burma such as Nagaland, Manipur, and Mizoram, where about 1.5 percent of adults were HIV positive, heroin was easily accessible from their neighboring country. There was also a particularly nasty form of addiction among young people who were taking a legal substance—Spasmoproxyvon (dicycloverine hydrochloride), sometimes prescribed for intestinal colic—mixing it with water and injecting it like heroin. It made their veins hard as the powder does not dissolve in water and accumulates at the point of injection, blocking the blood flow. I could feel their veins like stone pipes running down their arms and legs. They developed abscesses, had body parts amputated, and died from infection. And because possession of a needle was a criminal offense in India they also shared needles; thus many were HIV positive.

This was a *legal* substance, of dubious pharmaceutical added value; the government could easily have withdrawn it from the market. In addition, people were shooting other over-the-counter substances such as buprenorphine and dextropropoxyphene, as well as amphetamines massively produced in Burma. After a visit to the region with senior officials and members of Indian Union and state legislatures, the government promised to legalize programs for methadone substitution, and restrict the sales of Spasmoproxyvon, but implementation of the promise took years.

In every way, India was a far more responsive society to rational argument of this nature than Russia was. Albeit a bit slowly, democracy always got its way, with cross-party consensus through an All Parliamentary Forum on AIDS, which the always smiling and serene Oscar Fernandes, a yoga adept and catholic king maker of the Congress Party, had launched with a few allies from other parties. I visited New Delhi and many states of this huge country numerous times. Initially I was overwhelmed by the never-ending crowds of people and the loud pushiness of many Indians, but after a while I loved the country and its rich culture. The real problem became how to respond to the numerous dinner invitations from my growing number of always very hospitable friends and keep my weight under control. Thus in July 2003 I addressed the largest AIDS event ever in India, sharing the podium with the then Prime Minister A. B. Vajpayee, as well as Sonia Gandhi, the leader of the opposition, and Manmohan Singh, the future prime minister. Getting such consensus in the brutal jungle of Indian politics is no small achievement, but just as in the US Congress, AIDS transgressed political enmities. After initial strong denial of AIDS, the formidable machinery of the India Administrative Service got its act together by setting up NACO, the National AIDS Control Organization, supported by World Bank loans. It had some remarkable leaders: Prasada Rao, who gave it solid foundations and a strategy; S. Yacoov Quraishi, the great communicator on AIDS and later the chief election commissioner of India (I occasionally sing in his rock band); and the exuberant Sujata Rao, who solidly anchored the management in every state, working with community groups that had become very vocal, particularly the women's groups such as the Positive Women Network (PWN+). PWN+ was founded by a tiny woman from Tamil Nadu, Kousalya, who was infected when she was twenty years old by her husband, whom she had to marry to keep property in the family. Her story was typical of many Indian women with HIV, but she fought for survival and recognition of the rights and needs of women with HIV in India. When I first met her, her English was hard to understand, but she later became a board member of the Global Fund and regularly spoke at international events. Another key initiative in India was Avahan ("call to action" in Sanskrit), a very large HIV-prevention project among the most at-risk populations, led by former head of McKinsey in Delhi, Ashok Alexander, and funded by the Bill & Melinda Gates Foundation. These combined efforts led to real achievements, with a significant decline in new HIV infections and increasing access to HIV treatment. Better AIDS programs throughout the country also meant better epidemiologic data, and in early 2007 it became clear that UNAIDS had overestimated the size of the HIV epidemic in India: we now had empirical data from over a thousand sites in this vast country, as compared to just over a hundred before, and, equally important, we had data from India's huge rural population who turned out to be far less infected with HIV than we originally thought. I did not hesitate for a second to go public with this downward revision of HIV estimates, knowing that we would have to go through some difficult moments. UNAIDS indeed came under attack, and conspiracy theories about my deliberately inflating HIV estimates to raise more money for AIDS even made it to the front page of the *Washington Post*, when they managed to get access to an incomplete draft of our report. It was another tough moment, but our message to the world was that we put scientific evidence before political communication and, in any case, influencing epidemiologic estimates was a nonstarter, because the UNAIDS epidemiological data are generated in a process that involves literally over a hundred experts. Nothing was confidential in our work.

ADDICTION TAKES OVER the life of not only the drug user but often family and the environment as well. One of the most moving meetings I had was in Jakarta, the chaotic capital of Indonesia, in 2003, when HIV began to spread among drug users in the country. Because of the enormous stigma of AIDS, groups of people with HIV could not even rent a space to meet, so the UNAIDS office created a safe space for all kinds of community groups. One such group was made of parents—in fact mothers—of young injection drug users with HIV. Their stories of human suffering, of bribing the police to get their children out of jail, of financial ruin, were heartbreaking, and again I felt powerless, but also more than ever determined to fight for a humane approach to substance abuse. During that trip I also met another remarkable young Asian woman living with HIV, Frika Chia Iskander, who was seventeen years old when she became infected with HIV as a drug user in Jakarta. Frika was then shy and struggling with her identity as a person with HIV, but gradually became one of the world's best-known and respected AIDS activists, and a great spokesperson on AIDS.

THERE IS THE real world of drug users with or without HIV infection, and there is the often surrealistic world of drug policy makers, many of whom have never even spoken with a drug user, a social worker, a prison guard, or a doctor treating addicts. As much as I hated it, I felt that in my position I had to bring the human realities of drug use to the Commission on Narcotic Drugs—the world body that since 1946 annually reviews the global drug situation. It is the governing council of the UN Office on Drugs and Crime, UNAIDS' seventh cosponsor. In April 2003, it was that time of the year to go to Vienna, where this commission meets, with most members coming from law enforcement agencies. Justice and police versus public health. After I detailed the ravages of HIV infection among drug users and the scientifically proven methods to bring the HIV epidemic among drug users under control, I was attacked from many sides, except for some European countries and Australia. A Japanese deputy minister was very upset with me, and nearly yelled, "Would you give needles to your son?" That was the level of debate. Some "harm reduction" activists also challenged me because when I said that we must do everything we can to prevent people from using harmful drugs and to treat addiction, they felt this was code for a pure police approach against drugs. I thought, one tunnel vision against the other. The head of the UN Office for Drugs and Crime, the Italian economist Antonio Maria Costa, was ambivalent about harm reduction, because two of his major donors, the United States and Sweden, were firmly against this approach. Many countries still have not accepted harm reduction techniques and so suffer thousands of painful, entirely avoidable deaths. Scientific evidence without political will has little impact on people's lives, and politics going against evidence can harm people.

JUST AS FOR about anything in China, AIDS was a special case and required a specific approach. For years leaders failed to grapple with the reality of the epidemic, despite a huge cluster of contamination among people paid to donate plasma (this almost certainly amounted to well over 100,000 people, although the authorities admitted to no more than 35,000, in itself a high number) mainly in Henan province. HIV also spread among drug-users in southern provinces and via sexual transmission in the most entrepreneurial regions that were driving the Chinese economy: places that featured the "Three Ms"— Mobile Men with Money, as one man told me in a bar in Guangzhou. In the nineties Chinese AIDS patients were often punished or jailed when they were found to be HIV positive, and there was massive discrimination.

In June 2002, we issued a report entitled "HIV/AIDS: China's Titanic Peril," warning that China faced an epidemic of "proportions beyond belief." The UNAIDS representative in the largest country in the world, Emile Fox was a man of practical jokes from one of the smallest countries, Luxembourg, and had added as a subtitle a quote from Napoleon: "When China will wake up, the world will tremble." This hit a nerve, and we nearly had to close down our office in Beijing: in fact Kofi Annan called me (on a Sunday afternoon!) to warn me to change tack. He said, "Peter, you're a brave man, but nobody has ever won against China. So start building bridges, because we need China on board and that's not the way you're going to change anything." Annan was right and, in any case, our own epidemiologists were unhappy with the prediction that China would have as many as 10 million cases of HIV in the not too distant future—that estimate was not based on serious evidence. I went to China at least once a year, trying to establish a relationship of trust with various officials, urging a more robust and responsible approach, and basically acting like a fox terrier. I met with low-ranking officials at the Ministry of Health, then moved slowly up, many banquets later establishing a kind of friendship; in the meantime, I tried to become a familiar face at the Ministry of Public Security, the Ministry of Foreign Affairs, the Ministry of Labor, in several key provinces, and with Communist Party officials. Once you become a familiar face, you can build confidence and get a sense of who is calling the shots, to better understand what their main concerns are. My French friend in Beijing, Serge Dumont, was a precious adviser on how to operate in China. Serge is a fluent Mandarin-speaking gentleman who was considered the founder of the public relations industry in China in the 1980s before the current Western interest in doing business in China. As President for Asia of Omnicom, he seemed to know everybody who counted and organized the first private fund-raising event for AIDS in China; I appointed him as Goodwill Ambassador for Asia in 2006.

Things began changing on World AIDS Day 2003, when Premier Wen Jiabao visited a Beijing hospital and shook hands with AIDS patients. The SARS epidemic of 2003 with its huge economic cost (though very limited in terms of victims) was a wake-up call, and Iron Lady Vice-Premier Wu Yi was temporarily put in charge of the public health ministry. The Chinese government also announced that it would provide free antiretroviral treatment to AIDS patients who couldn't afford it, and promised free HIV testing, free treatment to prevent mother-to-infant transmission, free infant HIV testing, and financial assistance for AIDS orphans (known as the "Four Frees and One Care" policy). Still, these were mainly announcements, with few indications that the situation was massively changing on the ground. However, I gradually got more access to address sensitive issues. Thus after a meeting with Madame Wu Yi in the Great Hall of the People in May 2004, where she asked me to report back on my observations, I was allowed to visit a rehabilitation-through-labor camp in Guangdong province (near Hong Kong). It was a sobering experience: hundreds of women who were accused of prostitution or "antisocial" behavior were working in total silence in large factory halls, making small bracelets and cheap decorative ornaments without ever looking up. I was asked on the spot to give a speech to the women, and I asked the women a few question to learn what they knew about AIDS. Two replied with a decent answer, and all I could think of was to ask the commander to free the women before their normal time. I can still not look at small ornaments without wondering who made them in China.

There were groups of people with HIV in every major town, and I sat down with them at each visit. They were still very isolated in society, and at risk of police and other harassment. As everywhere, they were supporting each other and sometimes used art to express their existential feelings. One of them, Xiao Li, member of the Home of Loving Care in Beijing, gave me a moving calligraphy with a poem expressing his feelings about when he discovered that he was HIV positive: "I was lonely and confused / I finally understand a full answer to life is never an option / . . . it reignites my dignity and determination / when deprived of wings / we can fly with our vision / . . . so come by my side, fellow fighters and friends / together we shall conquer Mount Everest . . ." Another reminder not only of the universality of poetry but also of suffering and the desire to rise above crisis.

What 2001 was for the global AIDS response, 2005 was for the AIDS response in China. In June 2005 Randy Tobias, the US global coordinator, Joel Rehnstrom, the phlegmatic Finish UNAIDS representative in Beijing, and I went to Yunnan, the province with the highest HIV prevalence in China—an estimated 80,000 people with HIV out of a total population of 44 million. Yunnan is a beautiful mountainous region with great ethnic diversity and Kumming, its capital, has a population of over 3 million people in its urban area alone. Many of them gathered every evening around the lake of romantic Cuihu Park to drink the local vintage *puer* tea, sing, and dance in small groups in the open air. The province had introduced quite progressive HIV policies over a year before, as we could see in Gejiu City near Burma. We visited a methadone treatment and needle exchange clinic, a change from the traditional draconian cold-turkey-and-beating style of operation, though the latter approach continued to exist as well. The next day brought a rather comical surprise: on arrival at the Yunnan Police Academy where we funded an education program on AIDS and drug use, I had to review a parade of honor guards while a band was playing martial music. While I was not expecting such a ceremony, I thought that it was great that even security forces started taking AIDS seriously.

Most crucially, Premier Wen Jiabao had agreed to an audience on Monday, June 13, and this was to be one of the most interesting meetings of my life. It took place in Ziguang Ge (the Hall of Purple Light) in Zhong Nan Hai, the *really* Forbidden city, banned to ordinary mortals, which is next door to the old Imperial Forbidden City well-known to tourists. In this complex of buildings—a mixture of traditional Chinese architecture and a more Stalinist style, with an artificial lake surrounded by precisely manicured gardens—the top echelons of the Communist Party of China live and work. I was prepared for a rather difficult conversation. I wanted to raise the subject of HIV in prostitutes and drug users, as well as the ongoing serious human rights violations of HIV-positive people and AIDS activists, several of whom had been beaten up or arrested. So as usual I had a little note tucked up my sleeve with a number of talking points, all of them grim.

Without wasting time with the usual expressions of diplomatic nicety, Premier Wen came straight to the point—after all he is a geologist. He said, in essence, "I know what the problem is; just tell me what works to fight AIDS, and be specific. Forget who we are, I would like to know what works, and we will then see what can be done in our context. I realize these drug users are not only criminals but are also ill, and we should treat them as patients."

Instantly, my task became easier. After commending Premier Wen for his leadership on AIDS and praising Gao Qiang, the new minister of health whom I respected and liked a lot, I went for it, discussing the need for much more openness about the problem and the fact that although the virus is spread by behaviors that might be illegal or socially unacceptable, to protect society as a whole and ensure the much cherished *xiaokang* (harmony in society), you need to work *with* the people affected, not just jail them. For those who use drugs, you need substitution therapy, clean needles, and humane, medically proven substitute treatment. For prostitution, I said it was not my business what China as a nation decided to legislate, but I had been coming to China since the late 1980s and it was striking to me that in many hotels I stayed there were obviously several prostitutes, so it was essential to make sure that this commerce was done safely to protect the women and the population. I also pleaded for country-side training programs for police forces and the Ministry of Public Security, because although Premier Wen may personally have shaken hands with AIDS patients, policemen were still harassing them.

It was one of most open and direct conversations I had with someone of his stature. Premier Wen was an impressive man, he thanked me after one hour of discussion in front of a large number of dignitaries who had taken note of every word, and promised to follow up. Two days later on Wednesday I was scheduled to give a talk to the Central Party School of the Chinese Communist Party, something few outsiders have done, and nobody from the UN until then: they are the guardians of orthodoxy, and they train all the future top leaders. I spoke about AIDS as one of the great challenges to society and the need to solve such "secondary" contradictions as Chairman Mao had written in his famous essay and speech—I had done my homework for the school. At the unavoidable banquet after my speech, the director of the Party School made a final toast to my speech, concluding (that part in English) "party (has) two meaning [*sic*] in English, and we are good at both. *Gan bei* (bottoms up)!"

The following day, China's State Council issued a progressive new decree on AIDS that could not have been more concrete. Some pieces of it were literally translated word for word from UNAIDS documents, so it must have been put together very rapidly: it would be hard to present better evidence of our influence. It highlighted the need to fight discrimination against HIV-positive people, and the need for needle exchange programs and drop-in centers for methadone treatment, along with specific targets and a commitment to specific budgets. And all this, they delivered.

The cluster of medically transmitted AIDS cases in Henan was still a tricky issue. I had mentioned it to Premier Wen; I talked about blood safety and suggested a fund for compensation of those infected and their orphans. He admitted that "we have not been good at being open about this problem" and I got the distinct impression that he himself did not have a clear grasp of the statistics. China is a far less centralized country than many people think; regional governors are very powerful and in Henan they seem particularly secretive. No one significant was ever punished for it, and there must have been powerful people involved for the information to have been suppressed.

Much earlier in 2001 I went not to Henan but to Shinxan-Wuxi county in Shanxi province at the northern border of Henan, where the problem was similar although smaller in scale. In the mid-1990s people had been paid to give blood, some of which was returned after the plasma was separated out, in highly unsanitary conditions mixing blood from several people, some possibly infected with HIV. A very high proportion of the donors developed HIV infection and died. I met eight of them at the Warm Heart Center (hard to believe that such a name was chosen for a very cold and isolated cement building). They still had no treatment in 2001 and were condemned to death without antiretrovirals. The whole landscape of the area was blighted, an industrial wasteland of small coal mines and pollution; you almost couldn't see the sky for smog, and I could hardly breathe. When I had dinner with the governor back in the provincial capital of Taiyuan (again over 3 million inhabitants) I said, "Well, I'm here to talk about AIDS but I can imagine you have some other major health problems, with respiratory disease and lung cancer and so on." His response: "No! Why would you think that?" and lit another cigarette. It was total denial. Things that were not supposed to be simply were not. It was only in July 2007 that I was allowed to visit the villages in Henan province where most of the victims of the criminal blood donations had lived, and many died. I was surprised to see that the blood trade had initially brought prosperity to the community before bringing death. Greed in its most macabre form.

Despite all this encouraging progress, it was "one country, two systems" (as China says about its relationship with Hong Kong), for the AIDS response. In 2006 I visited another southern province, Guizhou, that had over 60 "rehabilitation and detoxification" and "methadone maintenance treatment" centers for a population of just under 50 million. In Zhijin County I visited re-education-through-labor facility, along with some officials from the Ministry of Health in Beijing. (None of them had ever visited such a facility.) It was a prison inhabited by pale young men in gray pajamas, nine in one cell with an open toilet in the corner. They were confined in their cell until 2 P.M. and had to study for six months the one-page house rules, which were the only thing on the wall of their cell. While we were talking I could see several of them shaking, possibly from withdrawal pains, and one fainted as I spoke. There was no medical treatment; if they became too violent they were strapped down. You could see the menace of the place: these men were clearly absolutely terrified of the guards. From there we went to a Western-style drop-in center for supervised methadone treatment, and needle and syringe exchange. Nearly all the drug users had spent time in a detoxification camp and were afraid of being sent back. One told me that it was a matter of luck or of police bribing capacity whether to end up in the methadone clinic or in prison.

But in general, China began moving forward quite swiftly with a much more rational response to the epidemic. The following year, when I met with the Chinese ambassador in New York, I was startled when he pulled out a copy of the speech I had given at the Central Party School, highlighted with yellow marker, and asked questions about the exact significance of various statements I had made. Apparently all Chinese Communist Party members were required to study this document: undoubtedly my most widely read speech.

BY MID-2005, SOON after China switched sides and joined the ranks of the rational, I found I could no longer hold off the pressure from UNAIDS board members who wanted an official strategy statement on HIV prevention, as this would then not only be official policy for the whole UN system but also provide authoritative guidance for countries. I had for years been ducking this task, because I feared that what would emerge in a board made up of member states with highly divergent positions would be a more or less meaningless and diluted document, when what we all needed was clarity. To be at all meaningful, a prevention strategy needed strongly worded positions on gay and women's rights, needle exchange and drug substitution programs, and interventions for safe sex, including within the context of prostitution. Purnima Mane, Jim Sherry, Ben Plumley, and I worked intensely behind the scenes to generate overwhelming support for our position, and particularly to neutralize the opponents to needle exchange programs, though that was interpreted as capitulation and weakness by harm reduction activists as I deliberately kept publicly quite silent while preparing the board meeting. The document was hotly debated for three days until late at night, but eventually all except Russia and the United States agreed to harm reduction policies, with countries like Japan and Sweden not objecting. Thanks to the flexibility of the PEPFAR leadership, the United States did not block the consensus, as long as we would add a footnote saying that it could not be forced to support needle and syringe exchange. For the first time the world had an agreed HIV prevention strategy, and the basic principle of "combination prevention"—that it takes multiple interventions to stop this epidemic—was formally anchored in global policy. I hoped that this would put an end to the fata morgana of the magic bullet solution for HIV prevention, but that turned out to be wishful thinking. In addition, as with so many things in AIDS, knowledge and technology evolved, thanks to continuing major investments in AIDS research, and more recently our armamentarium to reduce HIV transmission became far more extensive than in 2005, with circumcision of men, antiretroviral treatment as prevention of HIV transmission, and vaginal microbicides and preexposure prophylaxis (taking antiretroviral drugs before exposure to HIV). The challenge now is to customize the optimal combination for different populations.

HUMAN RIGHTS ISSUES were never far away when working on AIDS. They were not just part of our values, but we had learned that discrimination and stigma were major impediments for both prevention and access to treatment. Therefore AIDS-related human rights promotion was an essential part of our work. There were extreme cases of violence and even murder, targeting women or gay men infected with HIV. The brutal murder of Gugu Dlamini in her community on the outskirts of Durban, South Africa, in December 1998 after she had appeared on TV, where she talked openly about being infected with HIV shook the world, but it was by no means a unique event. As typically occurred in such cases, no one was ever found guilty of her murder. Another major obstacle to HIV prevention were laws criminalizing consensual sex between adults of the same sex, which is the case in 76 countries, punishable by death penalty in seven countries, including Iran, which has executed more than 4000 people for homosexuality since 1979. So I had to raise this issue in my meetings with numerous prime ministers and presidents—not always easy, to say the least.

Quite often UNAIDS had to intervene when once again HIV prevention workers or activists were harassed, arrested, or incarcerated—usually when they were working in the homosexual community, such as in several African countries, in Central America, or in Nepal, or with drug users and prostitutes. In China, AIDS activists were regularly picked up by public security agents, and we tried to find out where they were held to negotiate their liberation. We intervened with the authorities, and a few times even provided legal assistance.

In a truly surrealistic, but unfortunately very real, case, a Palestinian doctor and five Bulgarian nurses accused of having deliberately infected over 400 children with HIV in a hospital in Benghazi were prosecuted and repeatedly tortured. As so many others had, I tried to convince the Libyan authorities to free the medical workers; there was absolutely no evidence for their alleged crimes. But the madness of the Kadhafi regime was only fueled by the volatility of AIDS. Later, in December 2005, I thought I had found an opening during a breakfast with President Obasanjo in the Villa—the presidential residence in Abuja—as I felt an African-inspired solution might be more acceptable to Kadhafi than pressure from the West. Obasanjo immediately called the Libyan ambassador to Nigeria and asked for a discussion with Kadhafi on this, suggesting also some form of compensation for the children in return for the liberation of the health professionals. Nothing happened until July 2007, when French and European Union efforts resulted in the liberation of all six.

Another major issue I had to deal with throughout my tenure at UNAIDS was travel restrictions for people with HIV in over 20 countries, even for a brief visit, such as to the United States. This complicated our work at the United Nations in New York, as we always invited people living with HIV to participate in events we organized. Some had to lie about their status, and others were marked with a special status. It was so unfair, and from a public health perspective unjustifiable in a country with more than 1 million people already infected with HIV. As a result of this travel ban going back to the Reagan presidency, no international AIDS conferences could be held in the United States. Fortunately, following the lift of the travel ban by the United States in 2009, other countries followed. Even China abolished its travel restrictions in 2010, but Russia once again chose to remain on the side of obscure policies.

MUCH OF MY time was spent on better coordination of AIDS efforts among various agencies, and on the Global Fund to Fight AIDS, Tuberculosis, and Malaria, with its numerous board and other meetings. It was clear that without the Global Fund AIDS treatment and prevention was plainly inaccessible in many countries, as the US AIDS effort by necessity had to concentrate on a limited number of countries. So, ensuring its success and continued funding was one of my top priorities, and UNAIDS country staff spent up to half of their time working on Global Fund proposals and ensuring smooth implementation once a grant was awarded. The fund was able to jump-start HIV treatment in a minimum of time, and by 2011 it had committed $22 billion in 150 countries—a remarkable achievement by any means. These funds were also mobilized thanks to relentless campaigning by grassroots activists, the Global Fund, and public figures such as Bono, Nelson Mandela, Bill Gates, and Kofi Annan. As a completely new type of international organization, the fund had to invent its entire modus operandi, and it often went through rocky times managerially. After too long an interregnum, and two turbulent board meetings in which developing and high-income countries became very antagonistic, Michel Kazatchkine was elected as its second executive director in February 2007, winning the ballot with a very small margin from my deputy Michel Sidibé. A true Parisian intellectual and passionate AIDS physician with Russian roots, Michel Kazatchkine was an old friend from the days he headed the French National Agency for AIDS Research, and it was easy to harmonize our messages. We particularly worked together to raise money during a series of "replenishment" conferences to fill the coffers of the fund. I admired the fund for its transparency: you could find details of their grants, expenditures, and audit reports on their website—a model for the international system, even if their courageous exposure of corruption or poor management in some of their grantees sometimes turned against the fund. However, I was frustrated by a fairly dysfunctional board, with donor countries micromanaging the fund secretariat but not providing strategic direction and holding the developing countries hostage to their conditionalities, and because few board members had the guts to refuse to endorse the ever-escalating demands from activists for more money, even when those demands came from countries that had hardly started to implement the previous grant. I was further annoyed because, until recently, the Global Fund was financing AIDS, TB, and malaria activities in so-called middle-income countries that were well able to fund these activities from their own domestic budgets. This failure of governance, combined with management challenges and the international financial crisis, led to the fall of Kazatchkine. Safeguarding and fully financing the Global Fund is vital for defeating not only AIDS but also malaria and TB.

I was thrilled when the G8 Summit in Gleneagles, Scotland, in June 2005 committed to "as close as possible to universal access to HIV treatment and prevention," but my cynical half told me it would be difficult to promise more at a next summit—in any case it was the last time AIDS got such prominence at a G8 Summit, and the G20 did not seem to be interested in health or social issues.

It was in everybody's interest that the US President's Emergency Plan for AIDS Relief also be fully funded, so each year I urged members of Congress to continue to increase PEPFAR's appropriation, as well as to fund UNAIDS and the Global Fund, since we each had unique and complementary contributions to the global AIDS response. Global AIDS Coordinator Mark Dybul and I often appeared together at congressional hearings and at think tank events, even speaking in 2007 at Reverend Rick Warren's Saddleback Church in Orange County, California, as the support of Evangelical churches was crucial for the renewal of PEPFAR. Although I had given speeches in churches like the Cathedral of St. John the Divine in New York City and in the Church of San Francisco in Lima, Peru, they were always part of an AIDS event. This time, I was preaching for a real evangelical congregation, and I was quite nervous about it, especially having to talk about sensitive issues such as homosexuality. Before entering the stage in the vast hall, I took a deep breath, thought about Father Damien from my village, and spoke as I would have spoken in my home village of Keerbergen. After 30 minutes Rick Warren hugged me and said, "Home run!" (Maybe after all I would have made a good preacher.) The vote by US Congress of a $48 billion renewal of PEPFAR in 2008 was great news, and a rare moment of bipartisan consensus in an election year in Washington. I attended the signing ceremony in the White House with President George W. Bush, and the program continued under President Obama.

We had several severe setbacks, though. Perhaps not surprisingly, they appeared first in the countries that had shown the earliest achievements: Uganda saw a rise in new HIV infections after 2005, and in Thailand HIV was rising among homosexual men and injecting drug users, probably as a result of a refusal to introduce harm reduction programs and of the so-called War on Drugs, which was more a War on Drug Users under Prime Minister Thaksin Shinawatra. When, in 2007, UNAIDS gave Thailand a poor score card based on evidence coming from the Thai Ministry of Health, which had excellent epidemiologic data, the Thai delegate in the UNAIDS Program Coordination Board in Chiang Mai in northern Thailand objected strongly to our rating. He was in general a fierce defender of accountability and of independent evaluation, but obviously not when it concerned his own country. I was not willing to change Thailand's ranking as the facts were not disputed. It was just an illustration that as an "intergovernmental" organization, UN entities were always at the mercy of their member states when publishing honest reports about countries, particularly when comparing performance among them.

AIDS remained a global issue, with infections occurring every day throughout the world. In absolute and relative terms the HIV problem in high-income countries was clearly much lower than on a continent like Africa, but after the introduction of antiretroviral therapy, budgets for HIV prevention declined, and in most European countries there was a gradual increase of new infections, particularly among gay men. In England, despite its very high rate of HIV testing and free treatment through the National Health Service, the number of new infections doubled over a period of 10 years, nearly exclusively in gay men and migrants from HIV endemic areas. Parts of the United States remained confronted with a bad HIV epidemic. I was a frequent visitor to Washington DC, but was basically confined to a triangle between Capitol Hill, Georgetown, and Dupont Circle, with an occasional dinner at a friend's place outside this area. At one point in 2005 Michael Iskowitz, our man in DC, reminded me that with a 5 percent HIV prevalence, the District of Columbia had a worse HIV problem than most West African countries, and told me it was about time that I meet some people other than members of Congress, officials, academics, and white activists. He took me to The Women's Collective in an African American part of Washington not far from Howard University. It was as if I had traveled to another country. This was a group of poor, mostly black women living with HIV, founded by Patricia Nalls, a courageous woman who had turned her personal experience with HIV into positive action— a bit like what Noerine Kaleeba had done in Uganda. One woman after the other told her story of parental abuse, nearly daily violence, rape, drug use, broken relationships, hunger, and poverty. One tiny woman of forty, who looked like she was over sixty years old, showed me what was left of her toes—eaten by rats—and told me that she was now sleeping in a tent in her apartment to protect her from rat bites. Another woman showed a small plastic bag like what you use to put any small containers with fluids through airport security: it contained three small bullets—the harvest of a night of violence on her street. I was speechless, and wondered how much a human being can endure. From meeting Holocaust survivors and HIV-positive widows of the Rwandan genocide, I learned that our human capacity to survive and find meaning in life is beyond imagination, though not without limits. These stories from several continents suggested that we needed to sustain prevention and treatment efforts, and not cry victory too soon.

While the response to AIDS became more vigorous across the world, HIV had become *hyperendemic* in southern Africa, meaning a very high HIV prevalence with continuing new infections. I continued to fail to understand what made southern Africa so different in terms of AIDS from the rest of Africa, and the rest of the world, but in any case I was convinced that the region required a truly exceptional response to bring the epidemic under control. Besides numerous visits to South Africa, I also went to the surrounding smaller countries that had HIV epidemics that were at least as bad. In the tiny landlocked mountain kingdom of Lesotho 31 percent of adults were HIV positive in 2005, in some areas even over 60 percent! Life expectancy at birth had fallen to thirty-five years, down from sixty-five without HIV, but the international community completely ignored this country which had become a major sweatshop for mostly Chinese factories. The country was confronting an unprecedented triple humanitarian crisis combining poverty, malnutrition, and AIDS. So I joined forces with Jim Morris, the Indiana native head of the World Food Programme, and Carol Bellamy from UNICEF to gather international support and also to see how a pioneering nationwide door-to-door HIV testing campaign worked in practice. The uptake was surprisingly high, and you could feel the impact of AIDS everywhere. In community after community people, mostly women, were organizing themselves to cope with AIDS in the family, and there was a lot of openness about the problem, though less so about condoms. In contrast, the government had a fairly bureaucratic approach to the AIDS crisis, something I raised with King Letsie III, who was concerned about the very survival of his people and had declared AIDS a national disaster. Similarly landlocked, but somewhat wealthier, Swaziland—remember my mission from WHO in 1977 to "eliminate sexually transmitted diseases"—had the highest HIV prevalence in the world by 2004, with a staggering 42 percent of pregnant women being infected with HIV. The Swazi epidemic had "feminized," with over 55 percent of all people with HIV being women. Life expectancy at birth had collapsed to thirty-two years as a result of AIDS. In an alarming report, the UN Development Programme concluded that the "longer term existence of Swaziland as a country will be seriously threatened," reminiscent of the plague in the Middle Ages. It is hard to imagine that in modern times a virus can have such an impact but already in 2005 Swaziland had about 70,000 orphans out of a total (and shrinking) population of 1.2 million, with child-headed households common. In Mambatfweni village I saw how communities tried to protect these children from all kinds of exploitation, including sexual abuse, and support them while leaving them in their original family homes rather than putting them in an orphanage. It was impressive how, with very limited resources, the community joined forces without waiting for help from outside, though the drugs to keep them alive came from international aid. Several times I met King Mswati III, the last absolute monarch in Africa, who had banned women under age eighteen from having sex inspired by an ancient chastity rule, but then promptly married a seventeen-year-old girl as his 13th wife. There was a huge credibility gap between his policies and his own behavior. Given the continuing high rate of new HIV infections, and the lack of circumcision among Swazi men, the country was an obvious candidate for a large-scale male circumcision campaign.

Even if it was confronted with an equally daunting HIV epidemic, Botswana on the other hand seemed on the path to recovery thanks to the exemplary leadership of President Festus Mogae and his entire cabinet, the considerable and well-managed resources from diamond mining, and international support, particularly from PEPFAR, the Gates Foundation, Merck, and several US universities.

However, the country was less successful in terms of preventing new infections, and sexuality and gender relations were still very sensitive issues.

SINCE THE DISCOVERY of HIV in the 1980s we had all implicitly hoped that AIDS would go away one fine day and that technology—a vaccine, perhaps a cure—would eliminate HIV. No such luck. HIV is firmly embedded in both human cells and societies. I was very concerned about sustainability of our efforts: Who would pay for decades of treatment? Would we have new drugs when HIV became resistant to the current ones? How would second line antiretrovirals become affordable (Brazil's HIV budget for medicines was already doubling because of the increased need for second line drugs)? How would political and community leadership be sustained? Prevention efforts? Lifelong adherence to treatment and safer sex? Etc. As President Festus Mogae had rightly asked when we discussed male circumcision— why were we not emphasizing more circumcision of newborn boys, instead of only adolescent and adult men as this would protect the new generations? I liked his long-term view, but stressed that we need to deal with the acute and the long-term—unfortunately international policy remained limited to the short-term, which I felt was a mistake and missed opportunity.

So in 2003 I initiated several projects to think through what the long-term trajectory of AIDS could be, and in particular what we needed to do *now* to ensure the best possible long-term outcome. We started with AIDS in sub-Saharan Africa, as the obvious priority, teamed up with Shell's forecasting division in London, involving hundreds of concerned people in Africa. Under Julia Cleves's leadership this resulted in a 2005 report "Three Scenarios for AIDS in Africa by 2025," which made it clear that the worst was still to come in terms of impact of AIDS in southern and eastern Africa. It also made a strong case that it would not be enough to devote more resources to HIV treatment and prevention, but that supportive policies and good management would be equally key for achieving impact—nothing revolutionary, but important to state at a time when all attention went to raising money. Two years later I launched an initiative called "aids2031" (as the year 2031 will mark half a century since the first reports on AIDS in 1981). This was again an effort involving hundreds of AIDS experts and others, and was led by Heidi Larson, who had done work on the future of AIDS in the Asia region, and Stef Bertozzi. It turned out to be far more difficult than I anticipated to think so far ahead, perhaps because we were all struggling with daily crises of delivering HIV care and prevention. The highly politicized environment on AIDS might also have prevented people from daring to think outside the box, and some in the AIDS community feared that long-term foresight would deter from much needed action today. Not surprisingly it was young people who came up with the most innovative ideas, particularly during an aids2031 event at the Googleplex (Google's headquarters in Mountainview, California), which led to the creation of the Global Health Corps by Jenna and Barbara Bush and Johnny Dorset, then in their twenties—an initiative that twinned young people from the United States and a developing country to work together in a health project.

The aids2031 recommendations called for a redesigned AIDS response, far more tailormade to the specifics of the multiple and diverse HIV epidemics across the world, and proposing various ways to optimize HIV programs. By the time the report came out in 2010, most of its recommendations had already been taken up by several funders and AIDS programs, all concerned now about sustainability, optimal use of resources, and long-term impact. Thanks to enlightened leadership from people such as ministers Tedros Adhanom Ghebreyesus and Agnes Binagwaho, countries such as Ethiopia and Rwanda made smart use of dedicated AIDS funding to strengthen their health systems overall, but most countries strictly followed the rules of the donors, thereby missing an opportunity for a more sustainable response. In times of financial crisis all these issues became key, and will be so for years to come.

When near the end of my term in July 2008 I launched the traditional biannual UNAIDS report, just before the International Conference on AIDS in Mexico City that Ban Ki-moon attended, I could for the first time announce a significant decrease in both deaths from AIDS as well as in new HIV infections (except in the former Soviet states). Finally, I was the bearer of good news.

SUNDAY NOON, NOVEMBER 30, 2008, Ndjili Airport, Kinshasa. I had just come from an informal breakfast at the private residence of the young Congolese President Joseph Kabila with whom I discussed how to address widespread sexual violence and rising HIV infections in eastern Congo, which was still in full-armed conflict. We were waiting in the very loud and chaotic VIP lounge for a South African Airways flight to Johannesburg where I would give my last World AIDS Day address as head of UNAIDS, and the first one in South Africa since the resignation of President Mbeki in September. Then my BlackBerry vibrated: "Dr. Piot? The secretary-general would like to talk to you. Please hold the line." Ban Ki-moon thanked me for my input in the selection process for my successor (my mandate was coming to an end, beyond the maximum 10 years at this level in the UN), and he told me how impressed he was by Michel

Sidibé during his interview. The telephone connection was very bad, and the noise and music in the airport lounge were as loud as in a bar in Matonge, but through it all I heard Ban saying solemnly in his soft voice: "I have decided to appoint Mr. Sidibé as executive director of UNAIDS with effect of the first of January 2009. Can you please call him, and ensure there is a smooth transition between you and Mr. Sidibé" I felt great relief; UNAIDS would be in good hands. I immediately called Michel in Geneva, nearly shouting through the Congolese crowd speaking loudly in their cell phones: "*Mon frère, toutes mes felicitations!* Ban Ki-moon has just appointed you. We'll celebrate later this week in Bamako." (We had planned a while ago to visit Michel's native Mali together.) The connection broke off abruptly. The circle was completed in Congo, where my professional life had first taken off.

EPILOGUE

O
N DECEMBER 26, 2008, I closed the door of my now empty office and walked for a last time between the huge Mary Fisher sculptures in the nine-meter-high glass lobby of the Zen UNAIDS building, with its hanging and floating rocks. I would miss greeting the guards in the morning, having a quick word with the devoted women and men in my office who kept me sane during all these years—Marie-Odile, Sylvie, Karen, Caroline, Anja, Julia, Julian, Ben, Roger, and Tim—and rushing by the thought-provoking contemporary African art in the corridors. My successor Michel Sidibé would take over in a few days, leading UNAIDS and the global AIDS effort to the next stage. Just as he would arrange the furniture in his office differently, he would manage the organization differently and communicate differently, reflecting the rich heritage of Mali, France, and UNICEF under Jim Grant. I was proud that sometimes succession planning works in the UN.

I was not down nor relieved to abandon the influential pulpit of the UN, nor the snake pit of multilateral politics, and I had no withdrawal symptoms from the relative power and comfortable support that went with the job (except when once again those hopeless IT breakdowns hit me), because I had mentally and practically prepared my departure for a year. I must admit though that it was a great feeling to no longer be held responsible for anything that goes wrong on AIDS anywhere in the world. The moment I walked through the door it was all over, and my mind was set on the future. Just before the end of the year I would fly from Geneva to Harlem, New York, to start a new chapter of my life.

At a farewell dinner in December in Geneva, I asked Kofi Annan for advice on what to do in January. His answer was prompt and brief: "Sleep! Sleep as much as you can. When the responsibility falls off your shoulders, only then you will feel how tired you are." As so often, he was right. Every cell in my body had accumulated a decade of lack of sleep and constant jet lag—not to mention the never-ending stresses fueled by what were mostly pseudo crises. I often woke up in the morning and wondered which government would complain, which angry e-mail some activist would fire at me, which donor would announce the nth evaluation of UNAIDS, which UN agency would complain that UNAIDS behaved like an independent agency, which confusing or nasty newspaper article I would have to face that day. Just as in political positions, these are demanding jobs. Others may handle this better than I did, but I rarely could relax, even on vacation, when the US Government Accounting Office or a reporter would decide it was the best moment to launch another investigation. Work dominated life far too much, and my family paid a high price, which I deeply regret. Without their tolerance and support I probably would not have made it.

These are also lonely jobs, and there were very few people I could confide in and who understood what was at stake in terms of AIDS, how complex the environment was in which I had to operate, and how bizarre the behavior was of people I had to interact with. It was not easy to explain to friends and family how exactly I spent my days, as I was so often a victim of the 80/20 law, and it sounded like all I did was attend meetings, give three speeches a day, and sleep in planes. What I enjoyed the most was trying to convince people to act on AIDS and to strategize on how to move the AIDS agenda, globally and in each country. This required in the first place thorough preparation of each important encounter, a solid knowledge of the culture and political environment, and the background of the individuals I would meet, much more than the AIDS situation. Bearing in mind what my mentor Stanley Falkow told me about understanding how bacteria cause disease when I was working in his laboratory in Seattle, I tried to put myself in the position of the person I was going to meet. Trying to understand people's needs was also a guiding principle when developing policies—something insufficiently done in health policy.

Working in the United Nations system (it was an extended family with many very diverse members) was often not easy. Together with humanitarian aid, and very recently women's issues, UNAIDS was the most advanced attempt to "deliver as one" in the UN. Over the years I became increasingly skeptical as to whether the current UN coordination governance could ever be effective operationally, despite the goodwill of many, if not most, staff. The two main obstacles for delivering as one UN were the institutional interests of individual agencies—careers, political influence, budgets—and the incoherence and volatility of its member states, which not only had different, sometimes mutually exclusive, interests, but which also lacked internal coherence, as they promoted different agendas in different UN agencies depending upon which national department they represented. My conclusion on UN coordination was that it was a collective failure, and that the international community either goes for some bold mergers and acquisitions as the current plethora of institutions is too expensive, or that it accepts that pluralism is a strength, as long as only effective and well-managed institutions are supported and others closed down. The creation of new institutions outside the UN system to fix problems of the UN is not a solution, as much as I worked to make the Global Fund to Fight AIDS, Tuberculosis and Malaria a success.

Despite all imperfections, working as a senior UN official was a great privilege and allowed me to influence the global agenda in a way that very few positions offer—certainly when coming from a small country like Belgium. I also met an extraordinary group of smart and caring people at all levels of the system, and occasionally we even had fun during the otherwise dead-serious retreats of the chief executive board of the UN secretary-general. UNAIDS also provided a unique platform where the various AIDS actors came together globally, as well as in individual countries, and therefore could drive the agenda.

So, our achievements were not so much inside the UN system but in the world at large, which is what ultimately counted. I always thought that I was paid to make a difference against AIDS, and if along the way I could contribute to a better UN, all the better, not the other way around—otherwise it would have been "operation successful, patient dead."

The contrast between my formative years as a scientist-adventurer and leading a UN agency could not have been greater, but I thoroughly enjoyed the different lives I had. The transformation was gradual and took years, and rather than shedding the approach of a researcher, I worked hard to complement it with diplomatic, managerial, and political skills. My scientific background also gave me some credibility, but was most useful for analyzing the potential implications of new scientific information for policy. I had a double mantra: keeping AIDS as a global issue, not one of poor Africa, and keeping science, politics, and programs on the ground in sync. Science without politics has no impact, politics without science can be dangerous, and without programs people don't benefit. However, when I was appointed as head of UNAIDS, I had to learn everything the job required, except AIDS. My years as an activist in medical school were probably at least as useful as my actual medical training. When writing these memoirs, it struck me how many of the same people played a role at different moments in my life. Without their advice and support I would not have been able to function properly.

How unique was the historic context that shaped the AIDS response and how applicable is the AIDS experience to other health or societal problems? Around the millennium the economy was flourishing, official development assistance was rising, a generation "WE" of young people was connected globally through social media, and a relative optimism prevailed, despite September 11, the wars in Iraq, Afghanistan, Côte d'Ivoire, Somalia, Chechnya, and more.

In addition, AIDS was exceptional in that it was global, affected young adults who normally don't die, devastated entire countries, and often was associated with behaviors that are not approved of in society. This was not the flu or cholera that you can catch on a bus or from drinking contaminated water. Hallmarks of the response were the transformational role of people living with HIV and other activists, and a response that went far beyond the classic medical community. The combination of the unique features of AIDS and the global engagement of a wide spectrum of actors made AIDS the first *postmodern* epidemic, as Lars O. Kallings, the Swedish founding president of the International AIDS Society, once said. So it may be that the AIDS experience was historically unique, and there certainly was hardly a comparison between a short deadly epidemic such as Ebola hemorrhagic fever and the prolonged and equally deadly AIDS pandemic—even if the former makes better movies.

However, while AIDS was exceptional, it had broader impacts on how we perceive sexuality, on the doctor-patient relationship, on health as a global political issue, on the role of communities in health policies and programs, on the pricing of medicines, and on international development assistance. It was a catalyst for the emergence of "global health" as a major multidisciplinary field of study and practice, and generated major resources beyond AIDS to confront two old infectious diseases that were killing millions of people—malaria and tuberculosis—a major collateral benefit of the AIDS movement.

"Noncommunicable diseases"—cardiovascular disease, diabetes, cancer, mental health—are the pandemic of the twenty-first century, driven to a large extent by smoking, unhealthy food, lack of exercise, and environmental factors. This is an area that probably would benefit from the AIDS experience. For the first time in history a health threat to our survival as a species is not an infectious agent, but is due to the way we organize our lives and societies. Bringing noncommunicable diseases under control requires a coalition and resources even more formidable than what created the current achievements against AIDS.

We made good progress, but the end of AIDS is not in sight, and to this day, I remain haunted by the question of what I could have done earlier and faster. As for the future, I am greatly concerned about the sustainability of the response for the AIDS epidemic and for people living with HIV. HIV may be with us for generations and maintaining a high level of political engagement and commensurate funding will require a rethinking of political strategies, while making the new products of science available for HIV prevention among those who need it most, but are often those who are the least able to pay.

In my short life, numerous new pathogens have been identified in humans and animals, and new epidemics will undoubtedly continue to emerge, probably through the food chain as well as from animals. Can we anticipate these future outbreaks of new and unknown pathogens? To a certain extent we can, as for influenza, but surprises do happen, as with the emergence of H1N1 in Mexico, rather than in East Asia as was expected. Investing in a laboratory infrastructure, surveillance, and the training of relevant scientists across the world is a minimal requirement for early alert and action, but will not be sufficient, as difficult societal decisions will need to be made in times of great uncertainty around the potential spread of a newly identified virus. We must invest in improving such political decision making in uncertain times. Or did Louis Pasteur have it right when he said, "Messieurs, c'est les microbes qui auront le dernier mot" (Gentlemen, it is the microbes who will have the last word), even in our era of unparalleled science and technology?

Above all, the history of AIDS is one of refusing the inevitability of death because of lack of treatment, defeat, prejudice, and institutional obstacles, and moving mountains beyond familiar territory. It was—and is—the collective result of big and small heroes everywhere, a few villains, but also many who did not take up their responsibility. It brought out the best and the worst in human behavior. It helped me discover myself, and made me aware of my vitality as well as my vulnerability.

The global response to AIDS was a rare exception to the iron rule that international aid is fundamentally an extension of foreign policy and foreign trade, as illustrated by the long-term commitment to lifelong treatment in poor countries. The response was driven by a broad movement of people across the world and a sense of great moral outrage. As Philippe Kourilsky, the former director of the Institut Pasteur in Paris, wrote. It is perhaps the strongest example of global altruism out of a rational necessity in our ever-more interconnected world.

ACKNOWLEDGMENTS

Ruth Marshall has worked closely and patiently with me through-out the writing, including long hours of interviewing. In addition her research corrected the inaccuracies of my notes and the failings of my memory. Thanks to Charlotte Sheedy, Angela von der Lippe, and Laura Romain for believing in me and guiding me through the meanders of publishing.

I could not have written this book without the unfailing love, sup-port, and encouragement of Heidi.

My thoughts and my gratitude go to Greet, Bram, and Sara for their love, understanding, and care in often difficult times. Exciting developments in my life meant sometimes great turbulence in their lives.

Getting older also meant that I realized how much I owe my par-ents for a renaissance education, for offering the space to explore the world, and for supporting me even when I walked paths the sense of which they did not understand or approve. My siblings—Wim, Pol, and Lieve—were always there when I was in trouble and, of course, to celebrate life.

I have been influenced by wonderful and inspiring people who collectively made history, and who are the actors of this memoir. My profound thanks go in the first place to colleagues and friends at the Institute of Tropical Medicine in Antwerp; the International Commission for Hemorrhagic Fever in Zaire; Projet Sida in Kinshasa; the University of Nairobi; the University of Washington; the University of Manitoba; the International AIDS Society; the Society on AIDS in Africa; the Global Programme on AIDS of WHO; UNAIDS, the Joint UN Programme on HIV/AIDS; the Bill & Melinda Gates Foundation; the King Baudouin Foundation; and the London School of Hygiene & Tropical Medicine.

King Holmes, Stanley Falkow, Paul Janssen, Michel Carael, Jerry Friedland, Marie Laga, Mark Dybul, and Michel Sidibé were my mentors at various stages in my life, and without Marie-Odile Emond I would not have survived.

At the risk of unfairly not mentioning many, I would like to thank friends and colleagues for their support (+ indicates that the person is deceased): Zackie Achmat, Michel Alary, Ashok Alexander, George Alleyne, Roy Anderson, Kofi Annan, Louise Arbour, Dirk Avonts, Yvette Baeten, Bai Bagasao, Madhu Balla Nath, Ron Ballard, Stephen Becker, Frieda Behets, Paul Benkimoun, Seth Berkley, Stefano Bertozzi, Agnes Binagwaho, Bono, Tina Bonto, Ngali Bosenge (+), Caroline Bournique, Joel Breman, Mario Bronfmann, Richard Bruczinsky, Gro Harlem Brundtland, Françoise Brun-Vézinet, Jean-Baptiste Brunet, Bob Brunham, Piers Campbell, Lisa Carty, Andrew Cassel, Joe Cerrell, Suma Chakrabarti, James Chau, Julia Cleves (+), Hillary Rodham Clinton, Nathan Clumeck, Myron Cohen, Bob Colebunders, Awa Coll-Seck, Larry Corey, David Corkery, Sally Cowal, Alex Coutinho, Kathleen Cravero, Jim Curran, Achmat Dangor, Kevin De Cock, Paul DeLaey, Chris Elias, Brian Elliott, Hiro Endo, Gunilla Ernberg, Jose Esparza, Marika Fahlen, Anthony Fauci, Eric Favereau, Oscar Fernandes, Mary Fielder, Julian Fleet, Mark Foster, Skip Francis, Lieve Fransen, Louise Frechette, Geoff Garnett, Laurie Garrett, Bill Gates, Helene Gayle, Jacob Gayle, Tedros Adhanom Ghebreyesus, Geno Gysebrechts, Eric Goosby, Robin Gorna, Anand Grover, Meskerem Grunitzky-Bekele, Rajat Gupta, Robert Hemmer, Sylvie Herda, David Heymann, Mark Heywood, Lennarth Hjelmaker, Richard Holbrooke (+), Susan Holck, Karen Horton, Richard Horton, Chieko Ikeda, Michael Iskowitz, Aikichi Iwamoto, Carol Jacobs, P. J. Janssens (+), Francoise Jenskens, Karl M. Johnson, Noerine Kaleeba, Lars Olof Kallings, Joseph Bila

Kapita, Nils-Arne Kastberg, Elly Katabira, Michel Kazatchkine, Jim Kim, Michael Kirby, David Klatzmann, Philippe Kourilsky, Richard Krause, Mathilde Krim, Ulf Kristoffersson, Cristian Kroll, Jean-Louis Lamboray, Peter Lamptey, Debbie Landey, Joep Lange, Geert Laleman, Michel Lechat, Stephen Lewis, David Mabey, Kambala Magazani, Marina Mahatir, Adel Mahmoud, Mark Malloch Brown, Purnima Mane, Elisabeth Manipoud, Jonathan Mann (+), Tim Martineau, Arnaud Marty-Lavauzel (+), Marta Mauras, HRH Mathilde van Belgie, Souleyman M'boup, Frances McCaul, HRH Mette-Marit of Norway, Joe McCormick, Andre Meheus, Michael Merson, Ren Minghui, Sheila Mitchell, Hans Moerkerk, Sigrun Mogedal, Rob Moody, Stephen Morrison, Pol Moyaert (+), Pierre Mpele, Peter Mugyinye, Luwy Museyi, Warren Naamara, David Nabarro, Jeckoniah O. Ndinya-Achola, Ibrahim Ndoye, Peter Ndumbe, Elisabeth Ngugi, Anja Nietzsche, Herbert Nsanze, Nzila Nzilambi, Thoraya Obaid, Olusegun Obasanjo, Sam Okware, Mead Over, Stefaan Pattyn (+), Martine Peeters, Jean Pegozzi, Greta Peits, Jos Perriens, Joy Phumaphi, Ben Plumley, Frank Plummer, Carole Presern, Y. S. Quarashi, Tom Quinn, Prasada Rao, Sujata Rao, Geeta Rao Gupta, Olivier Raynaud, Helen Rees, Mary Robinson, Carlos Rommel, Alan Ronald, Christine Rouzioux, Jean-François Ruppol, Robin Ryder, Nafis Sadik, Roger Salla-N'tounga, Jorge Sampaio, Eric Sawyer, Jean-Louis Schiltz, Bernhard Schwartlander, Jim Sherry, Frika Iskander Shia, Werasit Sittitrai, Martina Smedberg, Papa Salif Sow, Paul Stoffels, Patty Stonesifer, Jonas Store, Jeff Sturchio, Tod Summers, Elhadj As Sy, Yuki Takemoto, Daniel Tarantola, Masayoshi Tarui, Luc Tayard de Borms, Henri Taelman (+), Marleen Temmerman, Lucy Thompkins, Randy Tobias, Mathilde van Belgie, Guido Van der Groen, Eddy Van Dyck, Simon Van Nieuwenhove, Jens Van Roey, Stefano Vella, Jan Vielfont, Mechai Viravaidya, Paul Volberding, Jean-Paul Warmoes, Judith Wasserheit, Jonathan Weber, Alice Welbourne, Jack Whitescarver, Alan Whiteside, Ross Widy-Wirsky (+), Marijke Wijnroks, David Wilson, Per Wold-Olson, Jim Wolfonsohn, Tachi Yamada, Elias Zerhouni, Debrework Zewdie, and Winston Zulu (+).

This book was initiated thanks to a grant from the Ford Foundation, where I was a scholar in residence in New York in 2009.

INDEX